New Rules for Healthy Living

A Better Understanding on Health
Will give you a Brighter Future
No Mistakes about that

By
EARL C. HARRIS

New Rules for Healthy Living

A Better Understanding on Health
Will give you a Brighter Future
No Mistakes about that

First Edition

By
EARL C. HARRIS

ISBN 978-0-9789013-1-8

Preface

In today's society, it is common for individuals to seek solutions and answers to the concerns of life through sources external to themselves. This tendency is especially true in areas related to medicine. Most individuals have been conditioned to accept the current teachings and research that have been developed by professionals in the medical arena. People have been educated to believe that what they may know or think intuitively, as non-medical lay people, should be discounted or ignored when compared to the teaching of individuals who have received their M.D.'s. or, PHD'S

However, throughout thousands of years of human history, until relatively recent time, this was not the case. In the past, sometimes out of necessity, people created their own remedies and cures. Increasingly, doctors and medical personnel have come to be viewed as those who have all the acceptable knowledge and wisdom pertaining to health. This is not to discredit the correct findings that they have presented, but only to emphasize that often new knowledge, which is advanced from sources other than the current medical establishment, faces significant obstacles to ever being made known to the overall population. What if many of the current teachings of the medical profession, that we were taught to accept, are wrong? What if much of the current research has been based on an incorrect foundation which is leading researchers to build a framework that is extremely weak? What if these present teachings have made us unable and unwilling to see new approaches that could help people to overcome the many health problems that exist or have existed for many generations?

As you read this book, I believe that you will discover that some of the ideas and concepts I delve into may at first appear to be foreign to the nature of thinking that we have been taught. It will require you to step back and to reflect on the new and different logic. By rereading certain sections, insights and understandings will begin to emerge if they do not at first glance. I wish only to bring to light new knowledge not currently understood by individuals in the medical field. Whether they are patients being treated with misguided therapies, doctors frustrated by inconsistent research findings, or businesses impacted by incorrect medical theories, my goal is to help everyone. I feel a deep sense of responsibility to share the knowledge that has been imparted to me in a way that insures it will reach those who need it the most. This book is the first of two that together will provide readers with information that will change their lives for the better in dramatic ways. The first lays the foundation for the second.

What can this first book do for you? A very critical question in light of the nature of how we live today. Many tasks and activities compete for what is the limited time we have each day. We all face the challenge of deciding into which ones we should invest our time and energy. Let's say a good friend shared with you that, "there is a book, just recently published, that contains tremendous insights and thoughts which are helping people to begin the process of moving toward a much healthier and disease free lifestyle." How would you respond?

Assuming you had confidence in your friend's judgment, your reaction might be, "I would like to know more, let's find a time when we can talk further." My goal for writing this book is to begin the effort of sharing this life-impacting knowledge in a direct and logical manner so that the reader can understand what is involved in developing the kind of healthy personal lifestyle and environment that has been sought throughout the history of mankind. This book lays the necessary foundation on which the second builds the strong, dynamic framework for as better life.

Table of Contents

Introduction

People are living as shadows, and not as they should be. Sadly most are unaware. We do not live up to our potential. This is the reason I have chosen write about "The Shadows". Our life existence is only a shadow; and we settle for a minute level of life and not for the ultimate potential of life. What is a shadow? Summarizing from various dictionaries helped to generate my working definition of a shadow as follows. A shadow can be described as a partial darkness or obscurity within a part of space from which the rays from a source of light are cut off by an interposed opaque body.

A shadow is a reflected image that cannot encounter danger or observation.

A shadow is also an imperfect and faint representation of an object.

A shadow is an imitation of something: copy.

A shadow is a dark figure cast upon a surface by a body intercepting the rays from a source of light.

We have several descriptions that teach about a shadow. They are showing that a shadow is a reflection from an object when a ray from a source of light makes contact with an object it creates a shadow.

Man's shadow is a reflection of his image, it's not man. It is only an image which can be seen but not touched or felt. A shadow disappears when the rays from the source of light abate. 1Chronicles 29:15 Job 8:15 14:2 Psalms 102:11 144:4 Ecclesiastes 6:12 8:13. The lives that we now live are only a shadow of man. We are not living within the full potentiality of one's body. It brings to mind that people are only a silhouette.

Seeing ourselves as nothing more than a higher class of a beast has contributed further to the misunderstanding of the potential of the human body. That assumption has led to the practice of trying to find answers regarding the human body through the exploration of the bodies of animals. The acceleration of technology due to the development of electricity has increased the amount of research being done with animals. The experimentation with animals has not given us the answers to what makes man tick.

The investigation of animals is like the human shadow, it only provides a general profile not the necessary detail of the human body. The shadow shows the profile of a body with a dark outline not capable of any recognition. This only lasts for a very short time, depending on the person's position. When a ray of light comes in contact with a body, if the angle is incorrect, it will not produce a shadow. The researchers are also following an incorrect angle or assumption. As a result, their attempts to understand the true functioning of the human body are falling far short of the significant insights they should have been able to discover many years ago.

It's the same with our bodies; the way we live daily. The body is only operating on a partial source of its strength. It's only firing on half of its cylinders if we can use the body like an engine of an automobile. Take a motor vehicle, with eight or less cylinders, that needs all its cylinders operating at maximum capacity to run correctly. As a result, the driver, and his passengers in the vehicle, can reach their destination safely without being discomposed. When eighty percent of the engine fails to run normally, that vehicle is not capable of getting anyone to work or not able to handle anything the driver has on his schedule for that day or time. Transportation has become a very essential part of people's lives in this century. It would be very difficult to avoid today's technology.

Compare man's potential to that of a motor-vehicle when all cylinders are operating correctly; it gives the owner or the operator satisfaction. When the engine only has one cylinder firing correctly, most of the time that engine will not start; especially if it is an eight cylinder engine. What the owner has to do he has to take the vehicle to a repair shop for repairs. When it comes to an engine job, the customer would first like an estimate. If the body of the machine is in good condition, and the customer is satisfied with the estimate to remanufacture or replace the engine, the repair shop will proceed to restore the same vehicle by customer authorization.

Man's shadowy life has more problems I think, in this era,

than any other civilization in the past. We know that a silhouette is something that's not real. Man is real. He is something we can touch, embrace, and never forget. Because we fail to embrace and touch each other, it shows that our lives are being lived as mere shadows.

We walk, talk, and live daily in prevarication. The only reason we behave that way; we claim we are alive and nothing is wrong with the way we are living. When we continue in these lies, the lies overpower us to make us believe this deception. We are like an automobile that looks great on the outside. When you find out the engine and the transmission are bad, the value of the vehicle is very low; only what the junkyard offers.

Man is a creature who is beyond price. But we do not behave like we are priceless. We exist from day to day like we are in the same category with animals. The value of a person should be exalted high above all the wealth of this world.

We need to stop being illusive, because a silhouette is only a dark reflection of a person. We see only through the lie when something horrendous has happened like 9/11.

Humans need to re-evaluate their lives. The way things are going these days, something drastic is the only thing that will make people change a little. A shadow is of no value to anyone. People don't pay their shadows any attention because there is no need. It appears and disappears not by the power of the individuals. It is the same with all humans. We do not have the power to come into this world or to depart.

Although we cannot control our beginning, there is no need for a shadowy life while we occupy this earth. The other thing that's possible is that life does not have to end as we came. We can change many things as we grow that the end will be better than the beginning. Many lives start as nothing and end up as they came. There is no need for a person to be shadowy from birth to death.

There are millions of folks globally that show tremendous interest in their automobiles, homes, and other earthly possessions; more than themselves. Take all the time many spend weekly to make sure all the things they take pride in so much are kept in tip-top shape. As soon as they feel something is not right, they will go all out to make sure that it is working perfectly.

If humans were in love with themselves, as they are with their jobs, sports, or other pleasurable activities, I feel we could all have a much better society globally. Especially, if people knew earlier how and what it takes to remove man's shadowy lifestyle; we would not need to be a silhouette from birth to death. Since no one was knowledgeable about man's shadowy life, we continue being a reflection, to ourselves and to everyone around us.

Being a silhouette at the time of slumber, the human body can only work partially. People's body is not functioning with its full potential. Since the understanding of the body potential was not knowledgeable before, it was difficult for our bodies to function normally even at rest, and not as a shadow. Our bodies also behave the same way when we are awake daily.

Regardless of the shadowy characteristic within humanity, there is a loving compassionate GOD who has been trying to remove the shadows of our life from us. We refuse to listen as He speaks. One of these days He is going to stop speaking to us; what then?

Early Experience

Chapter 1

My name is EARL HARRIS. I was born in Jamaica. I immigrated to the USA more than forty years ago. I have lived most of my life in America, a very beautiful country with great wealth and outstanding opportunity. A place where immigrants; and citizens have the opportunity to be industrious- where by, giving the individuals the power to excel far beyond one's imagination.

When I lived in Jamaica, life was very poor. For the poorer class, life was very difficult. Making plans for the future was not something one could grasp easily. Seeing what life was all about, I personally wanted to leave my native home to see the world.

Most of the things I dreamt about when I was a child I will never be able to obtain them in this life. In the life to come, the place where man will occupy there is no need for anything that we use in this life. I am thankful to GOD for the opportunity I receive to obtain a little of what I wanted out of life. It is not the greatest, yet it is not the worst. I have obtained great knowledge since I emigrated, I am not sure if I would have obtained all the knowledge I have, if I had remained living in Jamaica. I never entered any school of higher learning since I migrated likewise I never did before I emigrated. I did a corresponding course in Motor engineering. What would I have become if I had remained living in my native country? Possibly I could have been killed or something serious could have happened to me. No one knows the future; and what is ahead.

Poverty makes living difficult for all people, especially for the ones that live in wealthy countries or Islands. In-spite of the difficulties it's not really a bad kind of life. Now that I have experience the both worlds, I do love the life of poverty-in this sense: poverty has its advantages and some disadvantages. People of great wealth operate like they have all the advantages in everything in life. With poverty most of the time a person lives a very simple lifestyle, and being content, a person can be much more- healthy, than those that live in rich powerful Countries or Islands.

I do love Americans and all the people of the world. Yet I find-often times I miss my native Island. There are many reasons why I miss that place, not just because I was born there. I miss the things I did there and the people I did them with, especially the ones I worship GOD with. I love you all dearly, and I hope and pray we can have a great time in GOD on this earth before we go home to be with Him.

As I related before about poverty in Jamaica when I lived there, I find where many were unable to excel. I could be one of those individuals that remain in Jamaica, knowing that the day I left school I was still an illiterate. I cannot blame poverty. Neither should I point at my dad and stepmother, in-spite of their selfish behavior.

Man cannot see the future. We have to take it one day at a time. If by chance things turn out great we should be thankful. All my life I never thought I would address the world by writing. Having a mind as a child that one day I would speak to the world by preaching and writing, I would have taken time out to improve my English; and, as I write people would have less criticism to make. I am not ashamed of who I am and what I am. In-spite of my educational background I am thankful to GOD that, He can appoint me to teach the world many things our intellectuals have no knowledge about.

According to the Bible, GOD does not look at man's intelligence as his choice to be his messenger. GOD knows the hearts of humans therefore; it's the heart GOD makes his choice by. All the things that seem foolish to man that's what GOD uses to confound men all the time. Read 1Samuel 16:7 and also in 1Corinthians 1:19-29 2:14 3:18 &19 2Corinthians 2:14. It read in the book of Isaiah 55:8&9. *For my thoughts are not your thoughts, neither are your ways my way saith the LORD.*

I am thankful to GOD that He overlooked so many people and stopped at my door and took the time to teach me so much about the human body.

My life in Jamaica, and America, had its problems: I had ups and downs in both places. Looking at the problems I encountered, I realized that poverty has nothing to do with people's health. People get sick in rich powerful countries, as well as poverty stricken places. Death removes all from this earth, whether in rich places, or poor areas. Death respects no humans.

Financially, I had a very hard time making ends meet in Jamaica, I find out that despite all the wealth that's circulated yearly in America, it is much harder to make ends meet in the United States of America.

The poor behavior of humanity: shows poor characteristic in discipline, in the life of the people daily. For instance, in Jamaica voodoo was a method used by malicious poor people to keep other poor people in poverty. In the United States discrimination is the method used by the rich to stop a person from excelling. Looking at the both pictures, a person can see sin dominates humanity in both places.

One place uses voodoo: to stop another person from equality in the society, another place uses discrimination to stop equality in the society. This kind of behavior shows that people are bitter against one another. We down right do not care if other people live or die. We should love and care for others, as we love and care for ourselves. We are going to leave this world. If we leave this world as we came dead in sin we are going to be remorseful. We cannot carry anything with us when we part this life. All the wealth, and all the poverty we live with or in, will not bring happiness in the life to come, if we do not walk pleasing with GOD.

I encountered various sicknesses in Jamaica, and in America, It did not matter where I lived, I was unable to get genuine help from the medical professionals in both places. Jamaica was poor, and was not as advanced in its' medical technology as America. Being less fortunate with advanced medical technology would make a country less apt to help correct its health problems. The lack of medical technology should have made it very difficult to successfully help the sick and afflicted people. After careful evaluation, I see and understand that whether advanced, or somewhat behind with technology, this does not give any Country or Island more advantages or disadvantage in solving health problems.

Advancement in today's technology in the field of medicine has not made it any more successful in treating ailments. Physicians still are having a very difficult time curing folk's diseases. They are only doing a cover up job, and removing infected organs. When it comes to human bodies, man still remains an apprentice. They have not fully understood the body and how it functions and the process of how diseases develop in the human body.

The reason for my analogy, man is confused with the various diseases that keep popping up daily or yearly. Many of the old sicknesses that's been around for thousands of years, are still plaguing humans. This shows me, despite all the advancement in modern day technology, it has not given any more advantage in curing diseases.

Possibly, we might have more sickness occupying the population globally in this era than any other civilization. We can argue that the population is much larger today than any other in the past. Larger population should not give us the right for excuses. We claim we are much more advanced in everything. We talk about how intellectual we are, and all the knowledge we have acquired today. We think that puts us far more advanced than all the civilizations in the past.

The thing that we might have overlooked is the fact that we still are relying on the ancient legacy as our doctrine. We are unable to proceed beyond the knowledge that the ancient civilization left. I learned that many things that the early people were capable of doing, today, with all the modern day technology we have, we are unable to do many things they did in the past, simply because they never left behind the knowledge. They died with the knowledge, or the books got destroyed. Therefore we are unable to do what they have done.

Man today, with his education, needs to stop being overbearing with his pride. We look down on people when they do not achieve a higher degree of learning. We do not feel and think that some have to remain ignorant. Just as how we are all totally unaware of the human body and its facets; we can speak, and teach, how much we know the body. When it comes to the truth, much of the body still remains a mystery. We make up names of the body in our researches trying to convince people they are knowledgeable of the body, but in their dishonest philosophy, many remain ignorant to their death about the human body.

I have gained a lot of knowledge over the years, with my many problems I have encountered in Jamaica, and in America. I see and understand that all have to go through the same process to become a physician. A doctor does not study any kind of mechanical devices to become a physician. They study the body. All the technical work is done by the technicians. If the lab technicians make any kind of mistakes, the doctors are going to make even a greater one. They normally treat humans and aliments by the way they were taught. And it's not necessarily according to the patient's complaining. Humans are prone to make mistakes. If we notice, we have erasers on our pencils and other items we use to correct our mistakes. We are humans, and we have not the power to live without making mistakes; that is why we should validate what transpire first before we sue our doctors. They are subject to errors like anyone else.

Can we truly prove that the entire fault is the doctors? Our doctors study the body, and how to treat the body. The technicians study, either breaking down of the blood, or taking pictures of the body. If the machine malfunctions it will develop error. Treating by error can lead to death; same as the lab technicians, they too can obtain a malfunction in their gadgets, or faulty chemical. The doctors and the patients are the ones that are going to have unpleasant confrontation.

The opinion the doctor arrives at, causes him in most cases to require x rays, or blood work. Most doctors when they desire second opinion they will speak with another doctor or they will experiment with a drug before the result of the blood work, or the x-ray. They might change the drug they first prescribed, or they might continue with the first prescription if there is some kind of improvement the patient is having.

If the medication is unable to work in a satisfactory way, sometimes the doctors have to perform an operation, because they are unable to correct the problem that the patient is having. I am not saying that physicians do not understand the body completely. They are knowledgeable with some things. The greater is still perplexing, and will forever remain that way to humanity, if they maintain their research in the ancient legacy.

There is a transition that is not far away. With the knowledge I have obtained from GOD, there will be no more need for any doctors, or any more technicians. When there is no opposition, harmony will prevail. Humanity will be able to stand united in all things. There will be peace on earth, and no more war. Man is trying to enforce peace upon humanity. There will never be peace, until the prince of peace brings peace.

When peace begins to reign, sickness and death will have less control over humans. Many things that once made man behave repugnantly, will no longer cause people to live that way anymore. I am glad that a change is close. Life is too despicable to continue as it is going today. Something is needed in life that is much better than what we have today.

The perplexity of life sure makes people cantankerous. It does not matter which direction we are taking in this era, perplexity continues to plague us. I have encountered many problems in both the countries I lived in. I was unable to obtain an answer, or get positive results from doctors, from both the places that I lived in.

Who should I blame for my unanswered enigmas? Should I place the fault on the lab technicians, or the x ray technicians? Should we blame the men who are the creators of the equipment used by the technicians? What is the cause of humanity's pain and suffering? Why are we going through so many difficulties all our life? Why does nothing on this earth give genuine happiness? It does not matter if we are rich, or poor, life is the same for all. Having more money than normal, enables a person to have more of life commodities; and it does not give him or her complete happiness. Is it possible to have complete happiness on this earth? I think in the last dispensation, humanity will be able to have complete happiness for the first time, since we have become a multitude of people.

I have been to doctors in two countries. I was, unable to get satisfaction from the physicians that I visited when I had a problem. My problems started when I was a small child living in Jamaica. I am not sure if I should point at anyone for all the problems I encountered. Oftentimes I hear people say we should never use ignorance as an excuse for our mistakes. I am not sure if we should agree with that statement. When people: are unknowledgeable, they are ignorant of right and wrong. How can we behave wisely when ignorant of the fact?

The purpose of schools is to help remove ignorance from our mind, through the knowledge of our teachers, and the power of the individual faculty. Since humanity is unknowledgeable in so much, ignorance will forever remain in humanity.

Despite all the technological advancement we have made in the past several hundred years, ignorance is still a great part of humanity's daily life. As we travel this earth, we are going to encounter many obstacles. Why will we always run into trouble, because we have not taken the words of GOD very seriously? The day we begin to take all of GOD'S commandments with much more reverence, it's the day life can be much more pleasant. Giving total obedience to GOD will last from one generation to the next.

Because we have taken the words of GOD with little or no value, we have handed down pain and suffering, from one generation to the next. We are unable to find the answer how to seek GOD, and to walk with Him in spirit and in truth. Living and walking in sin, will forever keep humanity in ignorance as long as this earth remain.

I was a very ignorant person when I was a child living in Jamaica. I am not saying that I am not still ignorant in many things, now that I live in America. I am not knowledgeable with all things in life. I still have lots of blots. As long as I remain in this life, I will remain ignorant in many things that pertain to humanity.

Since I am only giving a partial part of my life that I lived in Jamaica, and America, I will only disclose my health problems. I will begin with my mother's death; I was a baby at the time of my mother's death.

My mother's death; took place when I was a baby, possibly at the age of three or four. I have no knowledge of my mother's life or death. What is it an infant can remember? They are the most ignorant of all. I do not know if I was a sickly child in my infant days, or if I was a healthy baby. I learned years later that my mother died when I was a baby.

I understand before my mother's death, dad lived at the same location where his mother lived. When my mother died, Dad moved to the place where his sister lives'. She could give him a helping hand with his kids, because of his work schedule. Working the kind of shift as my dad was working, made it very difficult to properly care for four small kids. Having a close caring relative, to help; helped our family, and our mental well being.

When we lived with dad at the same area with his sister, we had only one room, and that was a bedroom. That place was a tenant apartment. All the occupants of that location would use the same bath, and toilet. There were no kitchens. This building had a long veranda, or a porch, from one end of the building to the next, only on one side of the building. The occupants of the building would do all their cooking there, with an iron stove; that required coal. Cooking would take a longer time in those days, simply because of inconvenience. People will always find a way to make things pleasant in every situation.

When we lived at the tenant yard, and we occupied the one room, I know that I never wet the bed. No, not one ever complained, neither did I notice anyone had to do as I did when I lived with my stepmother. I do not know the day, the year, and the month my dad got married again. All I know we moved. After the move I was not able to sleep with anyone anymore; I started to wet the bed. I had to sleep alone. A cot was made for me. I had to wash it daily, and put it out in the yard to dry.

From the day I moved to live with my stepmother, I constantly kept running into all kind of health problems. I started to wet the bed. Then the next problem that started, I would vomit everything that I ate or drank. I was a difficult child to satisfy with food. I never once related my vomiting condition to anyone. They, not knowing what I was going through, gave me a nickname because I was eating too much.

When the vomiting would not cease, I turned the vomiting into regurgitation. It did not matter what I had, it would turn into regurgitation. What was taking place in my system I had no idea; all I know, I had to re-chew all the things I ate, even water I had to redo. I would get hungry very quickly, not long after eating. Upon the completion of the regurgitation, I would need something more to eat. The regurgitation and the bed wetting lasted for a long time. I never did count the years, as to know when they started, and when they stopped. I never visited any physicians for either problem. Dad was not the person that seems to care much about the children's health, as to keep them visiting doctors.

There was another problem that I had the same time, I had to always wear flannel undergarment, despite the tropical climate, is hot all year round. I became delicate, or anemic. I just could not stay healthy, as if to say, something, or someone was doing their best to eradicate me from the face of the earth. All the effort and their power were not powerful enough to kill me.

I had constant opposition all the days of my life, either when I lived with my dad, or I lived with my aunt, or I was on my own. Dad was not the kind of person that took his children to the doctors. He loved to experiment with making home remedies. I did not think he felt we should have any other ailments away from the common cold. Why keep going to doctors that need help themselves. They get sick, and have the same problems. I had problem after problems. They were on me at the same time. One never goes away, and then another would pop up; they all occupied my body all at the same time.

When I moved, the first thing that started, was wetting the bed, then the regurgitation, and then the anemic or being delicate, then I began to slowly injure my back by picking allspice. Dad purchased a piece of property that had allspice on it. Being a small undeveloped child, that strenuous activity was too rigorous for my body, it damaged my nerves in my back.

I do not know, when or how these ailments departed from my body. I never saw the need of recording anything I was going through in my life. I was very naïve when I was a child, or the pressure that I was growing up under stopped me from thinking that someday I might write a book, or simply write my autobiography. I would have recorded all the details; to the date of all occurrences in my life. Not thinking, or caring for novelties, I never write anything down.

I recently came to the conclusion that I should write about my unhealthy problems I encountered in Jamaica and in America. The reason for writing about my unhealthy problems, I am free of the enigmas, no thanks to physicians. I want the world to know, that I never did obtained any justifiable satisfaction in either country for my ailments, visiting doctors.

I never visited any physicians with any of my unhealthy conditions when I lived with my dad. Once, when I lived with dad, at his work location, I had a problem with my eyes. I do not know how I came about with the infection. I was the only one that had the problem in the home. I normally would go to the river daily and take my bath, even when I was going to school or church in the morning.

I practically lived at the ocean and the river. Since there was only one bathroom in the home, I could give myself a bath ten times and over sometime before the bathroom would be available.

One morning I went to the river, and I took my bath. I dove in and when I came up, I noticed one of my eyes began to hurt. I never paid much attention to the eye the first day. The next day it started to hurt tremendously. I visited dad at work on my way to school, and showed him the problem with my eye. He gave me an eye solution to wash my eyes. I being ignorant washed the infected eye first; I then used the same solution in the container that I used to wash the infected eye, and washed the eye that was not infected. The next morning both eyes were infected.

When we moved from St. Ann's Bay, to Roaring River, where dad worked, we had to pass the power plant daily when we were on our way to school. We had only three locations we could take, because the other location was the ocean. We were that close to the ocean. We had to always take one of the three areas for supplies we needed. The area where we lived, there were only seven homes. Four were close, and they were approximately a thousand feet away from each other. The other three were even farther, one or two were more than a mile away. When supplies were needed, we had to use one out of the three areas to get what we needed.

One of the areas was not accessible as two were. We had to walk four miles through the property to get to that town. If we drove it would not bring justice, because it was not a large city that had the population necessary for supply and demand. Many of the children from that area would attend school in St. Ann's Bay in-spite they had schools that they could attend in that town. The place we lived placed us four miles in three directions from each populated areas. When we were on our way to school, we had to pass dad's work place.

The next morning both eyes were infected, I stopped by the plant once more to talk with dad, showing him that my both eyes are now infected. He asked me how I washed my eyes with the eyewash. I related to him what I did. He rebuked me in my ignorance, letting me know I was stupid in washing both eyes without changing each solution for each eye. My Dad never spoke pleasant with me that morning. I attended school that day. The next day, I was unable to attend school: my both eyes were infected and very painful.

The pain in my both eyes became unbearable. I could not go outside, nor be exposed to too much light. I could not sleep and I was unable to relax day and night. In-spite of all I was going through, my dad would not take me to see a doctor. My number two sister read a medical book that we had at the home, and she experimented by washing my eyes with warm salt water, and then tied ice on my forehead. After a week of that treatment, my eyes' infection abated. A month later, dad, took me to see an eye doctor in Kingston. The doctor was unable to find anything wrong with my eyes, under such circumstances there would be no need for medication.

Telling my dad about any problem we had, was like talking to the wall. I used to relate to my dad about the pain and suffering I was having when I was reaping his pimento. What good was all the complaining; I ended up with nerves damaged that possibly would have remained with me to my grave. Nobody knows the future, and as the saying goes, it's never too late for a shower of rain.

We were possibly treated this way because our dad never got sick. All the years I lived with my dad, I never once saw him sick. I, on the other hand, seemed to be sickly all the time. When its not one thing it's another. Sometimes I would be weeding out the garden. I would feel like I was about to pass-out. I had to quit, and rest for a while; I would return later. I always had it very hard all my life; still I fail to understand why I need to work so hard in life.

Just as kids cannot remain living with their parents all their life, everyone had to make up their own bed. The difference with our life, we were forced to leave the home with nothing; not as much as one penny in your hand or anywhere. We did not have a job or any place to live. At first when I was cast out, a friend of mine, asked a friend to have me stay with him. Then I moved to live with my grandmother. Then my aunt asked me to come and live with her. I lived with my aunt, until I migrated.

I had a great time living with my aunt. She and her husband are two terrific people. I learned many wonderful things from the both of them. They were not the kind of parents that brought up their children in Christianity as my dad and stepmother did. Yet I find their home to be much more harmonious. I am not ungrateful to my dad and my stepmother. Their teaching of fasting and prayer still remain faithful in my life. A week has never past me since I rededicated my life to GOD, that I did not fast.

In-spite of my parents' misconduct, I have obtained something that I will never make anything take it from me. Death is the only thing that can remove prayer and fasting from me. That is something great I inherited when I lived with my dad and my stepmother. What I obtained at my aunt's, does help me to behave very wisely in many ways. The better of the both educations is prayer and fasting, because it brings us much closer to GOD.

When I lived with my aunt, I had no work to do as I did when I lived with my dad. I got my first job when I lived with my aunt. That job I had more fun than any other place I worked. Despite all the titillation I had: working at that job, it has given me my worse nightmare. How my problem started is difficult to understand, because there was no answer given for my problem.

My problem started like this: one day I had to remove an engine from a vehicle. After the removal of the engine, I notice I was having a pain in my lower back. I ignore the pain, because I always had lots of pain in my back even when I would fast a lot living with my dad, and my stepmother. I injured my back when I was a young child picking allspice for my dad. All because: he was thoughtless for his children feelings.

I remember when I lived at home with my father; sometimes when I was on a few days fasting, the severe pain in my back made it difficult for me to stand sometimes. I would not allow the severe pain in my back to stop me from fasting. I wanted GOD'S Spirit more than anything in this world; nothing was pleasant to me then, but GOD. I would not let the severe pain in my back stop me from fasting, and seeking GOD.

Although church was four miles away, and transportation was not accessible, I never missed one night service. Finding transport back and forth from home and church: was a difficult task in itself; still I never once thought of the consequence. The road, was pitch black at night, and we had to hitchhike a ride at night. When there was no ride, we had to walk home. I had great pleasure in those days when I was seeking GOD.

The day when I was baptized with GOD'S true Spirit, it was something wonderful to behold. But I never maintain many years walking with GOD faithfully. I got railroaded at my dad's and stepmother's home before they cast me out of their home. I never knew better, neither did I understand completely how to serve GOD faithfully in spirit and in truth. To this date, I still have a very hard time with the complete knowledge of serving GOD in spirit and in truth. GOD'S commandments require man to serve Him in spirit and in truth, and to love Him with all our heart, mind, soul and strength. We art to also love our neighbors as thyself. If this is what GOD requires of Humanity, who is pleasing Him?

When I was a kid, I learned so much about Americans, and the people that traveled the world evangelizing the people of the world. As a result I developed a belief at that point and my desire to move to America began. The attitude that I obtain, I would be able to walk more spiritually with GOD living in America. Since I lived in America, I find it to be a million times more difficult: walking with GOD, than it was when I was unknowledgeable in the laws or words of GOD, when I lived in Jamaica.

What I have observed in the United States of America, is that people tend to act like GOD is not genuine in the things stated in the Bible. Oftentimes I hear people call other people fanatic if they try to stand on the complete principle of the words of GOD. I also hear many would say that you are taking the words of GOD literally, because there is no need for literal acceptance of the scriptures.

The other thing I also keep hearing, is, that as long as you are speaking the name of Jesus, all is well. Because it's not of works whereby we are saved, it's the gift of GOD. Therefore there is nothing we have to do to be saved, but simply believe that Jesus died for our sins, and that's it. Therefore a person can always remain in his or her sin, and keep sinning as long as you believe, and confess that Jesus died for your sin.

I personally find that kind of doctrine to be preposterous. If it was that simple, why would GOD go through all that trouble, in a process of transforming Himself to become a man and live and die sinless for humanity? If literality was not required completely in all of GOD'S words, then, there would be no need for administering to the population the birth, death, burial, and the resurrection of Jesus Christ.

People of the world have taken Jesus' birth, literally, once a year. Almost all the world population celebrates the birth of Jesus. Even if it's being publicize as a method of merchandising and not being done to teach the world literality in Jesus Christ. We are not going to escape the wrath of GOD. We have not taken the words of GOD seriously. GOD is not playing. He is not going to change righteousness for sin, to please one human. We have to comply to His laws if we want to be saved.

I find even the singing in America, lacks inspiration. One group sings by nationality, because of being bitter against each other. We do not sing our songs as unto GOD, making melodies in our hearts only unto GOD. We go so far in our praise service, in a conforming way, making the music pleasant to the population, and not GOD. By the effort we place in making man love our service, we leave GOD out of our singing.

Americans and Jamaicans and the rest of the world have sold out. If the early evangelists were true to GOD in the early years of their evangelizing the world, they failed. Now they are the prophets of the Devil. The love of money has blinded not only the eyes of the people of America; the love of money got a major portion of the world's population in its control. Now we have only formality.

I have to save myself. If I do not conform to the words of GOD literally, it will be to my own destruction. When we know better, we need to do better. Right will never be able to change to wrong, and the things of GOD are right. They are true.

My pain in my back, I did ignore, because I always had lots of trouble continually, even when I was fasting. It is very hard to understand, why would someone suffer severely with back pain not having food or anything to drink? Ignoring my back pain after the removal of the engine, I proceeded to the playground to play soccer. After the game, I needed to use the bathroom. Sitting on the toilet, I came to the realization that something was wrong with what was transpiring. I looked into the toilet bowl; to my surprise; I see nothing but fresh blood, as, if to say someone cut me with a knife. At that moment I was terrified. A situation like that makes people panic.

The beginning of the passing of the blood that day was frightening. For more than two weeks, each time I go to the bathroom, I must have passed more than a pint of blood. It was a constant diarrhea problem I was having, and at the same time I was unable to obtain an answer for the problem I was having. I was not feeling sick, weak or anything. If I never had the pain in my back, and passing so much blood when I use the toilet, I would not know that I was having any kind of problem, and needed a physician.

This condition remained with me for more than two weeks, and all the blood I was passing each time I use the bathroom, I still was feeling wonderful. As I have stated before about my back problem that originated from allspice picking, I have always paid; little or no attention to my back problem. This time something needed to be done, and help was needed beyond my knowledge, or the way I was brought up.

My dad was not a person that would take us to doctors for every little kind of ailment that confronted us. Possibly he might think or feel that the body is capable of correcting its own problem it encountered daily. The use of man made medication, weakens the power of the body, and make the diseases linger in the body. I do not know for sure if that's the way dad believed. I am only speculating, because we were not taken to see any doctor when we were sick.

The perplexity of my condition ceased after two weeks, without taking any medication. The perplexity was not only on my part. Physicians were having the same problem I was having. They did not know how, or what to do for my condition.

After two weeks, the passing of the blood stopped, just as it started. It came without any warning, and it stopped the same way. It was not a little blood here and there. Normally a person would pass a little blood here and there, and then after a while it would completely stop. It stopped instantly, just as it started. The pain in my back abated in the same manner; it too never lingered on.

When the passing of the blood ceased I developed another problem that was much greater than when I was passing all the blood and the severe pain in my back. I then had a severe cramping pain in my stomach, which was much more horrendous than the pain in my back. This time, I was informed it's my appendix that causes the pain I was feeling in my stomach. I was not satisfied with one doctor's diagnosis. I visited several doctors. They all came up with the same answer, as if they all were in the office together or they all talked to each other on the telephone about my case.

The problem with the pain I was having, as long as I was working at the bakery, I would have the severe pain in my stomach. When I was off for more than two weeks getting ready to be admitted in the hospital, I never once had the pain. The first time I had the pain for more than two weeks, was when an enema was given to me the night before the operation. The pain I had that night was much more severe than the previous pain I had before. I could not take any kind of medication to use to relieve the pain. I had to suffer all night long with the pain.

The next morning I was taken to the operating theater. I do not know what they removed from my body. After several weeks out of the hospital, I returned to work. When I returned to work the pain came back. This time, it was much more severe. Now the doctors diagnose my problem as upset stomach. And for the first time medication was given to me. It was unable to alleviate the pain I was having. None of the medication I was given worked for me. For more than a week the pain would not subside no matter what was given to me by doctors. Not even sleeping medication was able to put me to sleep. After a week or more, I fall asleep one night. That night I had a dream, the dream instructed me that I should get some marijuana and cerasee, boil both ingredients in one, and then drink it.

The first thing I did in the morning when I awoke, I got some marijuana, and some cerasee. I boiled it, then, drank the concoction like you are having a cup of tea. I did not take the concoction just one day, I did it for years. I could get the both ingredients for free, and would drink it all the time. I would boil it daily, and carry it with me in a thermos everywhere I go.

After that first drink that morning, I never had the pain any more for more than twenty years. I had encountered more trouble with my back. Still I never passed any more blood when I used the bathroom. The blood I was passing was not from my penis, it was from my anus.

Although man has been studying the body for many years, the

body still remains a mystery to humanity. Humans always seem to develop some kind of ailments that keep our doctors, scientists, researchers, and our technicians perplexed all the time. I know that I have given the medical association a perplexing time in both countries that I have lived.

I was diagnosed that the cause of my stomach pain was my appendix. I was admitted in the hospital, I was there for more than a week before they gave me an enema. I never had any pain before I get the enema. The first time I had the pain, was the night before the operation. Next morning, I was taken to the operating theater. When I awoke after being taken from the theater; I had a bandage around me. After the bandage was removed I noticed I had an incision on my right side close to my groin. About a week later, the stitches were removed, and I was discharged from the hospital.

I later ran into the same problem again. This time I was told that I had an upset stomach. And for the first time since I started having the problem, they gave me medication. Each analogy does nothing for my suffering. Even when they said they removed my appendix, it did nothing for me. Should we accept that my dad's behavior; proved to be much more healthy, for humanity, than seeking a physician for every little thing that ails us? Our dad never practiced visiting doctors for everything. I started to do the opposite from how I was brought up.

I do not know if it was because of the tremendous pain I was having that caused me to seek medical help so quickly. I did not obtain any benefit when I sought help from man. I did completely forget all about GOD, and I never asked Him for any help. When I was in the hospital, more than one person addressed me, by saying that I should ask GOD to make the operation successful, and I would not die. I was not rude to the individuals; I just make them understand; that I could not ask GOD for His help, simply because I was not walking with Him. I related to the people that keep bugging me to pray, that I cannot pray, because I am not going to pretend like I am a servant of GOD. I was a sinner serving the Devil, and if I died, it was nobody's fault but mine. I turned from walking with GOD, unconsciously, not realizing what I was doing. I was not able to pick up the pieces again while I lived in Jamaica.

The thing that's very difficult to comprehend: is that I had no desire to attend churches. At the same time, as I drove on the road, going to work, or from work, I would always keep singing many songs I knew when I was going to church. As I sung those songs, I would always still feel the spirit of GOD move upon me. I could not understand what was going on, because I was not attending any churches. Because I was not attending any churches, I could not talk to GOD in prayer before my operation.

In all the problems I had facing me after I was cast out of my dad's home, I only once made a pledge to GOD. It had to do with getting me out of Jamaica. I kept thinking that it was a very difficult life in Jamaica. Through the hardship, it made it unpleasant for anyone to truly serve GOD in Spirit and in truth.

Looking at life in a financial way allowed me to be negative in my thinking about serving GOD faithfully. I could not see beyond my own ignorance. Therefore, I could not become positive, and turn from sin, and return to walk with GOD. Sin became a dominant force in my life. I did many despicable things as sin was my controller.

There are so many things in life that we will never learn nor understand. Man has being wasting years, and time and money, trying to learn, and understand many things about this universe, and all things therein, which will be none profitable to humanity. We are fighting for death and not life, gaining man's wisdom and knowledge does not bring hope for a better tomorrow. If humanity's life did end in death, it would be wonderful to think only for today. Death only ends man's existence on this earth. The life to come will be horrendous if we remain living in sin from birth until death. We are instructed of a new birth, which requires water and Spirit, to reign happily in the next life.

At one time I was one that was thinking only for today. Tomorrow was not in my vocabulary. The only reason why I was behaving that way, I was living in sin. As I lived in sin, I was a servant of sin. I was not always making plans for my tomorrow. Now that I have turned over a new page, I am sure that I will not leave this world as I came.

Transition to America

Chapter 2

My emigration took me from Jamaica to Western New York, the hidden beauty of America. I have not been to all the states; the few states I have been to, have not given me any interest; that I would leave Western New York. The only reason why I would leave Western New York: is because I am unable to handle the cold as I once did.

The economy has changed over the years in Western New York. It is not as prosperous as it was in the 1950s to 1970s. Many families left because of the poor stability of the economy. I know that we have to survive and also enjoy a little of life's pleasures. Life will lose its meaning if people only eat, sleep, and work.

If they lose vision, the people that live in a city, are going to perish. Life will become cantankerous. I left Jamaica because I did not see a bright future. Life was very difficult. Another reason for many people having a difficult time has to do with lack of jobs. Limited cash flow makes development stand still, which hides growth, and creates large unemployment.

When I lived in Jamaica, I personally never once was knowledgeable of discrimination. Neither did I experience partiality in treatment in the job market. I never once sought a position in the field known as the white collar. I took up general mechanics at the age of fifteen the year I left school. I always had blue-collar jobs. I never had any form of ill treatment. I personally always had a great relationship with people wherever I went.

Racial bias in America was unknown to me. People who; are racially biased behave despicably towards others that are not like them. I also found people that confess Christianity in America behave even more dishonorable. America is a place of great wealth. Millions of people left their native home, looking for a better opportunity in America than what they had in their birthplace.

I also realize that many immigrants regretted leaving their native home, because the picture painted to millions about United States of America, a land of equality for all. In my opinion, I feel that the United States of America; is the most bigoted country of all the countries in the world. As I traveled from one State to the next, I saw whites and blacks, treating each other dishonorably. The treatment I saw showed that one felt superior, and they made others feel inferior, as if all men are not created equal. I saw many ugly things that needed changing. Things may never change, simply because people have made money blinded their eyes, and stop their heart from being compassionate towards one another. We are commanded by GOD to love and care for one another. The true vision we should have in life is not there.

I understand the dream of most Americans, is to own a home. Therefore they visualize continually of someday they will own a home. The way: I see the vision of the people in America; is they have lost sight of reality. Fighting to own a home is the only thing they visualize. The cost is too much. Nobody truly owns a home in America-not if you continually pay such high taxes.

There is a double tax imposed on all property. The land is taxed whether there is a home or not. When a structure is erected on the property: the tax on the land changes, by reassessing the property. The value of the structure and the previous tax on the land escalate the tax, therefore making the individuals, or a company's taxes quadruple. In my opinion many policies administered by our legislative body over burden its population with too high taxes.

In my native Jamaica, when I lived there, it was poor and undeveloped. The majority of the people were illiterates. Despite the undevelopment of the country, and the lack of intellectuals, the tax-structure in Jamaica and the rest of the world is the same. Taxes are abused even though in the advanced countries we might think there are more intelligent people in government. Also the claim is they are more advanced in technology and stronger in their economy; taxation seems to favor the rich and not the poor.

I have observed many mistakes Jamaica has made over the years. Political revolution caused a set back in Jamaica's economy in a way that it never regained its economical strength it once had. I have seen many other nations do the same thing in their countries. This causes the economy to become weak, and in a recovery status. When I lived in Jamaica, in spite of poverty being so prevalent, I saw life was much more harmonized than it is today.

I know that millions of Indians died because of selfish reasons. Racial disharmony existed in the population of America. I am not trying to discredit America and its population. I am trying to show the mistakes we have all taken in life, simply because we are visionless in the most important things in life. Prosperity is pleasant, only if we maintain equity.

When I lived in Jamaica, people there also strove to obtain a home for themselves. In-spite of the hardships, they managed to build many beautiful homes. When they are completed, sometimes they are debt free. Oftentimes, when a church was built, the church building would be debt free.

In those days; people were more concerned about people. Money was not the main objective. Today, whether in well developed nations, or undeveloped nations, it seems that money is the main issue. If you are unable to borrow what you need from one of the many lending institutions, you will have a difficult time advancing in the things you would like to accomplish. Whether in rich developed nations, or poor undeveloped nations where poverty reigns. I find out that some nations call the helping of others bartering, and they make it a criminal offence if you are caught bartering. Man by greed, and poor insight, created an environment that's very much unhealthy.

As we behold the behavior of humanity in this era, we should all agree that the Bible is truly fulfilling. Man's vision sees only for today, despite we are commanded to live for today, and not tomorrow. Man does not know what the next minute will bring. Yet in a sense we have to live today with the expectation of tomorrow. Yet the tomorrow is not of this world. There is a life after this life. If we do not live our today pleasing as commanded by GOD, our tomorrow will be much more horrendous than our today.

The transformation of greed in our countries in our States, and in our cities is outrageous. It is getting more and more despicable. People truly do not care for themselves. By deception, all seems to be ensnared. We are unable to free ourselves from the trap of greed we are caught in.

When I lived in Jamaica, in-spite of its poverty, people would unite, and help others build their homes or churches, despite their profession. People never thought about losing wages when they volunteered their services. Life was much more pleasant in that era, than it is today. By being greedy, we have caused all things to escalate beyond man's control. We have not the knowledge or the understanding to reverse the problem that we have created.

We keep indoctrinating one another that education is very much important to stamp out illiteracy. If we are going to have an excellent future, all people need to be educated. The kind of education we are getting in this period, is not equipping us for a bright future. If a transition does not pop up soon, the future is going to be very unpleasant for all nations of the world.

Man's behavior is rapidly deteriorating by the educational system we are using today. We are only being educated for this life in schools, churches and everywhere we turn. Looking at man's philosophy shows that all keep looking to man for an answer that they think will strengthen them only for this life. Most people today seem to believe that the Bible is not any more an authentic book. There is no need for us to take anything it says literally.

We are told that GOD does not show respect to persons, As Eve and Adam sinned, they lost fellowship with GOD. All who remain in sin will likewise lose the same as did Adam and Eve. GOD in the beginning created all things beautiful, and made humanity equal. He did not put more perfection in some, and imperfection in others. All came through the same channel.

The problem I see with humanity, we are unable to maintain perfection. Many started out in a very excellent manner in life. As we continue living day by day, we allow the adversary to out-smart us just as he did Eve and Adam. We give up morals for immorality, we give up life for death, we give up happiness for unhappiness, we give up love for hate, we give better for worse, and we give up healthiness for unhealthiness. We maintain this horrendous life continually from generation to generation.

The statement I made about America, a place of outstanding opportunity, where many have traveled being very successful: in their success, they hamper the road for others. Today's opportunity is reduced to a minimum, which makes it much more difficult for advancement for millions of people that desire to move beyond poverty.

Adam and Eve fell. By their failure, they reduced life everlasting in happiness from the majority of the population. All humans are going to obtain everlasting life whether you like it or not. The majority are going to end up in the lake of fire, while the minority: are going to live with GOD in happiness continually throughout eternity.

Many refuse to open their hearts to the calling of GOD, as if to say GOD is only a myth. Man tends to heed the teaching of man in a greater regard, than the things of GOD, as if to say that man is much more knowledgeable. We are unable to see our own ignorance, simply because we have allowed the same serpent to trick us as he did to Eve, and then Eve to Adam.

The sin of Adam and Eve, removed from them a life of great pleasure, to a life of perplexities, and unhappiness. Driven from the garden, man had to encounter a much harder labor, and from that day, all women suffered greatly in child-bearing. In this age, man is trying to stop women from having any discomfort of children being born in this world. Despite their efforts, they are unable to change the law set forth by GOD. We have in this era all kinds of machinery that reduces most of man's hard labor, yet we are unable to stop laboring continually.

Man is disrespectful, not only to his Maker: man also dishonors himself. We have not noticed all the mistakes we have made. Adam and Eve are not the only ones that are responsible for the destruction of paradise. I do not know if we can apply America as the garden: of Eden or simply use America as coequal. The prosperity of America has become a thing of the past, simply because we have disregarded the laws of GOD.

Eve and Adam disregarded the commandment of GOD. Possibly they thought; GOD never showed them in full detail what the future would be like. It is the same with life in America, and all the powerful nations that once had great wealth. The truth of the matter, when we look at the prosperity of America, there is not one country throughout history that has reached the height on all things as the United States of America.

I notice the crumbling of America's power and success early on in my life in America. Today, the population continues to live a degenerated and immoral lifestyle. Most keep looking to the leaders to restore the power and its prosperity it once had. They are not thinking positively that they too have the responsibility to build or destroy the future of America. Most seem to only place the burden on a few people known as the politically elect. The people argue all the time the elected officials do not live up to their promises they promise, while running their campaign seeking either reelection or their first election. Failing to live up to the promises made during the campaigning, a recall might be necessary.

By the sins of millions, America will die, just as other countries did. Losing; the garden of Eden: it's a place where man can no long occupy, until it no longer can be found on the earth. It is going to happen the same way with America one of these days. It is going to be, a has been. The majority of the population will not believe that America will someday cease to exist. I am very fortunate that I have lived and experience many things that lots of folks will never experienced. I have seen millions that travel all over, and they have not learned much in their travels. Too many people travel, just for traveling, and their lives remain empty.

My life's experiences in Jamaica, and in the United State of America, have educated me in a very unique way. My English and my spelling might be very poor, on the other hand, the knowledge I have obtained I do not think I could have received it in any college. In my travels I have seen and learned all walks of life, I have seen great technologies, and I have seen little technology. I have seen great wealth, and I have lived in poverty.

Is there a much better life with the advancement of modern day technology, or with the people that live in poverty, and without modern day technology? Which of these worlds has a greater fulfillment of life? Are we trapped with modernization that much, that we are unable to differentiate right from wrong, better over the worst, truth over a lie? Do our educators have humanity in their full control, so that we now have to follow their every command?

Once in my life, being ignorant with the mechanics of the body, I would go along with our educators. Obtaining great understanding about the body, I no longer give an undivided attention to our doctors. It is the same with the men, and the women who dedicated their life, searching for answers to solve most of the aliments that have been plaguing mankind.

I have not escaped the plaguing of diseases, as many have. I have my share of problems, and they have been unsolvable by physicians. The health enigmas that I have encountered in two countries were mind-boggling to physicians and technicians in a developed powerful country, with its advanced medical technology. It was the same problem in a poor undeveloped country with less medical technology. In the poor undeveloped country, not having technicians reduces their ability to do in-depth research as the countries that have the advanced medical apparatus.

The medical profession throughout the world shares its medical research with the world of medicine. Whether it is a poor country or a rich country, this type of sharing of medical information helps the profession to solve global medical problems. When the countries with vast wealth are unable to find the answer for any kind of sickness, millions are going to suffer greatly; when their bodies are infiltrated with any disease that man is unable to treat successfully. By chance if the poor undeveloped country or Island should find the answer for one of the many diseases, they will not keep the answer as a secret. They are going to pass the answer to their medical colleagues.

There are hundreds of folks who study medicine; it has brought on controversy through perplexity of the complex human body. Developed and undeveloped nations are harassed by the study of the human body, which has not brought on agreement. Despite all the medical findings through research that has been published globally in connection with man's concept of how the human body functions, the medical world is not being honest when is comes to the understanding with how diseases develop in the body.

I am not trying to undermine anyone. In my opinion; I feel the public needs to be much more educated with the truth. There is a lot of emphasis being placed on removing illiteracy from the world population, and their feelings is that learning the basic general knowledge is not enough. The vast majority; are still in ignorance, in-spite of all the effort being enforced to stamp out illiteracy. It seems that it will remain that way as long as we remain selfish.

I feel that most of the emphasis placed in teaching: is being done to generate more cash for business. It is not done to make us aware of our ignorance and to educate us that we can move forward to a much better future. Our educators themselves run into the same problem, simply because they are still unenlightened with the true function of the body. Man has not been taught the proper procedure how to rest their body, and how to eat healthy. The diets that are being presented as healthy are just as unhealthy, as the people that are not on diets.

When we understand the formulation of diseases in the body, we will be able to truly educate the population. At the present time we are keeping people in ignorance. As we have a saying in Jamaica "when I live there, send the fool a little farther". That is exactly what has been transpiring for centuries. We keep hearing that if we eat correctly, and eat the proper way, we can avoid many ailments. Still the correct way of eating still needs to be taught.

When I lived in Jamaica, I never see people over indulge in eating like I see being done today. People are behaving like they have no interest for their own well being. They need someone to always hold their hands, and constantly correct them in everything they are doing in life. It's as if to say they are not responsible for their own being.

Looking at the behavior of the population, and our educators, we fail to see the strength of illiteracy that remains in people today. What I have seen, sluggard conduct has driven many to their death. In this era, we behave like we are above carrying our own food; and cooking at home is too much work, and that is too much time to wait for something to eat. We take everything in a sluggish way. We make someone else do all our driving for us. Then we can sit back and gossip all the time.

When I lived in Jamaica, I heard so much about the United States of America. I wanted to see it and the world. If I could reverse my life, and change it, and make it new, I think, I would not care much to live in America. The country itself is not a bad place; it is the people that are outrageously bigots.

I see the wealth of America makes the people feel they are above the rest of the world, and all the other nations are beneath them. I do not understand why someone would feel superior, and treat others inferior. We are all created equal. Wealth does not make anyone better in their human structure. All require the same daily, rich or poor. It matters not who you are, all need the same. You can only put on so many clothes daily and eat so much. If you overeat, you are just going to make yourself very sick. Whether you are rich or poor, eating too much will make you sick. It can kill you; our system was made one way, whether being black or white. It makes no difference if you are a king or a peasant. All people of the world require the same four essential items, or basic everyday needs. Remove one of the four essential things for life and man would cease to exist.

We need water, air, and food. Sleep should not be classified as an item, since it is not something we touch and feel. We do get tired and sleepy. That is a natural thing for everyone, as long as your body is operating normally. Abnormalities remove the natural behavior of the body, which place us in greater danger, and allow us to rely on humanity in order to exist.

The complexity of humans will forever plague man, because we have rejected our Creator. There is something that is so hard to grasp. This generation is not the first to ever deny the deity of GOD the Creator, and we might not be the last. When I lived in Jamaica, I personally never heard, neither did I see anyone confess with their mouth, that there is no GOD. I never heard anyone address that someone else made the statement that GOD does not exist, and that this world developed as it is today by the process of evolution.

I learned many things in America that's possible to learn I would never have learned if I had remained living in Jamaica. I had more encounters with sickness when I lived in Jamaica, than I had in America. All the medical treatment I received in Jamaica that was not helpful to me, being poor and destitute, has not made anyone a lesser person.

I have not seen, neither have I learned where any country's citizens reach immortality on this earth. This minute we are here, and the next minute, we can be cut off for eternity. What would we do? Where would we go for help? Man does not have the power to retain anyone's life. With all the power we have acquired; we still have not gained the power to extend anyone's life.

We behave today as if to say, man has surpassed all other

civilizations in all things, and that early primitive people were barbarians. Technology only makes life simpler, and at the same time, brings more death and unhealthiness. Being advanced with technology, we have placed good healthy living in the trash bin, for an unhealthy despicable life. The reason why we live the way we are living, we were not taught correctly.

I spent my childhood days in Jamaica. I was an adult when I left. I was knowledgeable about the various diseases that is known today. Where I grew up with my immediate family, we lived four miles from each town around us in three directions. Being secluded, we were unable to learn many things about the vast population. When I migrated, I was awakened to many unhealthy issues, which kept a vast number of the population in total reliance on the medical professionals. Despite millions that keep reporting the after effect of the medication they are taking, it has not stopped or slowed down people from relying on man for their help. To me, the help is doing more harm than good. Because we have no recourse, man has to maintain his only source of knowledge. Kill the only source, and that would only make things worse. People would be unhappy.

The problems I encountered in the United States of America; brought much more devastation to my body than when I lived in Jamaica. Possibly, one of the reasons for sickness to linger longer within the body might have something to do with the kind of weather, and the atmosphere.

Parts of the world, whose climate is tropical, keeps people's blood thinner all year. Being able to maintain thinner blood flow all year, makes it much easier to live healthy when we fully understand the function of the body. Being more informed with the operation of the body, we will be able to teach the correct diet to humanity that we will be able to be much healthier all our lives, while we live on this earth.

The areas of the world that are colder during the winter season, does have more profound effect on the bodies of the people that live in the colder climate. The colder weather changes the viscosity of the blood; it also removes a part of the body's power to overcome infections. When people's blood has become thicker, our distribution pump, otherwise known as our heart has to work much harder, and also all the other organs of the body.

The body being vulnerable to all the opposition in the world; makes it very difficult to live without contamination especially this epoch. All the modern day technology we have globally; places a lot of pressure in many ways that pressurize the human body to a degree of death if the body was not created with great fighting capability.

Take the fights we encounter daily and the addictions we add to our bodies, when we are sick; known as medication. Some medications help a little here and there. But some only create more problems. What a fantastic body man has. If the body was not created to withstand lots of resistance, many people would have died very early.

I personally have experienced the effect the colder weather has on a person's body; it takes a longer time to eradicate the invaders that invade the body during the cold weather. Please do not misunderstand what I am trying to make you understand about the weather, and the effect it has on our bodies. I am not saying that only the cold weather people are prone to illnesses. I am showing the difference in the weather, and the pressure that it places on our bodies by the cold climate over the hot climate.

I once spent about three weeks in Jamaica in the middle of winter. I felt great while I was visiting Jamaica. When I returned, after a few days, I felt like someone was in my back tightening it up with a wrench. I visited Jamaica before, during the colder seasons and I never noticed the change was as drastic as it was that year. Possibly the only reason why I felt it that much, it might have something to do with my age. As we climb up in age, the weather does have much greater effect on our bodies. The other reason why my back could function that way, is, I worked in the cold outside more that year than I did previous years.

The tightening of my body, made me feel as stiff as a piece of board. I regularly took real hot baths sitting in the bathtub. It never removed the stiffness from my back. I always had a lot of discomfort in the winter season especially in my back. I was unable to get relief, no matter what I did. Visits to chiropractors were valueless, as if to say a person has nothing better to do than waste time. The thing with humanity, we are not likely to be content with anything that ails us. The moment we begin to have the slightest of discomfort in anything

33

in life, we seek relief for the problem we are encountering. I was not happy with the pain I was going through. Therefore, I sought help in many ways. I was unable to obtain any help from physicians, and chiropractors, and all the various ointments prescribed for aches and pains.

How my unhealthy situations started, I made a silly foolish mistake one winter night by leaving a gas truck running inside a building. I was not thinking of the deadly gas that was filling up the building. Because it was winter and very cold I closed all the doors and windows. I returned to the building not thinking about the time bomb I had created by leaving a gas truck: running with the building closed up.

The truck had an air leak that needed repair. I never did what I did that night before. I would normally finish all my work before I would leave. That night I started to work, I left the building, I went and spoke to an individual to come and keep me company at work that night. Why I decided to do that, I will never know? Human behavior is something hard to understand.

If I did not stop to seek company that night, I would not have left the truck running that long. It would not have become hazardous to a person's health and become deadly. Seeking company, caused me to leave the building; with the truck running much longer: than normal. When I returned to the building, I did three things. The first thing I did was to get an applicator that I use to apply the brakes. Then, I proceeded to find the air leak. After finding the air leak, I removed the applicator. Then I turned off the engine.

I remember turning off the engine, and removing the applicator from the brake pedal. That night, I did nothing more on that truck. The next time I knew anything, someone was addressing me to relax, or they were going to sedate me if I did not stay calm. I was taken to the emergency room at Millard Fillmore Suburban hospital, where they revived me. I do not think I was in the garage ten minutes before I was overcome by the poisonous gas. The person I went and spoke with found me passed out. They quickly called for help. The quick response of everyone saved my life. I heard the nurses speaking when I regained some consciousness; if I remained in the building another ten minutes or more I would have passed from this life to the next.

One little mistake unconsciously and a person can lose their life. Man is truly a very frail creature. One moment we are healthy and strong, the next moment we can be like the grass, or like any other creatures that are powerless in maintaining life forever. We cut our grass weekly to stop over growth, that it might serve a useful purpose. Are we to say that the death of someone does serve a similar purpose as the grass?

I was graceful earlier in the day. Later that day I was almost cut down forever. Life is not a pleasant thing when it ends, especially if it ends without GOD, and without talking, and embracing each other. Many folks would feel much better if their loved ones were able to say; good-bye and they were able to hug and kiss each other for the last. That is what I heard many people say; while others said it would hurt too much to say good-bye face to face. Each person reacts differently in various situations.

We are created equal. Yet in our behavior, we are unequal. It is very difficult to understand why we behave unequally in so many things in life. It is not like our faculties are made with variations, the only thing that's different, we allow ourselves to be contaminated with erroneous teaching. I know that it is very hard to cipher between the different teachings that we have in our society; these can be mentally unhealthy. Dogma can keep people in ignorance all the days of their lives.

I am grateful to GOD. He opened my eyes to many things. He gave me many things that comforted me, despite all the contamination there is in the world. I could behave like the majority of the populations are behaving. Not that I am better or say I am more righteous than anyone else. Yet in every generation, from the beginning to this very day, there is always a person, or people that remain faithful to GOD. GOD always takes the time to relate to the ones that are true to His every command.

The question many might ask, why was my life spared? Why did things work that way that day? It might seem a little foolish or somewhat careless on my part, to leave the truck running in the garage all that time when I was away. The smart thing for me to do was turn off the engine, do what was more important to do first, and then, return to the job I started.

I have observed over the years, we always correct ourselves after the fact. We do not have the ability or power to see what the future holds. Not one human from the first to the last will ever be able to see what is about to happen the next minute. Many try to predict the future, and they fail. In their false predictions, many follow their pernicious ways to their destruction.

Many folks listen to the people that say they can predict the future. People, they are impatient and they would like to have a prosperous future. If people had the power to predict the future, I am sure that they would be the most powerful human that would be alive today. They would be able to control just about everything there is and the rest of the world would be fearful of the people that are able to predict the future.

Humans are deceivers. We love to play tricks with people's minds, because many are simple minded. Not everyone has the ability to lead. Not everyone cares for great wealth; some are content with just a little. Today, I think that the majority would be content, if they had a home all paid for and enough money to meet their monthly utilities, with sufficient food daily.

That's the reason why I say that not one person has the ability to see the future. Even though the Bible relates to us of the future, we have not taken any precaution for our wellbeing. Man in his pernicious ways speaks to us about the future. We tend to heed their ways, especially: if it has something to do with making lots of money. Money will make many people do; harmful things to themselves. When I lived in Jamaica, I used to hear this saying, "money make friends, money break up friendships, and money will make you take the life of your friends and love ones". It is a very sad thing to know what evil creatures we have become because of the love of money. Was I caught in the same category? Why did carbon monoxide poisoning almost snuff me out of existence?

Man should remain thankful at all times. Not knowing what the future holds, we are at risk at all times for many evil things. I never dreamed of the danger I was in that day. I too took life for granted, and was careless with my wellbeing. I am not the only person in this world that lives very dangerously and ignorantly. I think that the majority of the population of the world lives that way. Even when something drastic happens to us, we never even try to alter our life in a respectful manner pleasing to GOD.

Man is not placed here to live a life like we are living. What purpose do we serve to simply eat; sleep, work, and then we die. I do believe that man was created in the image of GOD. Since we are created in the image of GOD, there has to be more to life than eating, sleeping, working, and dying. The way our current educators are educating the population globally, is to say, life ends at the grave, because people are classified just a higher class of animals. I also see more people are accepting the doctrine of evolution.

Being unconsciously careless, I almost threw my life away; and possibly the destruction of my children. Since no one can predict the future, we have to speculate on the dos, and the don'ts. My death could cause my children to have either a cruel stepfather, or a good stepfather. It could also make them bitter in their heart because they lose their father at an early age. I am thankful to GOD. In-spite of my unconsciously foolish behavior: I live to tell it.

After I regained consciousness, they retained me in the hospital over a week, to treat me, and to make sure all the poisonous gas was removed from my blood stream. Each day within a six day period, I was taken to a decompression chamber, where I inhaled oxygen at a higher atmospheric pressure. Observation would also be part of my daily treatment to see if by any degree I was affected by the poisonous gas.

Upon the completion of my treatment, when they realized that the poisonous gas did not affect my brains, I was discharged from the hospital. It was not long after my discharge I noticed a few things began to happen to me that I never had before. I began to have colds much more frequently, and they would not subside as before. I would have to visit a doctor each time I caught a cold. My sinus would be infected, and the only thing that would work to relieve my sinus enigma would be antibiotic. Man's body is an out-standing creation. At the same time, it does have lots of flaws. The fault is not with the Creator. Man was given a choice, and we are the ones that chose suffering and death.

I would have sinus infections more than three times a year. I never ran-out of antibiotics because I always had several refills available. I suffered many years with the sinus condition, feeding on antibiotics all those years when I suffered with infection more than three times yearly. I remember once I ended up in the hospital, because of my sinus condition. They thought I was having a heart attack.

My problem that placed me in the hospital started like this; I felt like something got stuck in my passageway that drains the fluid from your head. I began to cough, and I was unable to stop coughing, I could not clear the area in my neck that seemed plugged up with some fluid or something. I kept coughing for a very long time. I was unable to breathe correctly and at the same time I was having terrible chest pain. I was in such a bad condition someone had to drive me to the hospital.

The examination in the emergency room by x ray, made the physicians working that evening, come to the conclusion that I was having a heart attack. The long time that I was coughing, placed a lot of pressure on my chest. They related to me the reason why they would like to keep me in the hospital for a few days that they could keep an eye on me just in case I was having heart failure. All the scars they saw on the X rays, made them believe I was having a failing heart and the possibility it might fail in a few days.

I was kept in the intensive care unit all the days I was in the hospital. That was about a week. When they felt I was not having a heart problem, they asked me several questions about my lifestyle; what I did daily such as eating and drinking, smoking, or if I did anything that they ascribed to heart failure. When they realized that I did not use any of the things they ascribe to heart failure, I was discharged from the hospital.

Each time I would have my sinus infection, I would feel like I was having a heart attack. I would have tremendous chest pains, and the pains would remain the length of my sinus infection. I kept on asking the doctors why I was having tremendous pain in my left lung each time I finished taking the antibiotics for my sinus infection. I never once obtained any answers why I would end up with lung pain when my infection of my sinus was over. Not one doctor was honest with me, one way or another. I am not sure if they truly knew the reason why I always ended up with severe pain in just my left lung.

The other thing I had to do each time I had an infection, even though I took antibiotics, I had to place several cough drops in my mouth all night when I was in bed. Then I could sleep without coughing all night long. I would always have a few pieces of cough drops in my mouth in the morning. I slept that way possibly more than ten years. We have our dentists, teaching that sugar, or sweets are unhealthy for a person's teeth. If that was the truth, all my teeth should have been decayed to a point where I would have none of my natural teeth by now.

Only one of my natural teeth was taken out of my mouth. The only reason why that tooth was taken out, I never knew better. The person that removed my tooth early in life, possibly never knew better. Otherwise he would have instructed me not to remove the tooth. I had sensitive teeth early in my life, possibly because I never had a tooth brush to brush my teeth.

As a child when we lived at our stepmother's home, we used a stick known as threw-stick. Maybe the hard abrasion over the years caused the gum to recede, and I ended up with sensitive teeth. My tooth would hurt when I had anything cold or hot. It was painful. The removal of the tooth did not stop sensitivity completely from my mouth. It reduced the severe-ness of the pain at first when my tooth was removed.

I had a few of my teeth filled. Still, I believe it was not necessary to do all the teeth that were done. Not being able to read the x ray correctly, we have to go along with what they tell us. I know that some business people practice dishonest gain to maintain the amount of money they would like to make yearly. The other thing that I see in our society globally, people are not pleasant when someone speaks the truth to them. We have become a people that enjoy lying, much more than when someone speaks the truth to us. To me: that is very sad, knowing that honesty is being placed in the corner. We behave like wealth is more important than anything else in this world.

I have seen this kind of behavior in millions of people globally. Even in the men and women that claim to be men of the cloth. The pressure placed on humanity for living, makes us become unconscious of the true reason for living. There should be no doubt in our mind that we have to exist. It is not easy to survive these days, because we all seem to be self centered in our attitude. The laws of the land sometimes make people change in their manners towards other people.

The other thing that might be the cause of why we behave the way we do to one to another, is that we take the commandments of GOD very lightly. As if to say GOD is only playing a game with us and we can keep on doing our own thing, and ignore the things of GOD: we act and behave like man is not failing man, when the problem is man and not GOD.

All the years I was going to the doctors for my sinus problem, they never did much for me. I knew that the infection would leave my body within two weeks or so. It never left me permanently. I would have several attacks yearly. They made my life very miserable. I tried more than once to find out the reason why I began to have sinus infections after the carbon monoxide poison infiltrated my body. To this date I have not obtained an answer why the changes began to take place in my body only after the poisoning took place.

If I was a person that always had a lot of trouble with catching colds, I might have understood that something may have been a trigger in my system that developed constant sinus infection. I am thankful that I am still alive in-spite of the few problems I once had after the carbon monoxide poisoning. There is a saying that goes like this, "as long as there is life there is hope." I am very glad that I am alive. Being alive brings me to a place where I am able to show millions the truth about many things that we possibly have been taking for granted all our lives.

The question I keep asking, if I die, then would these things remain hidden forever? Was I saved for this purpose? Once more we are stuck with the things of the future, and the things of the past will remain unchangeable to humanity. All we are able to do is take one day at a time. In-spite of the plans we have to make daily, in some way or another tomorrow always works its way in our walk of life; thus making our lives difficult because people are unable to take life on a daily basis. We keep making plans for the day to come, only with things that pertained to this life. The true life that we need to make plans for we keep ignoring.

The last time that I had a sinus attack, was once in 1997. Since then, I have not had any more sinus infections as I used to have more than three times yearly. I was persuaded within my mind that I was not going to any more doctors with my sinus condition. I decided to start eating some garlic. I would eat six cloves of garlic, and eat very hot pepper sauce daily. I also would use a lot of vinegar with what I prepared to eat. My sinus condition abated wonderfully. I have not seen a doctor since about 1995 with sinus infection. In the year between 95 and 96, I started to try some garlic tablets; these also did a much better job for my sinus than the antibiotics did. I never had anymore lung pain as I once did taking the antibiotics.

Now my body is able to fight off the attacks without even taking anything. I always knew when the infection was about to flair up. Now my body is able to stop my sinus infection without taking anything. The years I was going to the doctors, they were unable to help me for one year without taking any medication. I had to feed on medications all the time. I never ran out of cough drops. I would have to always sleep with them in my mouth, so that I would be able to sleep all night without coughing all night long. Now I can live without cough drops, and if I do eat any, it's because I love to eat hard candy.

I know that other people that suffer with sinus problem can also get the same relieve as I did. Not only sinus sufferers, the common cold condition that has been giving people more problems all their lives, they will be able to have less trouble. People will be able to sleep much better without taking any medication for their problem. I know what to do so that you can always sleep without having stuffy nose when sleeping. A stuffy nose can be a thing of the past. Sleeping can be much more pleasant for all people of the world.

Allow me to elaborate a little more on the things I ate with the hot sauce, vinegar, and the garlic. I spent many days and nights at my business location. Because it was inconvenient, I made my lifestyle very simple. I never went to restaurants, because I was having financial difficulties. Problems in life do have a profound effect on a person's life.

I am glad that I have always remained simple in my living. I never behaved extravagantly, and I have no intention of changing. The poverty lifestyle I had in Jamaica; it remained with me. I never over indulged myself in the behavior I see globally. I always think of other people, and how they are living, and what they are eating. I do love and care very much for people, therefore I live for other folks.

I was never a person that ate out a lot; I love home cooked meals. I do not allow food to control me. I was brought up on lots of porridge, and I love porridge to this day. I also did love to drink pot liquor, to this date I still love drinking pot liquor. In Jamaica we use to call the water after cooking, pot water. We would always add hot pepper sauce to the pot water, so that we would be able to enjoy the liquor.

Oats porridge was popular in Jamaica when I lived there. I do not know if it is as popular today as when I lived there. What I observed taking place in today's society, many folks feel that some of the olden days food is too poor to still eat. I still love all kinds of porridges.

We use to prepare oats more than one way. One way was hot. The other way was cold. I enjoy the cold preparation of oats very much. It is very easy to prepare. It is prepared like this. You get a bowl, then the oats, water, and some raisins. A person would place the oats within the bowl; add the raisins mixing it within the oats, then pour on the water. Allow the oats and the raisins to absorb the water for several hours. The raisins will help to sweeten the cereal you are about to eat. You can add ripe bananas, or any other kind of fruits that you like, or nuts to the oats that is now ready to eat. If you think it is not sweet enough, you can have sugar, or some condensed milk.

The preparation of the oats is simple, and very healthy. It required not much effort. Cows milk, gives it a greater taste than using water. I love it better using milk as the absorbing solution. There are folks that are unable to drink milk, and they enjoy using water making their cereal

Oats being prepared cold was what I had daily when I was eating the hot pepper sauce, garlic, and the vinegar. The only kind of meat that I ate was sardines. I also eat wheat bread, or some crackers. That was what I ate all day for more than a year, while I was spending all that time at my business location.

The one meal that I would eat daily, consisted of oats, milk, raisins, ripe bananas, garlic, hot sauce, bread, crackers, vinegar, sardines, or, some other kind of fruits. Although my diet was so meager for a year or more, I never lost as much as one ounce of weight. I would fast sometimes for a month just having bread and water. The bread was dry; nothing was added to the slices of bread, when I would eat them with the water. I never lost any weight even when I would be on just the water and bread for more than a month. The longest time I went with just bread and water once a day, was ninety days.

The time that I spent eating meagerly, I never took any kind of vitamins. I felt great, I never got sick. The kind of food I ate would not take ten or more hours to digest.   My system was able to get the rest it required. I was not over working my internal organs.

The way I lost my weight, I will be able to share with the world. It had nothing to do with diets and exercise. As I stated, I never lost as much as one ounce when I was eating meagerly. I lost all the weight when I was eating normally again. I am able to keep my weight down eating more today than I did for more than thirty years.

Many problems that once plagued humanity can also be a thing of the past. Most medications that are used today seem to cause some aftereffect. The other thing I know is many people die because of the medication they used to treat their illness. Many folks put too much trust in the medical professionals. They will never try anything else. They feel they are too educated to listen to anyone that did not study the human body through one of the many universities there are in the world.

Because a person did not obtain their ticket from one of the many universities,   does not make them uneducated in their knowledge of the body. The men and the women, who obtained their education in medicine through one of the many universities in the world, can only practice the way they were taught. Going any other way, will cause them to be ejected from the medical association.

There are procedures that guide all medical professionals who obtain their degree through the educational system. If one does not follow the guidelines, they will receive imprisonment for practicing medicine. The only reason for imprisonment, the medical association is trying to stop charlatans. In medicine, are these men and women honest with the way they are living? Are they unconsciously overcome by the power of their profession? Why do they act the way they do?

We need to be educated with the truth. The people that are responsible for educating society need to be educated themselves. A person can obtain all the degrees there are from one of the many universities in the world. That does not make him knowledgeable with all things. I was not educated in a university. That could be the reason I see many things that are lacking in our society today. At one time in my life, I was like most students; I would heed the teaching given to us by our educators.

Today, I find myself taking their words with a grain of salt. They have been giving us many incorrect ideas. I see and hear, over the years; our philosophers say many things about ailments caused by what we eat. Today, it is not uncommon to find them teaching something completely opposite. They are saying if you do not eat or drink some of the things they claim to be unhealthy, you will be able to reduce the causes of many sicknesses. They constantly keep changing their words. Why should we keep listening to the messages imparted to us from the scientists and researchers?

I have a very difficult time understanding man's conduct today. I am not sure if this has been the attitude of humanity from the beginning of time. All I know is we are despicable in this epoch in just about all things we do. I often see and hear many people doing things very dishonestly. They call it job security. Are we to say that our medical and pharmaceuticals association are responsible for the same actions as those who do a halfway job only for job security? The majority of our industries are guilty of poor production, just to continue making lots of money. The other thing why there is so much poor quality in every product on the market could be the waste. Lots of people yearly keep buying and throw out the old products.

How do we classify today's operation? People are at the mercy of our medical association. Our children are unable to attend school unless they have received their immunizations. Then they get to stick their needles into kids' bodies. This is a form of job security; same as how they advertise flu shots. People are gullible because we do not like to be bedridden. Not one person likes sickness. We all like to be pain free. We love happiness. When we are sick, we are unhappy. This is most common when we are infected with the simple common cold. Many people will fight hard to avoid catching a cold. Colds make our life miserable.

Today, trying to avoid all kinds of diseases, we often heed the doctrine of our educators. They in turn inform us that they have developed various kinds of inoculations that help to reduce many diseases that can affect us. They are not honest with their teaching. We will do harm to ourselves when we are immunized. By securing their status, they keep society unhealthy. Scientists claim we are ignorant of the body and that they are trying to educate us. They inform us that we need to be immunized for many different sicknesses. We find simple-minded people being gullible and giving heed to their job security doctrine.

I see many companies lose their shirts because of the flaws in their products. Possibly they were guilty of a scheme for securing their company for a long time. Look at the pressures there are today against the cigarettes companies. The medical board is making people aware that the cigarettes companies keep adding all kinds of ingredients to their tobacco. The ingredients are unhealthy and thus create a greater craving for cigarettes. Today, the medical association is keeping a minority of the people on their bandwagon. Their position is that smoking is the leading cause of many diseases, and we should all try and kick the habit of smoking. {Knowing many facts about diseases, I would like everyone to know that tobacco, and all the substance added to cigarettes, have nothing to do with any kind of aliments that are affecting people today.}

The misrepresentations of the medical board prove they are as guilty as all the other associations that deceive society to gain job security. These groups are so much into me, myself, and I that they are unable to see their unbecoming behavior. They allow the love of money to blind their eyes. As a result this leads to a lack of true care for others.

I began to have sinus infections after the mishap I had in 1979. I was unable to get satisfactory help from physicians. I lived on medication because that is the only thing they knew. Possibly in their classes, they were instructed how to maintain full control over people. Is it possible doctors know the causes of most diseases? If they should truly help people with their enigma, they would not make as much money as they do when they hide the truth from their patients.

I have not visited any doctor for the past sixteen years for my sinus problem. I have not had the problems as I had, when I was taking antibiotics that were prescribed by doctors. I cannot say that I even had one attack for the past sixteen years. Tell me why our physicians were not able to help me over the years. I would have several attacks each year when I was a medical patient. Since I have not had any more sinus infection, for more than sixteen years, I do not see the necessity to visit doctors any more. Now I am doing fantastic.

I wonder how many folks died because of the neglect of doctors to be honest with their patients. What can the medical board do to a doctor, when his patient is willing to fight for him? If a doctor: should truly stand for honesty with his patient, and for his patient wellbeing, possibly, his patient would stand behind him all the way. Can the unity of the people remove all barriers, and give strength beyond the medical board?

Possibly, it's a chance no doctor wants to take, because humans, patients in this case, are creatures that are unthankful. Most of the time we live very selfishly; especially in these days. Today, we have groups of people all over who stand in opposition to many laws passed by our government. We need to ask ourselves does the government due to love of the citizens pass the laws? Do they oppose the government, simply because someone loved to be in the limelight, saying they are trying to do what's right?

I have seen, and I heard, many folks try to do what's right. As soon as some people reach better financial status and they completely forget all the individuals they were once concerned about earlier now they are no longer in their mind. Likewise, Christians and non-Christians act in the same manner.

How do we expect to have a beautiful world to live in, when we are so inconsiderate? Most people expect GOD to always bless them. Yet we are not willing to obey His commandments. The majority of the population of the world honors the laws of their country. The minority dishonors the laws. They are incarcerated for the crimes they committed against the laws of man. If the majority was the lawless ones, not one country would be able to stand strong. How could any country survive if the majority of its citizens are lawless? How can we expect to be citizens of heaven, to live there if we are lawless to the laws of that land?

We honor man's commandments when we honor man's laws, and it has no control over us, because laws only apply to the lawless. The laws are not a judge to the lawful people, only to the lawless. The laws of GOD; do not judge the ones that honor, obey, and keep His commandments. In this life we have the lawful people encountering hardships because of the people that are willing to remain lawless. I see where people will continue to live a life of lawlessness, because they are at enmity with themselves. They behave like they are above the laws, until they are caught. Then, they look for mercy.

Is it possible we are having the same problem with our health? In some cases it might be possible. On the other hand, that's not the case. Sickness is not something a person can control. It does not matter how much we exercise and diet correctly. That is not going to stop us from being contaminated with some kind of disease, only if we were able to give the body what it truly required to protect itself.

I suffered a lot after I was poisoned by carbon monoxide. Not only did I develop sinus problems, but also my greater problem from the poisoning was with my back. I first developed back trouble when I was a very small child living with my dad, and my stepmother. I had to reap allspice for my dad. It was too strenuous for a young child, at that age. It possibly affected my nerves. The reason for my analogy, not once, with all the x ray's that I have taken for my back, did it ever show any kind of structural injury.

When I lived in Jamaica, I use to have lots of back pain. Even when I would fast, I would have severe back pain. I never could understand why I would have such severe pain in my back when I would be on a few days of fasting. Sometimes it was very difficult for me to stand up when I was fasting, because of the pain I was having in my back.

As a small child, climbing those allspice trees was not the

problem. The problem was the long time it took me to remove the allspice from the trees and the strenuous maneuver it took to reap the pimento. Being under-developed placed too much strain on my nerves year after year. The other thing that possibly affected my back also, was all the heavy loads that I would carry on my head for miles.

One reason why I say that allspice picking did more damage to my back, than any other work I did, was this. Each time I would stand, holding the large branches to break off the small section with the pimento, it placed a lot of pressure on my back. What would take place each time I was holding the branch for a moment, I felt like I needed to urinate. Sometimes I would climb down from the tree to pass my urine. As soon as I would stand to hold the larger branches to remove the pimento, I would feel like I needed to urinate once more.

Regardless of how I complained continually, it was of no avail. I was ignored, simply because, we had to continue reaping dad's pimento. I was not as important as the gathering of the allspice and the protecting of the trees, so that they would last for many years producing lots of pimento year after year.

I used to have a very hard time on those trees. Not only suffering with my back pain, but also working barefoot on the trees would hurt my feet tremendously for two reasons. There were a lot of sharp dry limbs that needed pruning. They irritated us continually because we were barefooted. Sometimes I would wear dad's work boots that he would wear when he would climb the trees. Reaping allspice was very much unhealthy for little children who had to climb the trees to remove the pimento from the trees. The people that sat on the ground, to remove the grains from the small branches, never encountered the problems as the ones that had to move the small branches from the trees.

I know that there were all kinds of weeds all over the property that was irritating if you accidentally touched them. Insects were another thing that was plentiful all over the property. On the ground we had to watch out for insects that could bite you. They also were located on the trees. It was hard enough to reap the allspice. Keeping watch at the same time for insects was another thing. When those creatures bit you it would hurt for a very long time. Not knowing what kind of a problem a person can run into when bitten we tried our best to stay away, being on the lookout all the time.

That's the place I first started having back problems. In-spite of the problem I had with my back, the first time I visited any doctor for my back was when I had an accident working for Kaiser Bauxite. One day at work, I was working on a truck. Oil was all over its platform. The shoes I was wearing were not suitable for that kind of work. I was still in my probation period. I was unable to purchase the shoes recommended by the company.

Kaiser supplied the proper safety shoes; however you had to purchase the shoes from the company. The truck I was working on had tires over six feet tall. The workspace I worked in was eight to ten feet high. I never measured the distance, because I never saw the need. If I was thinking about the future, and possibly putting my life story in a book, I would have been more precise in taking the measurement of the truck that I fell from.

I worked on several of those trucks before. They were not as oily as the one I fell from. The other hazard condition was my unsafe shoes. My shoes were not oil resistance shoes. Daily as you worked, because the area was so oily, it was very difficult to avoid stepping into oil all the time. That's why it is important to always wear oil resistance shoes. Shoes that do not have oil resistance soles get very soft easily. Therefore, it is unsafe to work around oil, with none oil resistance shoes. It was a combination of bad working shoes, and oily surroundings that caused my accident.

Kaiser Bauxite; had their own medical facility. I was taken to the company facility. X rays were taken and a complete examination was given to me. They informed me that I had no structural damage, and I would be fine in a few days. The only thing that might happen to me, I could possibly be sore for a few days.

My accident at Kaiser Bauxite Company in Jamaica was my first back x ray. My first ever x ray was taken as part of a company medical examination, for the job. That x ray was only to see if my lungs were clear. I also had to do another chest x ray at the American medical facility when I was about to migrate. I had two medical examinations done when I worked for International Harvester. All the x rays I have ever taken, none ever show structural damages to my body. Nerve damage is unable to be seen with man made devices.

January 1979, was the year, and the month that I was poisoned by carbon monoxide. That caused two problems to develop, after I completed the decompression chamber treatments. One was a sinus condition, and the other was my back enigma. The back trouble I had was much more troublesome than my sinus problem. My sinus would flair up, say four times a year, and it would always give some kind of warning, before it knocked me off my feet. My sinus enigma stopped me from working only once, because I was coughing so much, and I could not stop the coughing, I was taken to the hospital.

My back was something else. Many times I would go to bed, and was unable to get out of bed. The thing about my back which is very weird, working never affected my back. I hear many people complain when they are working, having back trouble. On the other hand, I felt better working. I have less trouble with my back.

I did not have any structural damage to my vertebrae; it was my nerves that I had problems with. Even thou my nerves were not pinched, what happened to my back, is this: When I was a child, I injured my back by strain. My body was unable to correct the injury that I incurred to my body when I used to pick allspice for my dad.

As I have stated, before I was poisoned, I would have severe back pain even when I was on fasting. I could not understand why I would have such a tremendous pain in my back when I live with my dad and my stepmother. I always found I had more pain, especially when I did fasting. At first when I migrated, I never had all the back pains that I had after I was poisoned with the gas from the truck I was working on one winter.

The most back pain I would have, was caused by standing in the same awkward posture, as I would have when breaking the allspice from the pimento trees. When I would work on an engine, that required the engine to be torque over two hundred foot pounds, and the room of the vehicles confined you to an awkward position, where one foot is higher than the other, you are placed in the same posture as when I used to reap pimento for my dad. The same pain I would have in my lower back, it's the same pain I would have when I am doing an engine rebuilding in the chasses of the truck, without taking out the engine.

That is how my back would bother me. I was able to fly and drive for hours without any discomfort. After the accident being poisoned, I was unable to fly as I used to. Driving was now uncomfortable. I was unable to travel as I did before. It was like I was incarcerated. I was unable to sit in any vehicle for any length of time. Only a few minutes I was able to sit, without being irritated, with pain all over my body. I was never a person that liked driving. Flying I enjoyed very much. I could not fly any more as I once did. The reason I could not fly as I used to, the airplanes companies' energy conservation reduced the size of seating. This conservation of smaller seating on the airlines caused an unhealthy condition for my back. All people's health is second place in the world of business. Money making is much more important than people's health. We fail to see and understand that money is unable to travel or move on its own.

Money is needed for humans to purchase their needs. When people are unable to get the money they need to purchase the items they are in need of, life is going to be unhappy. Having lots of money, with nothing to purchase with it, you can burn the money, because it will be useless. What; then is more important, people, or money? We need to stop caring so much for money, and put people first; we cannot eat or wear money. There should be no doubt in our minds that money is necessary for our upkeep today. Remove money, and would this dispensation end by killing each other? Humans are unpredictable; you never know what can happen from day to day.

When my back changed from minor pain to a major problem, life became unbearable. After the accident, I not only visited doctors for my sinus infection; I visited doctors and chiropractors. Doctors were the first I visited. They could not find any problem with my back, because there was no visual damage seen on any x ray. Man with all his wisdom, knowledge, and understanding, is unable to develop some kind of machinery that's capable of detecting nerve damages.

As I stated before about my back condition, it was not as irritating before I was poisoned. The problems that developed after the incident became mind boggling. I was unable to obtain an answer from all the physicians that I visited. The response I got from each doctor was as if I was trying to build a case that I would be able to sue someone for negligence. I was not trying to be deceptive; I truly was having a lot of back trouble.

Constantly having problems with my back, a friend of mine recommended that I should try a chiropractor. My friend always stated he got good help from his chiropractor, and thought I might be able to receive the same help for my back as he did. I made an appointment with my friend's chiropractor. We did the preliminary. He x rayed my structure. He informed me that he saw no structural damage to my body, not even any form of arthritis in my system. He proceeded by placing me on his adjusting apparatus, then he measured my structure.

He then informed me that one of my feet was longer than the other. He would be able to correct my problem, by the adjustment he would make as I kept visiting his office. Since I needed relief from what I was going through with my back problem, I was willing to try anything that would help. His first few adjustments; did nothing for me. I decided to stop going back to that chiropractor for a good reason.

I visited his office one day, and he adjusted my body; I never had any cuts or bruises on any part of my body. The next morning, the palm of my right hand was swollen very large. I was unable to close my hand or do anything that day. I could not use my right hand all that day; I called the chiropractor, and related to him my problem. He told me to watch it, rest that day, and see what happened the next morning. If my hand was still swollen, I should come right over to his office. The next morning I was fine; I was back to normal. I had nothing on my body swollen anymore. I did not call the chiropractor, and I did not visit his office anymore. Years later he retired. A young man purchased his business; he called me up, and informed me that he was the new owner of the practice, and if I would like to remain being a patient of his. I did try out his work. He was unable to help me.

Not able to get help from doctors and chiropractors, I stopped going to see those professionals. Years later I started to have a lot of problems with my feet and back. The pain this time was unbearable, with a discomfort of being very cold. I visited this physician and related to him the problem I was having. He informed me that my problem more or less it can be arthritis. The doctor recommended I should get blood work and x rays work done then; it will be more accurate in prognosis. The information that he gave me, he would better understand my problem when he get the result of the blood work and the x ray in a few days. He prescribed some medication for me to take until he received the results of the tests.

I took the medication for a few days. It did nothing for the problem I was having. What began to happen to me, I was unable to sleep, eat, and work? I was in complete torment day and night. A week later I called the doctor's office and informed them that I would like to speak to the doctor. The receptionist or the doctor secretary asked me what was wrong. I told her. She informed me that it takes a few weeks for the medication to take effect, and I should keep taking the medication for another week or two.

The more I took the medication, the worse I would feel. I could not sleep, eat, nor work. I remained in torment all the time, day and night. It did not matter what time it was. I quit taking the medication when I saw I was getting worse. After a few days of not taking the medication, I was back to my normal self. I was able to sleep, eat, and work. I was not in the torment stage as I was when I was taking the prescribed medication.

A month later, I returned to the same doctor's office. I wanted to know the result given to the doctor about my x ray and the blood work test. In the doctor's examination room, he did his normal routine examination. He proceeded to inform me that the x rays and the blood tests both show that I have arthritis in my system. He said that he could help me in some way, since my problem is related to arthritis. He wrote a prescription and gave it to me. I asked him if it was the same prescription as the first one that he gave before. His reply was yes.

I replied by asking him this question, had his office people informed him that I called and wanted to find out why I was having all the discomfort taking the drugs he prescribed for me. He did not hear; he replied, and walked out of the room where we were. He never returned to talk with me or make any kind of suggestion what I should do from that moment on.

I did not pay him for my office visit, because he was rude for leaving me in the examination room, without making any kind of suggestion. He never gave me any kind of prescription to fill. The paper he wrote the prescription on he tossed into the waste paper basket. When he was walking out of the examination room, he never recommended seeing another doctor, or a specialist.

I continued having the problem with my back and my feet, and being cold. It was not pleasant what I was going through. The coldness was not much trouble to me, because it was summer. The problem with the coldness I was having, continued to fall. I was speaking to one of my customers one day, and relating to him the problem I was having with my feet and my back. He informed me that he had a very good doctor, a podiatrist, and I should go and see him. He made the appointment for me to see his doctor. I kept the appointment. After doing the necessary paper work, he proceeded by taking x rays of my feet. The result was negative. I would recommend this doctor to sick people that are looking for a good physician.

The result of the x rays and other normal tests done by the doctor, did not show anything wrong, or necessary for any kind of treatment. He made a recommendation that I should get blood work done because it's the best way to see if I have any kind of arthritis condition in my body. The x-rays that he took were negative in every way. It was not necessary for him to do any kind of treatment to my body.

The Doctor informed me that he would like to do experimentation with my feet for a few days. If it worked, then he will know what he would like to do. What the doctor did, through experimentation, made things even worse. I returned to his office several days later, and I told him that his experimentation was more devastating to me. The doctor did not say much when I informed him that his experimentation did not help. He then gave me the results of the blood work, which came back negative. I had no problem with any kind of arthritis in my system.

How could it be possible a month earlier, another doctor was treating me for arthritis? Then a month later: another doctor by x rays and blood work could not find any disease of arthritis in my body. The doctor was very honest in truth. He let me know that day he was unable to treat me. He could not find anything wrong with my system, according to all the knowledge he obtained from school about the human body.

He never left me hanging like the other doctor, who left me in his examination room. The podiatrist did not charge me. He said he was unable to do anything for me; therefore he was not going to charge for any visit. He recommended seeing a chiropractor. He even went so far as to make the appointment for me. Fulfilling the appointment; the chiropractor did the same preliminary examination like all doctors do. The completion of the paper work goes to the next stage. The first thing he did before he started to question me, he took x-rays of my bodily structure.

When all the x rays were developed, he took me to a room where he would examine the picture of my bone structure. Each picture he would go over with me. He shows me and explained what he saw needed to be done. He would speak about each X rays picture he would put up to look at, and he says I have not started to develop arthritis as yet and all my bone structure is in good health. I just needed to be realigned. It was going to take lots of adjustments on my part to correct my situation.

When someone is ignorant, people will take advantage of the ignorant people. I needed help, because I was suffering. This chiropractor recommended three visits per week, until he felt it was not necessary anymore. Then he would change it to once a week. This chiropractor was very dishonest. Each time I visited his office and he adjusted my body, I was in more pain than when I walked into his office. The information he gave me, showed I would have pain for a while. Soon I would be fine. The more he adjusted me, the worse I became. It did not matter what I was saying to him. He was not listening to what I was saying. The other thing was this, also. He had a very hard time adjusting my body. The doctor would perspire profusely when he tried to adjust my body. One would have to say, that chiropractor was exercising, the way he was perspiring.

The problem with my feet and the constant pain in my back continued about nine months. I visited doctors and chiropractors.

Only one was truly honest out of all the medical professionals I visited. All the others were just out for my money. They never were truly honest with me.

The amazing thing is this. The same time I was having all the pain in my feet, and my back, and feeling cold here and there, my wife was expecting a baby. I never once heard of a man feeling any pain when his wife is in child bearing. Not thinking of the possibility that could be my problem, I kept seeking help from humanity. They, being dishonest in the knowledge of the possibilities and the impossibilities, kept feeding me medication or adjusting my body to correct what was not the problem all the time.

The day my wife had the baby is the same day all the pain I was having with my feet and my back ceased. I was back to normal only with the pain I had that developed after I was poisoned by carbon monoxide. As the pain subsided, I realized that man will never be able to fully understand the bodily functions. Being dishonest because of pride, knowing that people are going to talk about their lack of knowledge in their practice, they seem to love to always act as if they know what they are doing.

Not thinking that they are doing more harm by not being honest, they continue this chicanery on people. There are so many people being hurt. They are able to maintain their deception for a very long time. Many folks are getting educated with the deception of the medical professionals. They are reaching out to other methods.

Some things might last for a long time. They are not going to last forever. Our educators have been doing a very naughty job for hundreds of years. Now, they are going to run into a lot of trouble soon. It is nobody's fault but theirs. It is good to educate people, but don't forget to educate yourself first.

Somebody someday, will be able to open even a minority of the people's eyes. That will eventually help the majority to see where they have been going wrong. I have not studied with the intellectual professors of the world. Still the knowledge that I have obtained simply by observation possibly may surpass most intellectuals. Because they live in books written thousands of years in the past, they remain looking for answers that will profit nothing today.

The exultation of ones intellectual ability brings folly to the individuals. When a person humbles himself, and is being exulted, life will be much more pleasant for all. The folly of a fool; only establishes more and more foolishness. This in-turn destroyed many strong nations. As long as people remain to be superior, we are going to have a topsy-turvy world. We need to stop this superior, and the inferior behavior we have in our society. Remember we are all created equal. Someday, we are going to account for one another, whether we like it or not. Being rich is not going to prevent you from giving an account. Being poor, is not going to prevent you from accounting likewise. The status you acquire while you occupy this earth will have nothing to do with your accounting in the life to come.

I stopped for a short while from seeking help from the medical profession with the sicknesses enigmas I had. Nothing that the doctors gave me worked to free me from the use of man made medication. I tried all kinds of remedies for years, and nothing worked but antibiotics. The years I used medication, I lived at the doctors offices. Spending so many years visiting doctors, and not being truly helped, I became dissatisfied. Being annoyed taking antibiotics, I tried garlic with hot pepper sauce, with vinegar, and I was able to reduce my sinus problem much sooner without any after pain effect. Today I have not had any more attacks as I did in the past.

My back, in December 1989, gave me the same problem as I had in Jamaica working at the bakery. I was working on an engine when I started to have this very severe pain in my lower back: same as I had in Jamaica. This time, I needed to use the toilet much sooner than when I was in Jamaica. I went to the toilet. To my surprise, the same thing happened to me once more.

When I started to move my bowels, I feel the same sensation as it was when I first had the problem more than thirty years before. I eased to one side, and looked into the toilet bowl. All I saw once more was fresh blood. Like someone had taken a knife and cut me, I was bleeding to death. All the blood I was passing, I never felt sick, nor did I feel weak. Each time I would use the toilet, I would pass fresh blood like someone cut me with a knife. It seems like I was passing a pint of blood or more each time.

The first time, I had that condition, it lasted much longer. It stopped with a cramping pain that placed me in the hospital to remove my appendix. This time, the passing of the blood lasted only four days. Once more, it was the same with the doctors in the United States of America, despite having all the modern day technologies. The doctors did all the possible tests known to man. They remained perplexed with the passing of the blood. The knowledge I gained with my health enigmas, man's actions is the same everywhere we go in the world. It does not matter whether rich or poor, educated or not, we are still ignorant to many things in, and of this world.

This time when the blood stopped on the second week of December 1989 I had a serious diarrhea problem that was unstoppable by any of the over the counter drugs. I had to get a prescription drug to stop the diarrhea condition I had, it continued until about the third week in January of 1990. The stoppage of the diarrhea in January did the same thing to my stomach as it did in Jamaica.

In Jamaica, I had a serious cramping pain that lasted much shorter than it did in America. I was able to stop my problem much earlier in Jamaica the second time, which was much more horrendous the second time than the first. The first time, the doctors said my appendix was the cause of the cramping pain. The second time was an upset stomach. Nothing man made was able to help remove the pain. I had a dream one night that I should use marijuana and cerasee boil the both ingredients, and then drink it. I did, as I was instructed in the dream. It worked to alleviate the pain I was having for many years.

Living in America, I was not able to get good marijuana, and fresh cerasee. So I had to live with the pain for more than six months. I visited doctor after doctor. One recommended that I should go to a specialist. He made the appointment for me, and I fulfilled the appointment. As we all know what is required by all medical professionals, you have to complete the preliminary before anything can transpire.

The completion of the preliminary; took me to the examination room. He did his normal routine check, and asked me a few questions. He made an appointment at the hospital for x rays to see what was going on with my system. That result was negative. He then ordered upper and lower GI, which once more turned up negative. He then used a scope up through my anus to look in my bowel to see what was going on with the problem I was having. All the tests, which were done, all were negative. Not once did they prescribe any kind of medication for me. They could not find anything. They did not know what to do. They were not honest to stop me from visiting their office. Each visit at the specialist was a hundred and fifty dollars.

Not able to get any help from the doctors, or the hospital, I quit going to the doctor. I think he was glad I stopped coming to him, knowing that he was perplexed. Or maybe he felt I was once more lying, like when I was going to other doctors with my back problem after I was carbon monoxide poisoned. I stayed home for about six months or more, unable to work or do anything. Most of the time, I was in the bed, sleeping like I was in the womb, so as to help relieve the pain. Some days I would try to go to work. As soon as I would start to drive down the road, I would have to return home, and get back into bed, because of the severe cramping pain.

Looking back in Jamaica, when I lived there, more than thirty years ago when I first encountered passing all the blood; they were unable to solve the problem. More than thirty years later, living in a country that has all the modern day technologies, they too were unable to solve the same medical problem I had. We need to see and understand modern day's technologies have nothing to do with solving people diseases.

Not understanding the body and how it functions, forever will keep man in being ignorant of the body. Man keeps behaving like he has complete knowledge of the body. It keeps lots of people in their ignorance as they are.

Sometimes, the only way I would be able to get out of bed, I had to have someone massage my vertebrae, joint after joint for me to get out of bed. I would go to bed being fine, and then be unable to get out of bed. For years now, I have no need of any more chiropractors. Nor do I need anyone to massage my vertebrae any more. I never get out of bed with any more pain. I am not saying that I am pain free. The little pain I have does not mean much. If I do not have to sit down in the morning when I wake up, I have no pain all day long.

I kneel down to pray daily: morning, noon, and at night. Then I sit down to read my Bible. Most of the time, I have a slight pain in my lower back, left side. By experimentation, I was able to correct most of the problem myself. GOD gave me some great understanding about the human body that was able to help me with my problems. I will be able to pass this knowledge to the world very soon. Then all might be able to understand how the body works. It is easy for the human body to fight off diseases without the aid of medication and vitamins we are instructed to take daily. Man keeps on teaching, that they understand the human body and the requirements to be healthy, and we are not getting enough of the things we need in our foods daily.

I am showing the world the problem I had in Jamaica with sickness. Our medical doctors were unable to help. I am also showing that I have the same problems years later. The doctors of the United States of America were unable to solve them likewise. The sinus condition I had, that I never had when I was in Jamaica; that kept me on antibiotics by the medical doctors in America, I no longer have, and I do not use any medication.

I previously stated that I used garlic, hot pepper sauce, and vinegar to treat my sinus condition, because I was not being helped by the medical professionals. When I became despondent with years of being medicated, I diverted from medicines to experiment. The appropriate answer for me not having any more sinus infections was not corrected by using garlic, hot pepper sauce, and vinegar. In this issue, I will not disclose how I was cured of sinus infections, flues, and even the simple every day cold, that affect so many people yearly. I also want you to remember, I once used to have lots of back trouble that is also a thing of the past.

I am in a position to teach the world the truth about the body and how to even lose weight without the hassle taught by our educators on how to lose weight.

Overcoming Major Hardships

Chapter 3

My first job in America was with International Harvester. The first day I went out seeking a job, I was hired. It was the first door I entered into looking for a job. I was new to the area, and the people, and I never knew my way around.

I was not familiar with the weather or the area of Western New York. I was the person that the company sent out the most on road service. When winter started, because I was not familiar with the cold weather, I did something that was very foolish the very first cold freezing winter of my life. I am from a country that has tropical climate. I never saw snow all the years that I lived there.

That year in the frigid cold and snow, I encountered a few problems. Being inexperienced with the cold, and because no one instructed me on the dangers that can occur not being properly attired, I did something very foolish.

I do not know if the men at work were trying to educate me with the winter weather, or they were trying to discourage me from working with them. There were other foreigners there; which never did any road service at all, possibly because they were just learning to speak English, and their English was still very difficult to understand.

I, on the other hand, feel I still do a very poor job when it comes to speaking and writing English. I never took time out to study English after leaving school. I never saw the need then. Now that I am putting together the knowledge that I have obtained from GOD, I somewhat regret that I never furthered my studies in English.

I am not completely remorseful; in a sense I am delighted that I never entered any school of higher learning. Looking at the understanding I have obtained from GOD, I ask myself, if I had entered a school to further my education, would it have been pleasing to GOD? Could I become complacent in life? I have seen so many people speak against the older written English versions of the Bible. People do not only speak against the older versions of the Bible they also do not like to read the older Bibles.

I heard lots of people express their opinion in regards to their feelings with early English. The majority seems to be in favor of the advanced English used today. I could have been one of those person's that despise the old for new, and the truth for false. By rejecting the truth to satisfy my own educational background, I could have stopped GOD from giving me the understanding of the body. GOD also instructed me to maintain my poor English to the world. I should not make intellectuals do too much changes; in my writing. He would like the world to know, that He does not choose people to work for Him by man's wisdom, knowledge, and understanding. When He makes his choice, He is able to equip the individuals to His liking. He does not equip people to simply please people. It is according to what GOD needs in a person. Man does things to please man. We normally leave out GOD in everything we do.

I never imagined I would someday speak to the world by writing. Possibly it is a very good thing that humans are unable to see the future. We have to take it one day at a time. Mankind does not know what the future holds. I left home one day feeling wonderful; I got to work one day, and they sent me out to repair a vehicle that broke down on the road.

That particular night it was very cold. I had no knowledge of wearing gloves. That night working on the road, I almost froze my fingers. Not knowing right from wrong, being new in a strange place with strange people, I hurt my hands because I never knew better. The vehicle I was working on was close to the shop. I never realized that it was that cold that evening. I was working on the road for a short time without any gloves, my fingers became extremely cold. For a minute I thought I was going to lose my fingers.

I returned to the shop when I completed the job I was doing. I headed straight to the bathroom. I turned on the water and ran the water until I thought it was hot enough. I proceeded by putting my hands in the hot water to reduce the pain I was feeling, because they were so cold. The hot water was able to reduce the pain I was feeling in my fingers quickly.

Being ignorant, I did more harm to my body than good. Oftentimes I hear people say that we should not use our ignorance as an excuse. I am not using mine as an excuse. I was the one that suffered for years, with being foolish, by trying to remove the hurting of my fingers too quickly.

After I did what I did, I was told the right way to remove the coldness from my fingers. I should have done it much slower, and used my own body temperature to slowly remove the coldness from my fingers, by rubbing my hands together, and blowing warm air from my mouth on my hands.

Using hot running water the way I did, it was unhealthy. I hurt the joints of my fingers in a way, which each fall my fingers would always feel like they were freezing. My nails would become red, as the fingers would be icy cold. That's how my fingers would be yearly in the fall. When it is winter, my fingers would not hurt quite that much as it did in the fall.

I had that condition for many years, which progressively did worsen. I never did seek help from any physicians, for the problem I was having with my fingers in the fall. At first I would only have the condition where my fingers would be freezing in the fall. As soon as the weather got colder, my fingers would not be as cold, or give me all the trouble it did when it was not as cold. As soon as the weather got colder my fingers would be normal once more. Why my fingers would act up in the fall, and in the winter it would return to normal? In my opinion, I feel; that I should have had more problems in the colder weather.

Humans are a frail creature, yet powerful. We are unable to withstand ignorant treatment to our bodies, yet powerful enough to endure great oppositions. Man would not have to confront all the barbaric opposition daily if we did just one thing. All should know that we are creatures that are flesh and blood, and our bodies were not made to be abused as we are doing to ourselves daily.

Take my ignorance in my foolish behavior when I placed my freezing fingers in the hot water. I was looking for quick relief from the cold pain I was having in my fingers. By not knowing the remedy for frostbite, I hurt my body. That caused further grief. My body would have remained much healthier if I had patiently waited and allowed my body temperature to restore my fingers to normal.

Due to my lack of knowledge about frostbite, and the inexperience of pain and suffering cost me a lot. I have encountered lots of sickness in my life, and I am thankful to GOD, that He as shown me the potential of the body and the power of the body in healing itself. I see and understand lots of mistakes people are making. The constant mistakes we are making are destroying us. GOD has given us understanding as to what is needed to stop people from killing themselves daily.

I have made all kinds of mistakes since I relocated. They have caused mental anguish; physical pain is another. Both anguishes; are painful. The one that is hurtful the most is the one that is unable to medicate my cure. Man made medication, does help in someway to alleviate people's pain and suffering. It might not work in all cases still it helps a little here and there.

GOD is the greatest medicating source there is, we sometimes are unable to reach Him. There is a source that provides medication for all ailments, whether it pertains to physical or emotional pain. To reach that source we find it most difficult, because we are creatures that fail to see and to understand what is best for us. I am not sure that emigrating is for everyone that migrated. We do not have the power and the ability to see the future. We are unable to see what is ahead, because we are creatures that will constantly keep making frequent mistakes that will forever place us in much anguish.

I should not blame my ignorance because of the cold weather, and moving to America was not an inappropriate move because of the mishaps. What makes it become hurtful; is it my inexperience with cold weather? The problem stemmed from my lack of understanding of what the cold can do to a person's body that is continually working in the cold without prior knowledge of how to dress for the cold. Sometimes when you look back, it makes a person wonder why they do the things they did.

Many a times I wonder about being in the cold, knowing that I was just a few days earlier in a warm climate. It seems sometimes like I was only in a dream. I am unable to relinquish the dream, like the story of Peter Pan that lives in never, never: land, which is only a story. My life in the cold seems to be that way for a long time. I know that I was not physically asleep. Neither was I dreaming. To dream in truth, a person needs to be asleep. People often speak of daydreaming, which is completely different than what I was experiencing.

Taking stock of my life in the early years of my migration, I am glad that I was more or less semi-conscious. Oftentimes I wonder what my life would be like; if I did maintain the kind of life I was living in Jamaica when I migrated. It did pay to be in the state I was in. That could be the reason why I did what I did with the hot water on my fingers. It could be the same thing that happened when I was poisoned by the gas in the garage.

Each time I had some kind of mishap, it left a problem behind. I have never run into a situation that left without a mark. The gas poisoning left me with sinus and back trouble for many years. My fingers at first which were cold, or frozen, left me with two problems for many years. One of the problems was pain in my finger joints for many years. Each time we hit the fall season, my fingers would freeze all the time.

The pain in my finger joints would progressively worsen, from the fall season to all year. I never took any medication for the pain with my fingers. Neither did I seek help from any physician. I never saw the need to take every little problem I have to man. I am able to bear a little pain here and there without anyone knowing what I am going through.

As the years went by, things kept getting worse. The pain in my fingers kept increasing, and adding more and more problems day by day. It progressively increased in a way that I was unable to work as I did many years ago. I started to have pain between my thumb, and my index finger. I was unable to hold things long in my hand when working, especially being a mechanic. A mechanic holds a wrench with their thumb, and their index finger. When there is pain within those two fingers, you have to rest for a while, then go back to work.

Most of my problems would occur when I was working. Not only when I was standing, also when I was on the creeper. Most of the time, you had to work with your arms above your shoulder, or chest. I would put down the wrench, and fold my arms on my chest, until the pain would leave. I would do that all the time until the completion of the work I was doing.

I also had severe pain at my elbows all the time. Once I had a dream that I should use some garlic, placing them by strapping

65

them on the location of my elbows that were hurting. I did try garlic according to the instruction in the dream: it did not work. The bandages I used to strap the garlic to my elbows, stripped some of the skin from my arms, and made them sore for a while.

When I saw I was not being helped by the garlic to alleviate the pain, I quit using the garlic, because of the problem the bandage was doing to my skin. The pain, in my elbows was a continual pain daily. The only time I would not feel the pain, was when I was sleeping. I tried all kinds of exercises for my arms, and my fingers, and my back. It did not matter what kind of exercise I did, not one was able to give me any comfort with my pains. I hear so much about exercise and what it can do for a person, that it will make a person try anything to free themselves from pain and suffering.

I never visited any doctor for my finger and elbow pains. It should not matter whether I did or not, because I was going to doctors and chiropractors for back pain and sinus condition and they were unable to help.

Daily as I went about my business, I kept seeing and hearing lots of other folks were having similar problems as I was having with my finger joints, and with the pain between my thumb, and my index finger, and also lots of pain at my elbows. They had been visiting all kinds of doctors, looking for an answer that might help them. Many operations had been performed to no avail. They made the individuals worse off.

I got to understand that millions of people all over, are suffering with an ailment they call tendonitis, and carpal tunnel. I personally, have seen several individuals that were suffering with tendonitis, and carpal tunnel, and they had to wear a hand brace after the physicians had done many treatments. What seems to happen, the treatment does more harm to the patient than good. They are unable to work anymore. They have to be placed on permanent disability.

This condition is not only with women; men are having the same problem. They are unable to get satisfactory help from our medical professionals. Something is wrong with people today. Why are we refusing to listen to our own selves? We are the ones that keep having the problems. All the doctors that people keep visiting for their health problems most will never truly help. Doctors are killing us with their intellectual degrees. We fall in the trap of being intelligent, is the only way to go in this epoch. We continue visiting these professionals to our own destruction.

I see people today are caught up so much with the philosophy of obtaining a degree from one of the many universities. They do not care to hear what anyone has to say, if they are not educated through the policy set forth by man's standard of education for today's people.

Looking at today's doctrine, I see only prevarication in every dogma. Whether it pertains to schools, or churches, or medicine, all seem to be on the same track. The name of the game is money. When you refuse to play the game, you are going to be an outcast. The people that handle all the keys are going to lock you out. We are unable to find any person that's willing to fight and overturn the boat of destruction.

It is very sad to see the behavior of humanity in this era. The things we do for having a little cash on hand. A person will kill whoever stands in his or her way, just to have some of life's commodities. All that we keep fighting for does not give anyone, longevity on this earth. As I travel this earth, and as I observe people today, I am hurt. The reason why I hurt so much, has to do with what I see happening. What is taking place is not a very pleasant thing.

I speak of my life in the first several years that I migrated, as if to say that I was in a state of semi-consciousness, as if to say I was partially asleep. I also make mention that I never regret being partially asleep. It might have done me more justice than injustice. Despite my analogy, I was not ridiculous in my behavior as I go about my daily routine. I was able to maintain the correct track a person needed to take during their life on earth.

I have seen millions of people daily: intellectuals, illiterates, or people that are living on the streets, which are unable to behave positively. Because they are demonic possessed, all seem to walk the same. There are similarities in people's behavior today. We can find the majority are selfish. It matters not who we are, from the preachers to the ones that confess that there is no GOD, to the ones that are insane, that we claim are unable to fend for them-selves.

Are we so sure that these people are unable to provide correctly for themselves? Is it possible they are so intoxicated with the policy of today's society; that they are hiding under the cloak of insaneness? Lots of folks today are fed up with life and the way things are being handled.

I was never instructed on how dangerous the cold weather is to a person's body. I had to experience it for myself and in a very hurtful way that did remain with me for many years. I saw millions have encountered the same as I did, with different treatment: mine was instantaneous. Others had a slower process over the years, which possibly did more damage to the individuals, than what I did at first.

What I have learned all these years, because the winter weather does have a profound effect on a person's body, we should take better precaution to prevent pain and agony in the later years of our lives. I could have prevented many years of pain and suffering, if I did know better. If someone that lived all their life in the natural ice box had instructed me of the deadliness of the cold snowy weather, I would not have made the foolish mistake that hurt my fingers for so many years.

I have been trying for many years to show other folks what to do to remain healthy in the years to come. I know that the Bible teaches us that we should not take thought for tomorrow, because we are unable to control the future. In-spite, we are unable to control the future, it still does not give us the right to completely ignore the future, which is tomorrow.

I think, what the Bible is trying to relate, is this: we should not completely dwell on carnal things, as if to say, our life depends on the things we use daily. I read in the Bible that man should not live by bread alone, but by every word that proceedeth from the mouth of GOD. St. Matthew 4:4. How is it that a person should live more by words than food? Words are not a physical thing. Food is something a person needs to sustain life on this earth. Why is it then much more vital for the words of GOD for people to live by, than our natural daily rationing? Seeing the truth within the words should awaken us to the more important facts of life.

Being selfish, we are unable to live as we are instructed to do. Looking back at the way I used to do all the road service, it does make a person ask a lot of questions. Was it a form of discrimination: being black, and being a foreigner? I never knew my way around. Each time I was sent out on a road service, I got lost, which would always take more time than normal. The company, whose vehicle is broken down, paid from the time the mechanic leaves the shop until he returned. The longer it takes the mechanic to return to the shop, the more they are able to charge the customers. Was it a policy of discrimination, or were they trying to discourage me that I would quit? Was it a method of making more money for the company? We might never know the truth; we can only speculate on the issue, and leave it there.

As the years went by, my fingers began to give more trouble. They did not only hurt all the time, they would be stiff. It was like people that have chronic arthritis, when you see their fingers are swollen and stiff. My fingers were not swollen. They were stiff and hurt all the time in the joints.

I was never a pill popper. I lived with the pain all the years that I had it. The only time I would take any kind of medication, was when my sinus would flair up. Aspirin was not something that I would take. For the past thirty plus years, I doubt if I have taken twenty aspirins. When I have any headaches, it too will pass. The only time I can recall ever taking any aspirin over the past thirty three or more years was February of 2003. I ran into a very serious problem; that almost took my life.

The problem started something like this: I had a fire in the building that I rented, or say leased. The fire was due to negligence on a person's part. People often say: what is to be, it cannot be reversed. It does seem that it is true. The way things have been going in my life, it is very weird. I have been having one problem after another. It does not matter what I do. It does not look like any man can stop it. The more I tried to make something change for the better, the more it got worse.

My life for the past eighteen or twenty years has been slowly deteriorating. It matters not what I put my hands to, all falls apart. A few people made recommendations that I should go to people that are necromancer, to free me from a curse that someone put on me. If I do not seek help, I am going to lose all my earthly possessions that I have acquired since I migrated.

More than once I replied to the individuals that if GOD sees fit that I should go penniless, there is nothing anyone can do to stop it. When GOD blessed someone, they are blessed. Man and the Devil are unable to reverse the blessings of GOD. All soothsayers, sorceries, necromancers, and witches, or whoever we can dream of, are unable to reverse or stop anything that GOD started.

I am determined that I will never seek the aid of humanity with any kind of magical power. All the power that is used for helping people the way they are doing is not of GOD. GOD is displeased with humanity when we practice the art of necromancy, soothsaying, or sorcery. All of those proceeded from the god of this world, which are the Devil and his confederates. What we might have overlooked, the Devil and his confederates have not been able to do any good work with the power that they have. They can only do the opposite of good, despite that they are acting like GOD. They are just deceiving people with their evil. They are unable to work on the good that is of GOD, Being evil; they can only do unrighteous acts. When men use the influence of the Devil: to do all kinds of workings: that is Devilish.

People keep speaking about me, that I am stubborn. Possibly it is because I refuse to seek the help that they keep recommending. I do not object about man's help when it comes to loans, or other kinds of help that we should give to each other in time of need. The aid that is used to conjure evil spirits is a no, no. Despite all that I put my hands to that keeps falling apart, I know that GOD is able to correct and restore trillion of times the things that I have lost.

If man should be the one that helps me, through the source of the Devil, what will be my answer some day when I shall stand before GOD to account for my actions living on this earth? I know that we all need the substance of this earth to exist; that does not say we should sell ourselves to the devil to live on this earth.

As I study the pattern of my unstable life, I see a hand of evil that has been trying to waste away my life for many years. To this date, the evil force is not successful. The only reason why he is so persuasive, he must know something that is very important that I was born to accomplish. He has been trying all my life to annihilate me that the work of GOD might not be fulfilled in my life.

All the problems that I have encountered all my life, I should have ceased to exist a long time ago. I can remember when I was a small child. I got burned all over my body with hot porridge. I was taken to the hospital, and remained there for a long time. The scar on my hand remained the longest and possibly left because of the cold climate. I dove in the ocean once, headlong, and got stuck on the sand where I could have drowned.

I lived with my dad and my stepmother at her home in St. Ann's Bay; at that time, we used to gather wood for cooking, my stepbrothers and I. This day we were close by the roadside. By an accident, one of my stepbrothers almost cut off one of my feet. The cut was by my instep and my ankle. Fortunately for me a car came by and we stopped the car looking for help to take me to the hospital. How wonderful it was a doctor, and he worked on my foot there, the best he could. Then he drove me to the hospital and finished what he started on the road.

Knowing what happened to my foot that got cut; I could have bled to death. If help was not given to me as quickly as it was, I possibly would have to have an artificial limb for my right foot. Thanks, be to GOD that the doctor was passing by when he did and stopped also to help. He could have continued his journey to where he was going without stopping. So many things happen to us that we are unable to answer correctly what happened.

Take the fire that destroyed my business. I was standing in the solution when it exploded. I tried to extinguish the fire. I could have been killed. I have to say that I am a very fortunate person to be alive and to talk about what happened with the fire. I need to be thankful to GOD for being alive today. The enemy failed once more in his conquest.

Not long after the fire, I ran into another problem. This time death was also close at my door. The winter of two thousand two and three was exceptionally cold. I was in the building trying to work, and to organize things in some way that I could clean up the place and finish working on the vehicles that I had there that did not get destroyed in the fire.

Not thinking that it was that cold, because I was not feeling cold at first, I continued for a while working without any heat. The fire did destroy a lot of the things that were in the building; I am still fortunate that all things were not destroyed. Only a few vehicles got destroyed in the fire. Not one person got injured. As long as there is life there is hope to regain all that got destroyed in the fire.

Working in the cold building, I started to feel like my insides were freezing. Normally, a person's outer layer would be the first thing to start to get cold; I was not feeling that cold externally, it was internally that was giving me the problem. Then I noticed my forehead began to be very cold like my head was also freezing up. Then my whole body began to feel like it was freezing, I related to my friend who was there with me, that I was going home because I felt like I was freezing up.

I drove home; the vehicle I drove home in the heat was not working. Soon as I got home I jumped into bed. I was unable to eat or sleep for weeks. I spoke to friend of mine in Canada about how I was feeling. She suggested that I should drink some alcohol, mixed with some lemon juice. I did that. It never did me any good, I still was unable to eat or drink anything for more than two weeks. I was not getting any sleep at the same time. One day I felt like eating some fruit. I called a friend of mine, and asked her if she could get some fruit from the store for me. They were not able to get it on time.

In my home, I had some canned peaches, pears, and applesauce. I ate some of the pears, peaches, and the apple sauce. I was stopped by a horrendous pain in my stomach. I went to lie down. The pain continued for a time, to about one hour and a half. At the end of that time, I felt my intestines, or stomach open and let the food I ate past through.

Not long after the opening of my stomach that let the food pass through, the pain I was having in my stomach ceased. The alcohol that I drank three days before, I tasted in my mouth and felt it in my system after the food passed further into my stomach. I then realized that my intestines were closed, and it reopened. I related to many folks about the tasting of the alcohol three days after I drank it. I do not think too many people believed that I tasted the alcohol three days later. It is very hard for people to grasp what happened to me. They wanted to know, where the alcohol was staying in my system

72

that I would taste it three days later. Many folks thought that I was lying. Nobody is able to consume liquid and three days later be able to still taste it. There is no need for me to lie or make up a story to impress anyone. I know what happened. I was surprised myself when I began to taste the alcohol once more that I drank three days earlier.

After the opening of my stomach, I was unable to eat solid food for more than two weeks. I tried to eat some rice and other firm foods. What would happen each time I had some solid foods to eat, I would have severe pain in my stomach. Especially at the area where I felt my stomach open and let the foods pass from the night before. I would also feel sick to my stomach when I ate solid foods.

For more that two weeks I remained on a liquid diet, then slowly I started to have solid food once more. During this problem, it was the first time in over thirty years that I did take some aspirins. I was having constant headaches, night and day. I was unable to sleep, night or day. For a while I had no appetite.

At the same time, when all these things were happening to me, a lot of sore like bumps were popping up all over my head. They hurt all the time. I was unable to lie down on my back or my side. It mattered not which side I laid on, there was always pain, because of the sores that were all around my head.

When I was unable to eat or sleep, I was dragged to the hospital. They kept me there more than a week. Before I was taken to the hospital, I was sick at home over a month. I was unable to hear anything out of my ears. It was like I was deaf for several weeks. My left ear came back before my right ear. My right ear remained a problem for a long time.

I also had a lot of problems on my right side. From my head to my foot, it was like I had a stroke. I had a tremendous headache all the time just on half of my head. It felt like my head was about to split open all the time. That was the reason why I took the aspirins.

The first night I was able to get some sleep I had a dream that informed me that a portion of my brain was dead. If I had visited the hospital earlier when I first got sick, they would kill me with all the medication that they would some how inject into my system. Nevertheless I should not worry myself, about the section of my brains that were dead. GOD would take care of my dead brain.

When I got some sleep, I would possibly sleep for about ten minutes or so. That was all the sleep I was getting. Being dragged to the hospital, the doctors questioned me, and I spoke to them about not being able to sleep, eat and the sores that kept popping up in my head. I also related to them about my hearing, and the dream; I held back nothing from them.

The doctor ordered blood work, and x rays. When they were not pleased with the x rays, they ordered a cat-scan for my head. They did all kinds of examination on my body. They checked my ears to see the cause of my hearing loss and the cause of all the problems that I was having. All the tests they did turned up negative. They thought I was faking the sickness. They recommended that I should remain in the hospital over night. I was kept there against my will more than a week. Despite that I was in the hospital, I was unable to sleep. I was given sleeping pills, and they did not work. At first they gave me a hundred milligram. Then they changed it to one hundred and fifty. Those did not work.

The biggest problem I was having in the hospital was being tortured on their hospital bed. Whatever I was given to sleep on was very uncomfortable. Their mattress was too hard. It was like I was in a torture chamber. How can a person ever sleep when they are being tortured? Hospitals I understand are supposed to be there to help the sick people recover from their illness, and not get worse.

The knowledge I acquired over the years, with my last visit to the hospital, opened my understanding much broader than before. It truly showed me that people are not really being helped in a very healthy way in the hospitals. It is very sad to see that the people that are educated by our educators are still ignorant of helping the people that are sick.

At first, I was very upset when I was forced to stay in the hospital against my will. What I observed while in the hospital, taught me that the people we look up to as trained medical professionals of the human body, in truth, are still backward in a very great way. It is very sad to see and know that billions are in the same ship of ignorance. Yet they are teaching billions how to be healthy when they still need lots of teaching. Having a ticket from the university they graduated from has not given them the true knowledge how to help the sick and afflicted people.

Looking at the various pieces of our modern day machinery used in the hospitals, and how the men and the women are still working in trial and error method, hurts very deeply. The thing about this kind of practice, people are relying on these men and women with great expectation for their health to improve when they are sick. In my opinion, people put their life in the hands of these men and women. We have been brain washed with lots of propaganda.

I feel people should stop putting so much confidence in accepting the medical philosophy in this era. Physicians obtain their knowledge about the body by a procedure set forth by each country's educational system. After satisfaction in their studies, they receive a piece of paper with their names, stating that they are now qualified to meet all challenge of the profession they acquired while attending the University of their Choice.

I observe in man's behavior that they somewhat ignore the people that are suffering. They use their knowledge according to the way they were taught when they were studying to get their degree. Since man is unable to see correctly what a person is going through, they have to practice according to how they were educated. This takes us back to trial and error. One little mistake is detrimental to the individual. Because the majority live in the ship of illiteracy, when it comes to the human body, we follow the leader of the people that claim they have expert knowledge of the body because they are graduates from a medical school. Because they are graduates, does not make them know fully what they are doing.

We get upset with mechanics when they use an un-skilled method like wire to hold a vehicle together. The unsafe procedure using bailing wire can be deadly. Not only to the operators: it also can be deadly when it comes into contact with the people in the surroundings because quick fix has no guarantee. The law of the land prohibits all unsafe repairs on all motor vehicles. It does not matter how rich and powerful anyone might be, they are not permitted to repair any kind of transportation and put it on the highway, being unsafe.

Motor vehicles are a mechanical piece of machinery made from a material known as iron. Iron comes from the earth and is made through a process with fire. Metal does not have the ability to think or feel. It cannot speak. Neither can it move itself. Where-ever we place it, there will it remain forever? We make lots of laws, governing the way these mechanical devices are made that it will be safe when in use, hoping; that the unsafe equipment would not take people's lives yearly.

The body of a human is much more delicate than any piece of machinery. Man is flesh and blood, which is very soft, and very easy to be destroyed. Man's body does not have the capability to withstand harsh treatment as a piece of metal. Put man against a piece of steel, and the steel will cut and destroy the flesh. The metal will not be wasted.

We put more effort into procuring our feeless substances. The things that can feel, speak, move around, and can truly care, we have less feelings and care for. We go about our daily routine like humans are less important than our machinery. We refuse to take our cars and trucks, to any mechanic shop that works in trial and error.

People like to take their transportation to qualified people: Ones that are capable of making you satisfied with the service performed on their vehicle. Take the trial and error being done daily by our medical professionals, and we accredit them as being very skillful. Should not we as flesh and blood creatures be more outrageous with the kind of practice being done on human bodies daily?

Look at what our medical professionals are doing daily with humans. People are creatures known as flesh and blood. We eat and drink to stay alive. We are unable to survive without sleeping. We take wire and metal, and we tie up man's flesh and bones. We congratulate our men and women that they have performed an outstanding and excellent job. When they are finished with their job they say well done. They send you a bill for thousands of dollars, and we being pleased with their botched job, pay without opposition.

When an individual's equipment is being botched up, some people will go so far, as to kill the person that botched up their vehicle. Daily in the courts all over, you can find people who are dissatisfied with jobs they feel were a botched job that they receive from whoever performed the job. All kinds of professionals are being sued daily, because the clients feel they are being gypped. Many doctors are up in arms today, because they feel they are being taken to the cleaners daily and that their insurance premium is outrageous.

I see a lot of flaws in so many things we do today. The reason we have so many bad things in our society is that we have destroyed the mine set among the people, and they are unable think. Take the artificial cadaver invented by man; they are trying to make us aware; people who desire the medical profession will be able to complete their medical studies in a shorter time by getting away from the study of the real flesh and bone structure of human cadavers, and use the artificial mechanically made cadaver.

I read in the newspaper, our researchers would be grateful, if they were able to have access to more than a hundred thousand of people's computers one day. Access to that large amount of computers, would give the medical association the power source needed to find the answer that they have been looking for hundreds of years. Once more I see within the medical occupation, continual deception as when I was in the hospital. It is the same thing I see they are trying to coax people to let them have the use of your computer in a day to solve humanity's health problems.

A computer does not have the power and the ability to think on its own. It can only revert to what is programmed. It cannot formulate, and then reply. If it is not there, it cannot give you what you are looking for. Whatever you are looking for has to be implanted.

Look at man. With all the power we have to think, and to create, if the knowledge is not implanted within the brains, no matter how hard we try we will never be able to create anything. The ability and power has to be there first. That is why we go to school so that the teachers can work to get out what is deep within a person's brains.

There are millions of people all over the world that never learned to read. The reason they remain unable to read, their faculties were not developed, which make it difficult for them, and others to help in educating them. All the instruction they have been given all their life was not powerful enough for them to understand what people were teaching them. Since man is unable to educate everyone, so they have the power to think, feel, and reason, how are they going to make a machine do what they are unable to have people do?

Scientists teach that people developed genetically. Yet, we find that while some parents are very backward their children are intellectually smart. The thing is this; not everyone can be outstanding in life. We have some doctors who are more qualified in their skills than others. It is not that there are better schools which are able to give anyone a greater understanding; it has to do with the individual's faculties.

Our schools help individuals to develop what is within, by starting to work with our children when they are very young. Waiting for old age makes the process longer and harder. If a person's comprehension is very slow, greater effort is needed to help develop that person. That is what I see in the medical field that I have experienced. I am not speaking of what I hear someone said or someone write about. I am addressing what I have encountered with our medical professionals. Whether it pertained to MD'S, psychologists, or chiropractors, it does not matter. I see the same behavior in all. I also see similar behavior in many other professional people.

Looking back on my recent admission at the hospital; I want you to know that I came out of the hospital in a more unhealthy state than when I went there. I was not getting any rest, because I was being tortured in their beds. While I was a patient in the hospital, I was fortunate to experience three different rooms. Changing rooms did one thing for me; it opened my eyes to see, that all the beds in the hospitals are just torture chambers.

It did not make any sense to complain. Whatever bed I was placed in, would have done the same thing to my body. I was given sleeping medication. They did not work. If it did work, I would still only get about half an hour sleep time. Oftentimes during the night the nurses would keep checking on me to see if I was sleeping. I was not going to make them know that I saw them each time they came to see if I was sleeping. They never did walk directly up to my bed. They would simply open the door and peak in. The light was always off. Standing far away was not good enough to know if I was asleep.

What was happening with me in the hospital? I noticed I was in a lot of pain, especially my feet. They were very stiff. I never really did look at my feet when I was in the hospital. The reason they were so stiff was they were swollen. When I got home, somehow I looked at my feet and they were both swollen.

At first, when I saw my swollen feet, my reasoning was negative.

I felt it was the sleeping pills, or other possibilities, because I was not sleeping, or because I was drinking too much milk. With the knowledge I acquired about the body, I can tell you straight up it was the bed that tortured me so much.

I have so much that I want to tell you, something that is very important for you to know. I am very sorry that the time is not right as yet to tell you. The time is very near. It is sooner than you might think. All you have to do is wait a little bit longer. It is not years away; it can be months.

I am trying to open your understanding. I know that I have a very great task on my hands, especially because I know that millions of people all over the world today, feel or believe that the only way to understand the body is to be schooled by one of the many universities in the world, otherwise you are an illiterate when it comes to the body.

Our men and women profess that they are very knowledgeable about the body, because they have been through intensive study and research. We need to ask ourselves, why are they so perplexed with so many diseases? Look at the many new ones that pop up yearly that keep men in their trial and error game all the time. What about all the old ailments that have been around so long that man is unable to stop or even treat correctly?

All the problems that I had all the years, I was unable to be helped with all the knowledge that our men and women have acquired. This makes me understand, that they are still void of understanding many things about the body. I just did not have one problem all my life; I ran into many difficulties that were unsolvable by doctors in two countries.

I made a statement somewhere in this writing, "May GOD help us". The reason I made that statement had to do with what I recently experienced with doctors and psychiatrists. I would like the truth to be known. As I see it, many might not have seen it as I have. I think it is a very sad story. If I was treated that way, I am sure that everyone is being treated the same way.

We need to always understand that man is human. They are not powerful enough to penetrate the inner being of humanity to know what is there and how to fully treat anyone. Therefore doctors will forever work with a practice of trial and error. We need to always understand that about humanity. Man is fully being controlled by the Devil. As long as we are being controlled by our enemy, we are going to have all kinds of problems that will be unsolvable by humanity.

Whoever we serve, and obey; what he has to give, that is what we will have to receive from him. What is it the Devil has to give? The Devil; only has deception to offer. He does not have the truth. Therefore he cannot give the truth. If he should ever give the truth, he would be destroying his own leadership. His confederates would in-turn oppose him. He would not have anymore kingdom of his own, that he gave up heaven for, so that he could take over this earth from man: to be lord over humanity.

Mankind has given away what was theirs for nothing, to become the subject of a tyrannous leader. We just sit back without any resistance to such a cruel leader. He keeps us in agony all the time. He uses the ones that are our intellectuals to keep us in deception all the days of our lives. They tell us that they know so much. In truth, they are just being used by our enemy.

When I was taken to the hospital, the doctor that examined me was not able to find anything wrong with my system. According to the way he was taught, he thought I was only hallucinating. According to the ability he had obtained by man's knowledge, nothing was physically wrong with me. His educational background let him come up with an answer that I needed to see a psychiatrist.

The doctor asked me if I would speak with the hospital psychiatrist to see if they could evaluate me. He was lost in his knowledge, only because he is a servant of the Devil. The Devil has full control over him. He thinks that every person a doctor is unable to find anything wrong with needs to be examined by another puppet of Satan.

I see what is happening to humanity today. We have placed so much confidence in our education that we are unable to correctly think on our own. I see that education has placed a huge blindfold over humanity's eyes. Education has kept us more ignorant than any other civilization.

You might think that I am being cruel to our educators. You might be thinking that I should not be so dogmatic against the people that are responsible for educating people. Let me show you something. I am not so much against the formal educators, in-spite that they are the ones that encourage millions to proceed to higher learning. That turns out to be destructive to the majority of the population globally.

The educations that I am totally against are the ones that keep teaching us that we need to diet to remain healthy. If we add exercising to our dieting, we will be able to fight off all kinds of invaders that are trying to invade our bodies to destroy it. They keep feeding us lies all the time, saying that they are educating us. Because they are blinded and cannot see themselves, they do not know that they are the instrument of Satan.

That is why; it might appear that I am cruel in my writing against our educators. If I am cruel with my writing, I might just help a few folks to wake up, and remove the blindfold before it is too late. As we take stock of the increase in diseases internationally, we should realize that man is helpless in the stoppage of even the economy that is getting out of hand. How then are they going to stop what they are unknowledgeable with?

I spoke with one of the many hospital psychiatrists. I do not think he listened to one word I was saying. He took the words of the doctors, and other people, and treated me on their words. To me that did not make any sense. When I objected, and tried to walk out of the hospital, they called for help. About six, or more men came. They forced me onto one of the transporters that the hospital uses to take patients from one section of the hospital to the next. They held me down on the transporters, strapped me down, and then injected me with some kind of tranquilizer.

The other thing was this. I was informed that if I did not take the medication prescribed by the psychiatrist, I would remain in the hospital more than a month. It was imperative for me to consume the medication. Then I would be able to be discharged earlier from the hospital.

I played along with their evil maneuver, by taking the medication from them. They saw me place the pills in my mouth. That was it. I never swallowed the medication. I was determined that I was not going to make those evil monsters destroy me. I was not going to lose my sanity, become insane, and remain being a puppet the rest of my life.

I wonder how many people, who were sane, lost their sanity because they were willing to heed the men and the women that informed them that they can help. Since the medical professionals have a one track mind they can only prescribe drugs for their patients. The truth will remain hidden forever. Most folks listen to the educational teaching as the only source of knowledge. If you are not within the bracket they accept, you are going to be treated shamefully.

Since I do not accept society intellectuals of today, I was able to save myself from the erroneous unhealthy treatment while millions were being swindled out of their sanity. It is sad to see what evil creatures we have become. It is because we have allowed the wrong educators to educate us. It might be late for some; it is not late for everyone.

I hope and pray that as many people that read what I am saying may try to turn their life around for better things to come. I can teach you the appropriate ways to be much wiser than you are doing. That you might stop; giving so much heed to the doctrine of devils. At this stage in life: look where we are heading. Is there any help, real help that man has to offer? Look what they were trying to do to me by their education.

I was not pretending that I was sick. I was having a lot of problems. I really and truly almost froze to death. I was so bad that my stomach would not allow food to pass into my intestine, to my digestive system; as taught by man we have to eat to retain life: we have a notion that we have to eat to live.

I am sure what I am saying is accurate. What happened is my body shut itself down. As a result, my body was able to keep itself alive. By stopping food; from being digested that produces the necessary nutrients needed to live healthy, my body was able to work in another way that was much more powerful.

When a person is sick and they keep eating all the time, their body is unable to work as it can. It has to keep digesting the food we keep stuffing in our system all the time. This behavior stems from the poor understanding our medical professionals have who lack the understanding of the body's full potential. Our educators keep teaching us that we need to have three balanced meals daily and that we should have snacks in between meals. I know that if my system did not shut itself down, I possibly could have passed on and gone to the next life. The weeks, in which I was not eating, my body was working in a manner far beyond man's knowledge about the body. It is shameful to see, and to know man's deception, and to know of all the people that give a listening ear to these men and women daily.

I am not trying to be subterfuge in my writing. Neither am I being deceptive in any of my speech. In this book, I am not going to show you what your body is capable of doing when you are sick. I have my reasons. In the near future you will find out. You will not be regretful you learned when you did. I am not playing games with your life, or trying to make you become my merchandise.

I know that we have developed a society that requires money to purchase our daily ration. Without money these days, we are going to have a difficult time making ends meet. Despite the demands, I do not see the need to lie, to cheat, or to kill others to get rich. Being rich is not a sin. Neither is being poor sinful.

My ambition is to help people; if possible we might be able to unite and try to take back from the Devil what he has taken from us in the first place. By this time, the knowledge that we find within all the books written showing man's behavior from generation to generation, should have made this generation, with all the technology behave wiser than all the previous civilizations that have come and gone.

After analyzing man's behavior in every possible way, it is very hard to grasp man's movements, and to understand why we live the way we do. We are devastated at the time of a person's death. It does hurt when someone departs this life. Yet we fail to see and understand what it is saying to the living when someone dies.

As we address man's behavior, it is so hard to figure out why we act the way we do. We speak in contradictions in almost everything we do daily. Humans are confusing creatures. Even the things that we teach one another that are correct, we do not maintain them continually.

Take for instance the foods that are being served in the hospitals.

They are very unhealthy for the consumer. Yet we find they are provided by the same people that keep prescribing to the population that junk foods are unhealthy. When I was admitted in the hospital recently it was a shame to see the poor quality of the foods being served daily.

I do not think our medical association has the right to publicize, healthy and unhealthy foods. They are guilty of feeding sick people with the same unhealthy foods. I think the first thing they need to do is to maintain their own philosophy. They should not be allowed to censor a product, and then, have some company mass-produce the food that they used to feed the patient in the hospitals. How is it, on one hand it is unhealthy, and on the other hand it is very much healthy?

It seems, as long as money is involved, we are going to create a double standard in many things that we do in this life on this earth. People are being made puppets for no good reason. Something needs to be done about the evil pathway that we are treading.

I cannot speak for everyone. I know that I can speak on my behalf, and possibly, I might be able to speak for a few citizens. The majority is difficult to address. In this era I feel that the majority does not care in a moral honest way. Being puppets, the majority are in a ship of death. Because death is the controller, they maintain that kind of lifestyle as long as they remain walking this earth.

We are going to hear that the medical association does not have much to do with regulating the food served in hospitals nation wide. They also have nothing to do with tobacco distribution, and the foods that they keep publicizing on TV, and with all the monthly publications that get publicized globally each month. They can get millions of people's attention internationally, on cigarettes, and other food products that are unhealthy for consumption. People are listening. Why are they not doing anything against the unhealthy food being served in the hospitals?

It is not only food that is being served in the hospitals that are unhealthy; many things a person is knowledgeable with, and will find deadly and unhealthy, are being used in the hospitals all over the world. Since I was recently admitted into the hospital, I came out of the hospital much worse than when I went there. I am awakening to millions of people that they're being killed yearly in the places where they go to be treated.

To me that does not make any sense. In every direction a person looks, it is senseless. The only reason why people keep flocking to these places is that, they are puppets to our educators. When our medical association speaks the majority listens to their own destruction. The only reason possibly that people heed the words of the men and women that addresses man's health, is that there is no recourse. Since there is only one source, when people are being afflicted with ailments, they have to run to the only source that is available.

I, would like all the world's population to know that we now can create a genuine source, that will give you a recourse. The source you will have within your hands will be able to give you great peace of mind. You will not have to run to the doctors for everything that ails you.

When you obtain the source that will be able to give you this recourse, you will be able to understand many things that have been hidden from your understanding most of your life. I say most, because you will learn about them before you die. I have been learning many things that have been hidden from our wise and prudent men of today. This is why I am writing to you; I am willing to share with you what was handed to me. It is not pleasant to maintain what was given to me only for myself. If I do not pass it along, I will part this life with all the knowledge that was given to me. Millions are going to remain suffering all the days of their life.

As you read about my partial life in Jamaica and in America, you have seen problems that I had been through health wise. Medical teams in two countries were unable to truly help me with my medical problems, whether there are modern day technologies or no advanced technologies.

I am not being subterfuge. I am speaking the truth. You will be able to be helped just as I was helped. Now I do not need to visit chiropractors any more and I do not need to keep visiting doctors as I once did for a sinus condition. As I might have stated somewhere along the line, I will be able to show you how to lose weight without any exercising, and to diet differently than our educators are teaching dieting.

Just relax, take off your shoes, and sit back in your easy chair. Make your body do the work for you. From this day forward, at that time, all you have to do for you body is feed it and put it to sleep. Your body will be able to do the rest for you much better than you can.

Slumber

Chapter (4)

After careful evaluation I realize that humanity from the beginning to this present day fails to discern the importance of sleep. I look to my upbringing and I was never taught how one should sleep correctly. Not knowing the importance of sleeping healthy, people have taken sleep for granted by looking upon slumber as just resting by going to bed.

The other thing that's transpiring is that when our body automatically becomes tired, and is trying to shut itself down, we just place it anywhere it's convenient. One would simply fall asleep anywhere, on whatever is available, and at the time as long as they are getting some rest.

To this date, I realize that the vast population of the world has not the faintest idea how to sleep correctly. The other thing I realize is that all the educators of the world do not know the proper procedure to teach the correct way to sleep. If they did people could get the total rest they are entitled to all the days of their lives. Lack of proper and healthy sleeping approaches should show humanity that our educators fail to have the knowledge and understanding to educate the population on the importance of sleep. Because we are not knowledgeable about the importance of slumber we place ourselves in danger. Even our scientists, along with the researchers, fail to see the destruction the world population is doing to itself.

Scientist doctrine states that this universe has existed for millions of years. Man has been trying to find all kinds of answers about man and this world. Millions of people from various parts of the globe take time out to lend a listening ear to the scientists and educators who received their certificates from one of the various universities. In their doctrine they keep informing us they are very knowledgeable about plants and animals. We find the same claim is being made by them about humans, and also the universe.

Yet, we hear many sounds of perplexity in the teachings of men. They state that they are learned people with plants and animals, as well as the creation of this world. Finding great conflict in their teaching shows that we fail in harmony all the days of our life. One group, over here, says there is no GOD. Another says there is a God, but he is not the one that created this world. Some believe that GOD is the Creator. Yet, they are in irreverence to Him.

All the people who ascribe to this world through the process of evolution, which is self creation, do not believe in a supreme being known as GOD. They accept a theory of teaching known as the big-bang.

By a massive explosion things came into existence. Theoretically, from this start, man, animals and all vegetation were able to develop to what we see and touch today. All of man's wisdom, knowledge, and understanding, obtained so far have not done much for us over the generations of man inhabiting this earth. Man with his understanding has turned many things upside down and inside out, looking for all kinds of answers in conjunction with the diseases that is man's misery.

Seeing man's prevarication awoke me to these words "Wisdom truly excelleth folly as far as light excelleth darkness". (Ecclesiastes 2:13). Believe it or not, generation after generation we just keep on failing to understand there is a very simple procedure to finding many answers in regards to man's many illnesses.

Teaching of diets seems to be common in today's daily living. We behave like food is the essence of life. We know that food is vital and very necessary for human survival on earth. Sleep is just as important as food. One cannot survive for long without food. Likewise, we are unable to last long without sleeping.

Take away from mankind things like food that they love so much, and life might come to its end. If the individual did not die, he would not be able to move as normal or eat as much. His stomach would shrink. He would have to eat like a baby, only having liquid for a time regardless of his/her age.

Not many individuals take a journey into life by not eating or drinking for thirty days and thirty nights. Going that long without food and water, requires great self discipline. That is not found in many folks. Most humans do not have a character within their minds to endure such rigor. Not many individuals see the need of such a rigorous maneuver. Most people do not like to be disciplined.

Throughout history, only a few have I learned of, have gone without food and water for more than thirty days. I have not seen or learned of many humans going without food and water over thirty days. Since food is vital for one's existence, what about sleep? A person can go for thirty days or more without food. Can we go thirty days without sleeping? Eventually one will kick the bucket, described as death, by not sleeping. Take away sleep from someone and I know they cannot exist for too long.

Take both food and sleep from a person at the same time, and I am positive that, that person's life would be very short. Death would be imminent for all people if they withheld food and sleep from themselves. Having food only for thirty days, what would be the condition of one's body after going that long without sleeping? I am not encouraging any individuals go without food for a long period.

I have learned from our educators that we should not go for days without eating and drinking. I have not heard, neither have I seen, where we place great emphasis on sleeping over eating. Is it possible for a person to maintain their life not eating for thirty days? Can a person maintain their life without sleeping for thirty days?

All my life I have never seen nor have I heard of anyone going for thirty days or more without sleeping. Examine the life of one who does fasting a lot. We will find out they never miss any rest. Slumber to a person who fasts a lot is very important. People that diet a lot need their rest. They never give up their sleep.

We don't have lots of people capable of doing strenuous fasting and doing significant physical work at the same time. People that do a lot of fasting normally make sure they never lose their sleep. Most start their fasting during the night as they slumber, because it's not as strenuous for them. Some can go for days without any intake. Others need some liquid intake to keep them from dehydration. Some feel they need to heed man's teaching that they will encounter dehydration going without some kind of liquid for days.

Someone that spends most of their life fasting will normally make sure they get their rest. Slumber is not only for sleeping. Eating food is not only to satisfy one's hunger. We should eat and drink. Our bodies require food as a means of sustaining life. Sleep works hand in hand with all the food we eat daily. At night sleep should take care of the rest of the essential needs for a healthy life.

What so many of us overlook, including our educators, is that we can overdo our eating and sleeping. Either of the two can be harmful by living an unrestrained lifestyle. We have not found out the proper procedure of eating and sleeping correctly because our intellectuals are unknowledgeable about the body's full potential.

Failing to understand the full potential of the body, even with all the modern technology we have in this era, millions daily go through severe agony. We have not found the simple answers to why man really needs to sleep and to why it's so important for humanity to get the proper amount of sleep daily.

The advancement in technology today requires men to work twenty four-seven everyday of the year. Under modern day work schedules, people do not work just one shift. Many have to work one of the three shifts designated by the company they work for. Therefore each person's sleep time will vary by their appointed schedule. Whether they work hours during the day or at night it does not matter; one needs to always get their sleep. Day or night a person's body does not recognize only night for sleeping.

When a person's body begins to change from conscious to unconscious, we should try and give our bodies the best comfort possible. Human behavior with slumber, work, and other activities keeps our days and nights filled to its maximum. This prevents us from nourishing our bodies as we should. Failure: to understand the appropriate amount of food and sleep for our bodies to remain healthy; stops many people today from getting the correct daily amount of required sleep and food.

Because we either get too much sleep and food, or not enough, we cannot meet our appointed schedules. Punctuality, for whatever we have to accomplish daily, is very important for a pleasant routine. Many people use alarm clocks to wake themselves so they can get to work on time.

When our alarm clocks malfunction, in most cases, people miss some of their normal daily activities. It does not matter whether it pertains to work or to other appointments. Sometimes we take an extra little nap because we never got the appropriate rest our body required during our slumbering hours. The other thing that is possible is that many times we simply hate getting out of bed whether at night or during the day.

Failing to understand the importance of slumber in this era, many of us place entertainment and pleasurable activities over their health. Not realizing what the most appropriate thing a person needs to remain healthy for many years, we sweep it under the rug until our health starts to fail. Many think differently when they lose their jobs because they were constantly late. Constant lateness would call for dismissal.

There are reasons why so many of us are always late. We find too many things that occupy our waking hours. Man will always keep putting off sleep for some reason or another. Many people throughout their lives seem to believe money, food, and other items should be placed before sleep. It seems many keep trying to postpone their slumber by finding a way to live without sleeping so as to have more of life's wealth.

Wealth and all the pleasures have little or no value when sickness starts to control your body. I once had a very good friend, who had a few dollars. Inappropriate as it may seem, many of us only look upon a person as wealthy simply because they are worth a lot. My friend once said to me that if it was possible to purchase good health from a healthy friend, he would have that done, because he learned the system of how to make lots of money. Regaining new life as a child, with an adult understanding, would make it easy to obtain all the wealth; he would simply use days or months earlier to purchase better health. Doing that would also give him a longer life span also.

He and others eventually found out that it's not possible for anyone to exchange their life, in the same manner they use money to purchase our daily needs. I also realized that man cannot use money to purchase good health when it's too far gone. Going over my friend's words helped me to realize that his desire, to purchase a new healthy life for himself, had awakened me to many things that I seemed to have overlooked.

Each person's life is without price. We cannot place a value on a person's life because it's unchangeable in all forms. If that was possible, only the poor would die and be the ones who would remain being sick all the time. People who have great wealth would always purchase from the poor both their health and their life. I realize some that are poor would not give up their life for all the wealth in the world. Others would not care what would happen to their life as long as they could get something to eat and drink, as well as lots of sex."

GOD is the only one that can give man an extension of his life. Still it's not money one can use with GOD to obtain an extension of great health. All it takes for a person to receive great health and a longer life from GOD is to simply remain faithful to him in all the things he commanded. He will do the rest that he promised humanity.

Knowing that we are unable to purchase longevity and good health, why are we fighting so hard for money, homes, cars, and other perishable items? In this era people allow nonessential items to create a hindrance to their daily slumber. I do realize the days we are living in and what has been adopted as our normal way of life. We allow the teaching of our philosophers to blindfold our eyes and minds. We see and think only of this world's substance as being of vital importance. Only when sickness and death is at one's door that they see the importance of one's health and life, then they try to place it in the correct perspective.

My friend's love for long life and good health awakened him to life's importance. He had made a great living for himself by making lots of money. Seeing the importance of life, he wished there was another way he could take to remove sickness and death he saw hovering over him. Months before his death, my friend and I had a very long conversation in his car. He made me understand it was too late for him to make a change in his life that would make a difference with GOD and man. Even though I saw the pain my friend was undergoing, I was unable to help him. I see where millions are in the same boat as he. I know that many would like to alter their lifestyle.

The problem is this: man can only see today. People that lived in the past have always used hindsight over foresight. That continues in the present. It seems to be that hereditary sickness is transmitted genetically generation after generation. I do not see anything else that has transmitted hereditarily. The other thing that's possible with humanity is that our poor knowledge, in conjunction with man's well-being, could be the true reason we lack foresight all the days of our lives.

Observing man's comport, even through books, I see that the majority of humans all over the world do not show much interest in their real health until something drastic happens that affects them. It forces them to do some alteration one way or another. I also see over and over where many do not care one bit what happens to their life. They simply keep living dangerously all the days of their life.

Humans are very difficult creatures to understand. They fight so much "to keep up with the Joneses", as the saying goes, that they constantly fail to see what life is all about. I have not seen, nor learned, where one person ever fights to become sick "to keeping up with the Joneses".

When the Joneses are sick we fight to stay away. People hate to be sick anytime in their lifetime. Diseases rob a person of the things they love to do and what they enjoy. Most humans will end up in their beds. People whine a lot when they are sick. It should make one ask the question why is it we complain so much when sicknesses confront us. Since we do not show any real interest in our health until we get ill, we should not whine as much since we never restrain ourselves when we are feeling great. Over and over we keep failing to see the evil we are doing to ourselves.

We keep emphasizing that we are adults. Adults place lots of emphasis on newborn babies that they should always get lots of rest daily. They are much more delicate than adults are. When babies lose their daily sleep, it is very unhealthy for their structure to develop correctly. Death will overtake that child. A newborn child does not have the power to nurture their body. It takes a caring individual to correctly nurture that child to have good health as they grow up. When a parent fails to spend quality time with their babies; many times it scars the child for life.

During their infant days, many times, those babies end up with various sicknesses which affect them all of the days of their lives. A person should never laugh at any kid who is obese or has some other illness that will follow them from their infant days. It is caused by their parent's neglect throughout their babyhood. Since babies are unable to feed and clean themselves, we should always make sure that they are getting their daily required needs. Therefore, someone should make it very important that the baby's needs are being met each day.

A person who is a good parent will always make sure that their baby receives what it needs as its comfort daily. It is not only food and a bath that comfort a baby daily. Babies also need the warmth and loving affection of their mother and father as they cuddle them all the time. Sometimes, that's what the child needs the most. So many times we just give them a bottle or a pacifier for them to stop crying. The baby needs comfort in some form or another. The bottle or a pacifier does that for them. They have to learn to be comfortable with what they obtain from their nurturer.

Because they only speak by crying, we never truly try to understand what the children are saying in their crying. Lots of parents these days are too busy with the affairs of this life to bring up their children in a way that should be most important. Having cars and a beautiful home are much more important than a child's upbringing. We can find lots of kids that turn out to be hooligans or vagabonds.

It's not always the child's fault. Still each child has a responsibility for their own well being in life. We cannot always cast the blame on parents.

The essence of sleep is also vital for the child's proper growth. As the infant develops, we always reduce their sleeping hours. The child, just as an adult, tries their best sometimes to reduce their hours of sleep daily. This is a great concern that caring parents have. They will make it a priority of their duties to see that their child gets their daily required rest.

As a baby increases in their growth, they reduce their amount of sleep. Also, the pattern of their feeding changes as they progress in growth. They now start to get a little more solid food. Not all liquids are given to the child daily. Adults do not need as much sleep as newborn babies up to the age of about three or four years of age. Adults are more developed with stronger bodily structure. Even the food they eat is made different than babies.

Looking at adults' comport, I see that they change in many ways that are more unrestrained than children. Good parents monitor their baby's eating daily. They are precise about feeding their child. In all things in life we have good and bad. There are good, loving, and compassionate parents. There are evil, inconsiderate parents who have no feelings at all for the well-being of their offspring. It is difficult to understand how and why someone's parents would be so cruel to their own kids.

Many parents that live selfishly behave the same way with their children as they develop. It can be the reason why many kids end up with uncontrolled eating habits. They eat as they are being taught at home. Good, caring unselfish procreators always show their kids self-restraint with their own eating habits. The fault I see these days is that our adults need to change the way they eat. We have reduced our sleeping hours, and increased our eating habits. As we reduce our slumber periods, we should likewise reduce our food intake. It is not necessary for anyone to consume the large quantity of food they have daily.

Adults behave worse with their eating habits than infants. Is it because they have the power to get whatever they crave? Infants, and the next stage up from infancy, are unable to get what they want. They have to always ask by crying or some other method to get what they want. The other thing that might be possible is most adults hear teaching that one should eat three balanced meals daily. Each time people feel hungry they should have something to eat. Thus having snacks until their correct mealtime, such bad habits are difficult to correct.

It's very hard to grasp that kind of teaching: that an adult should keep eating that much. We place restrictions on children's daily intake because of their pediatricians' teachings. If they think the kids are over developing at a rapid pace, that will affect the kids as they mature.

When parents heed the doctrine of their pediatrician, they place their babies on the diet the doctor gives for the baby. Adults, after a certain age, do not grow anymore. They just expand all around by body size and not by height. Adults do not need to have all the energy that children do. That should teach us that we need to eat half as much as we do each day.

We fail ourselves by heeding the teaching of our educators which makes us believe that we should always eat between meals and that fasting is very much unhealthy for humanity. It's sad to see what evil creatures we have become. We fail to see and to understand that what is good for our kids is also good for us. All the things that are bad for our children are likewise bad for adults. In reverse order, things that are bad for adults should likewise be bad for kids. What is good for adults should also be good for kids.

The once caring, loving procreator can stop having the caring, loving feelings for their child. They no longer look at the child as tender. They leave them now to fend for themselves, without any restraint, believing they now are capable of doing for themselves. Many kids now behave the way they see their parents behave. Not only in eating habits, they follow their nurturers every movement. Whether it's sleeping, or other things that adults do that are unhealthy, kids also will do unconsciously. All because our educators say they know so much. They do not realize that they are doing the same bad things with themselves and their kids as they raise them.

It's very hard to indoctrinate others when you, yourself, do not know any better. I will continue saying forever that the hereditary transmitted diseases we have within humanity are bad habits we pick up from each other.

The teaching we find worldwide, that sickness is hereditarily transmitted is only hogwash. There is no such thing as ancestral trait, only the dirty habits we adopted from our families. As the child grows, they too fall in love with many things that they find great pleasure with. They are willing to start giving up their sleeping time, so as to play with the things they are now in love with. Sleep is no longer of importance to them any more. They now find it hard to get the rest they still require.

Just as many adults refuse to put aside nonessential items, so that they can get the rest their bodies need daily, their kids behave the same as they do. All the things we use to occupy our days that are not beneficial, we should try much harder to reject from our lives. Then, we can get the slumber our bodies are in need of daily. Too many kids would stay up all night if they were never forced to go to sleep. Many kids have so much energy, that they never get to use it in the appropriate way they should. They usually outlast some of their parents. Some procreators have to take a nap daily while their babies are taking a nap. Otherwise they will end up getting sick.

The problem I see with people these days is that we are too impatient all the days of our lives. Each day we would like everything we look forward to, to be fulfilled. That is impossible to happen. As the saying goes, "Rome cannot be built in one day". Most of the time; we only stop when our bodies are completely exhausted. We cannot overpower the unconscious state that is overtaking us. Many times we try to fight off the tired feelings that are working to shut down our bodies for its resting period. The only reason we stop sometimes is because we no longer can overpower the shutdown stage our bodies reach.

Personally, no matter what I do, I cannot prevent sleep from taking over my body. Sometimes sleep overpowers us so much we sleep in places unheard of: here, there, and everywhere. Over and over I hear many people say they are so tired. They fall asleep in the bathtub while taking a bath or they never reach their beds. They fall asleep on their sofa and spend the night there. Many never make it home anymore; they fall asleep in their vehicle and end up dead as a result of an accident.

Humans are creatures that do not know and understand what is good for them. We take things for granted all the days of our lives. Why do we behave the way we do? Our leaders and educators were never knowledgeable about the correct understanding of the body's true potential. Lacking knowledge, they keep man in ignorance all the days of their life, even from previous generations. Until just recently, we are learning what the body is capable of doing.

I also see the need for people to take time out one or more days per week to give their bodies rest from eating. We are killing ourselves by not allowing our organs to rest. We are not going to die if once a week we do not eat or drink anything.

The way we are living daily, by constantly eating without resting, it is more harmful to us than a day here and there for our body to rest by not eating.

Giving your body a day of rest, by not eating or drinking, is not a form of dieting. A person's body should also rest from day in and day out eating all the time.

We need to understand that many of the foods we eat take more than ten hours to digest. The constant eating never gives our digesting system any days off as in resting. Our body needs more than sleep as its rest. Withholding food from your system at least once a week is a very healthy thing for your body. It is not unhealthy as you keep hearing teachings that you some not go without eating of drinking any thing for twenty four hours.

What is a very good life style to practice, when you eat late at nights, or evening, do not eat anything when you wake up in the morning. It is a healthier to wait until about noon to eat or drink anything. I realized it is not going to be easy for a person to change their unhealthy way of eating for a healthy one. Never hearing this kind of healthy teachings before, people does eat constantly; morning, noon and at evening, or say nights.

Not hearing or getting teachings that your body will adjust healthily when you change your unhealthy eating to a healthy eating practice. At first you might feel discomfort, just ignore that feelings for a while and your body will adjust itself in time.

Look at the time being spend or the discipline made to exercise because there are teachings that it is healthy, and you will be able to avoid or reduce many diseases from infiltrating your body. It far better and healthier for you to reduce your unhealthy eating habits that to do physical exercise.

Our bodies have the ability to protect itself better far above all our understanding that knows about our bodies. Our bodies do not fight against itself. It work keeping us a live for a long time, and that is what we need to know, and to understand.

Controversy on Sleeping

Chapter (5)

With the stratagem that are available from business that relates to sleeping, a person does not know which philosophy to accept. One says this and another says that. Others will say it matters not where you slumber, or what you use to get your rest as long as you obtain some kind of rest. Why do people need time for sleeping? Is it because there are days and nights? Is it because of man's sin and we die? Is it because we are flesh and blood creatures? Being like us man cannot exist without a sleeping period.

Since man needs to sleep, is it possible there is a correct way we all should sleep? If there is a correct way we all should sleep, then there must be an incorrect way we can sleep likewise. If we are sleeping incorrectly, what harm are we doing to our structure? When a person's body begins to reach its point of rest, one should not fight to stay awake. Many times our opposition to nature's beckoning will hurt us later in life.

Think about the law our government enacted for truck drivers. Was this law made with man's health in mind? Why was this law made? Was it only for reducing accidents on the highways? Was it made to teach man the importance of sleeping? What was it our sovereign heads of State saw or heard? Why did they pass a law trying to make truckers reduce their long hours of driving without any slumbering? Was it made in consideration for human lives? Was it because of the constant complaining about highway deaths? Was this law enacted to teach humanity their ignorance of the way they are killing themselves for nothing? This shows men's comport is full of impatient behavior because we are greedy for nothing. We have questions after questions. How and where can we find the correct answers for all the questions we have?

Today's people place a lot less value on their lives. Money and other commodities in this world have been given a greater value. People's conduct shows they disregard their lives, and place it as nothing. Things like homes, cars, clothes, food, and bill paying are placed first and foremost over their bodies. The thing that is so striking about people comport is that man will be the only thing that will be judged for their life on this earth. Nothing else will receive a just compensation for living on this earth but man. That is the reason we should place a greater value on our heads than vanity.

The law for drivers was enacted for humanity to care for themselves and others. Many find it to be preposterous because it reduces the wealth they fight so hard for. Reducing the hours drivers spend behind the wheel, also lengthens the time one takes to reach their destination carrying whatever supply they are delivering.

Before this law was enacted, I learned that truck drivers would often take medication that was developed to keep people awake. Both men and women used these drugs to stay awake. They enabled them to make their delivery much earlier, so they could make several trips in a week. Reducing the hours of the drivers, and lengthening the time of delivery, brings less money for the truckers. It possibly cost more for the consumers. Many laws enacted by our government have been profitable to some. Others end up going out of business. I do not think man will ever find the perfect solution for all things to work in favor for everyone. The other thing that might be possible, with the law the government made, is that it could reduce some of the trucks on the highways. The intention is to make the streets safer for cars and other small transports.

What most of us possibly overlooked is the long-term effect that someday will shut down our bodies for good by sickness or by death. Most humans do not believe in making plans for tomorrow. They live a reckless life daily until some serious accident or sickness is encountered that moves them from their life of being lax.

Not many make plans for life after death. Neither do they make plans for this life. We can find millions who believe that death ends man's existence forever. Some people believe that man is just a higher form of animals, since they have some similar characteristics with animals. Men and animals die; both eat to remain alive, and both species multiply by copulation with male and female ejaculation that produce offspring.

We have so many different teachings or beliefs that are very confusing to the simple minded. Individuals that are weak are unable to think on their own. We find many who do not know what they should accept as their philosophy. They try to be neutral as to say they do not like what is taking place.

There is no neutral ground whatsoever. We might think and feel that one can be neutral with this life and the life to come. Similar behavior is found in people who speak as if they are fearless of death until sickness begins to knock at their doors. The moment one starts to feel some kind of discomfort, they will visit the doctor complaining about the changes their bodies begin to make. We visit our physicians because we are fearful of pain and suffering. Don't ever forget death. Death is man's greatest adversary. It brings us to our knees all the time. It matters not how arrogantly a person lives on this earth, he or she has to respect death.

Many only think of their health at the point of death or sickness. At that stage many never receive satisfactory help from their doctors. Ignorance is a deadly thing. When people are not knowledgeable of danger, they live, walk and breathe danger until death snatches their life right out from underneath them. Failing to know the reality of how a person should walk in this life, we carry ourselves dishonorably because we do not know any better. I am not saying that all walk this earth the same. Some try very hard to do better before sickness strikes. They show respect for the laws, while many walk lawless. Not many realize that the laws are for the people who are lawless.

The laws only affect the lawless. People who live lawful lives; the laws do not affect them. Should men change their ways? Lots of truck drivers feel the law enacted against truckers is unfair. I understand that some do not abide by the laws made for their health. I am not sure if the things I hear about the truckers are correct. Not everything we hear someone says means that is the way the story goes. Is it possible that we can live healthier for a very long time if we listen to man's doctrine? What many truck operators do, I hear, is cheat with their logbooks. They constantly falsify their records so they can continue driving and making lots of money. Gossip is one of humanity's weaknesses. Sometimes a story is passed along incorrectly.

Analyzing man's conduct, I see inconsideration for one's own welfare. Not knowing the truth about the law enacted by our government, we can only speculate until we obtain the correct answer concerning the truck driver's limitation in driving on the road. Since we do not respect the quality of good health until we find out death is knocking at our door, at that stage, we quickly find a physician we think will be able to restore our health back to normal. Most of the people that visit doctors never totally follow all their instruction to the letter.

The reason why many never follow all the instructions to the letter is that they work, sleep, and often forget to take their medication with them. Humans are creatures that are disrespectful to laws that should always keep us in check. Like the road users who most of the time only think for themselves and are very inconsiderate of other road users. The possible question, with any law our government makes, is it a sham? Do our elected officials truly care for their subjects well being? I learned that large corporations are the decision makers. Many times what they say goes. The company that has the most cash keeps things running in their favor. Businesses that do not have lots of cash have a very hard time surviving. They cannot rub shoulders with the aristocrats of their society.

Thinking negatively we will always remain in ignorance all the days of our life. Its past time for all to know that money is the controlling power these days. Daily, all over the world, people keep losing their lives over money. Look at the ratio with crime globally. We need to be awakening from our slumber that keeps us from learning the truth. Even in our justice system we see partiality. The influence of the rich gives them greater leeway to get away with more crimes. The poor always suffer shamefully more in almost everything in this life.

We are so greedy for vanity. We treat the poor very badly and call them all kinds of unpleasant names. In this world we have many sluggards who care for nothing. They refuse to make things better for themselves. Many poor do not have the resources for advancing in many things their souls lust after like the rich. Just as the rich are killing millions daily to stay wealthy, we have the poor trying to do the same to become rich or to change their life around.

Most rich are able to educate their children much better than the poor, so they can have a much better life. Most poor are unable to send their children to good schools so that their kids might have the daily requirement for today's standard of living. I find in this era many look down on people that are less fortunate to be in the standard we set as intellectuals. Looking at mankind's comport, as regarding education, some feel they are somewhat more advanced than those who have not obtained any tickets from a university. Such persons are looked upon as illiterates.

As we analyze the people addressed as the illiterates and the intellectuals, it is clearly seen that there is not much difference in this area. Not many seem to think about an illiterate or an intellectual in this manner. All seem to go about their lives without having the facts of reality. As we reason and think of the overall picture that stands before us all, we can see that all are equal in this. Whether ignorant or educated, sin is still the dominant force within humanity. All seem to behave the same way.

I see illiterates lie, steal, get drunk, and kill each other all the time for a few dollars. Our educated people live in the same category as the uneducated people. They too lie, steal and kill each other. It might not be for the small change the poor uneducated folks kill for. The educated kill for much larger amounts.

Whether large or small, killing is the same. Those who are educated and feel within themselves that they are above the dummies should think again. Their education has not given them any more power over their thinking than the people they look down on as below them. When a person obtains a certificate from one of the many universities globally, it does not mold the character to be honest at all times and in all things that we put our hands to do these days. Pride and respect are no longer being taught anywhere.

Even when people are in colleges trying to be intelligent, that is where many learn to be intoxicated. Bad education practices are in universities. Many learn a lot of evil in the institutes of learning. All the evil they learn, while attending college stays with them many times to the grave. Many end up in the pen sometimes for a very long time.

We need to stop looking down on other people, whether they are educated or uneducated. All the quality of evil is still in control. I see that education, as we call it, does nothing within the heart of humanity as to say, since they are counted as an aristocrat because they are educated, they live flawless. People should live as though education not only improves my reading and mathematical skills, and other subjects taught in school, it should also teach them to be honest in all things.

People's conduct all over the world is the same educated or not. I find even the people who call themselves Christian, have morals that are very much undesirable. This shows that people behave very foolishly in all walks of life.

According to rumor, regarding the law enacted by the government for truck drivers, the drivers keep breaking the law daily by falsifying their logbooks. They see only money they are losing. They never see more haste, more waste. Many people over the years lose their lives because of haste.

What I have seen and understood on the highways is that all the accidents are not always the trucker's fault. I feel that cars and smaller vehicles cause more of our highway accidents than trucks. All are guilty of long hours without sleeping. It is not only the truckers that are tired while driving. It's the destination many folks keep thinking about. Why do so many refuse to stop and slumber for their safety and others?

An, impatient trait that dwells in mankind only shows we move without grace. When we hit the highways, many never drive the speed limit. We normally drive faster then the speed limited posted on the highways. I do not think that it's the fast drivers that necessarily are the ones that normally cause accidents.

We could have much higher speed limits on the roads and still have a lot less death as we travel daily. It's not speeding that is the necessary thing we need to control. What we need to control should be man's total behavior.

It is hurry, hurry all the time once we hit the highways. The same restriction for truckers should apply for all road users. All should pay a fine. Many lose their lives yearly on the highways. The reason why so many lose their lives could be the fault of poor understanding for what is more important for one's welfare.

Time after time we place our destination, or something else, more important than ourselves. Not understanding the essence of sleep we go on with life as if to say nothing can befall us. We will remain that pathway, until something happens to wake us up. I also know that it's not always possible to react to one's bodily beckoning at the time for whatever the body is calling for, whether sleep, food, or to dispose of one's bodily waste. Sometimes where you are, it's not always convenient to give the body what it's asking for.

Over and over, we are at places where we cannot satisfy the cravings of our bodies. Our bodies do crave for a lot of things. There are four things that one's body will not allow one to deny from it for too long when it is in need of them. One is sleep, another is waste matter the body would like to dispose of, food is the third, and water is number four. Two out of the four the body will not wait for long. When the body is calling to get rid of number one, we have to stop whatever we are doing and go relieve the body. The same goes for a person's waste from their bowels. Putting off for some time the discharge of urine and excrement from one's bowels; will in the end create serious health effects to a person's body? There are some things we can put off that are not deadly to our bodies. Some are very deadly.

We should know that there are many things that are very essential for one's body. We need to learn the ones that are most important. We should always try to make the body at all times get these vital things over all the others our body craves. I know that one's body needs to be washed, stay clean and smell beautiful at all times; not just a few times here and there. Too many times I see where many of us put more effort into the cleansing of our bodies than sleeping, I see and learn that a person should brush their teeth after each meal: we should also floss after each meal.

I hope and pray we could, from this day forward, place a lot more emphasis on sleeping over all the other things that we do with our bodies. The reason so many types of ailments exist with humans is that we are not sleeping correctly. Our body cannot work the way it should. Many people try to put off slumber for another day. The fault is not the unconscious state of one's body that we are never able to be more healthy. The fault has to do with our poor knowledge that has been withheld from humanity all of our lives.

When a person's body calls for rest, he should always try to give the body what it's asking for. Just as how we feed the body food when it is hungry and we go to the bathroom to discharge waste, we should try our best to do the same for our bodies when sleep is beckoning. Allow the body to have free course for your health.

I know that sometimes our bodies at work, or church, or at some of our daily routine show some kind of fatigue. We need to place our body where it can shut down for a little spell. Many times the body is very tired. It's because the body has not obtained the rest it needs. It thinks we should do better than we are doing.

Failure to give the body the required rest it needs daily, in the end will be devastating for a person's body. Starving the body of the things it needs, will someday make it hurt all over. In the days of pain and suffering man will not be able to truly help the people who will be suffering.

We need to understand that man is not knowledgeable about the essence of sleep. Wise men would not have made things to keep us awake. I know there are pills made for making people fall asleep. That might be not all that bad. On the other side of the coin, it's not that good. The thing we should do is to try to teach people to relax and stop looking after worldly goods that have no real value in the end. They can learn to have much better health in the future. The love of money makes mankind become a barbarous creature. We keep killing each other for vanity.

Starving the body, of the most important thing it needs, will shorten many other things the body is capable of doing. When we give the body too much sleep, the body will also lose some energy. Over and over I hear many people say that if they have a very large meal their body is about to fall asleep. The reason, why many individuals' bodies react that way, they are feeding their body all that food when their body is slowly working towards shutting down their body for rest.

A person's body does not instantly shut down the body for its sleep. It slowly shuts it down. The way we feel and think we always give food to our bodies when it calls for food. We should be much stricter with our sleep, than feeding our bodies with food. Our bodies need to be fed daily with sleep even more than food. I hear lots of people say they feel wonderful many mornings when they get a good night's rest. I have seen many people on many a morning after their night of rest, look like they aged a lot. This is simply because they never get any sleep, or enough sleep.

I have never seen a person look like they aged one bit if they go without food or do not use the bathroom for days to discharge their waste. Neither have I seen any person look like they aged because they have not washed their face or combed their hair or taken a bath or a shower in days. This shows me that of all the things that our bodies need sleep is still the most essential of all. Sleep is the least thing we give our bodies out of all the vital things our bodies require.

Give the body the appropriate sleep it requires, and at the end of slumber the body will feel wonderful just about all day until it starts to draw near to the time of sleep. Then the body starts to work to bring the body into an unconscious state once more. We are killing ourselves by the way we are sleeping. Our bodies know that they are dying. The bodily instinct knows nothing more than to always try to revitalize itself. The body just keeps trying day in and day out to stay alive.

I know that the body does not have the ability to teach and to speak directly to us about the things we are doing wrong. The weirdest thing that's hard to understand with the body is that one's body can detect all the bad things we are doing to it. Yet it's unable to speak to us in a correcting way so that we can improve our poor treatment to ourselves.

The body is a great creation. In-spite of all the abuse we do daily to ourselves, our body never becomes discouraged. It just keeps right on trying to remain alive and rescue us from the danger we encounter daily. Seeing all the things we do to stop from sleeping, the body never stops from trying to put us out unconsciously. Many take drugs to keep themselves awake. Many times we just simply fight hard, by physical labor or in an active way, because we want to accomplish something we are doing we think is much more essential than resting our bodies. Sometimes we can overpower sleep from our system. Other times, it matters not what we take or do, we are unable to stop our system from going out like a light.

Even when we go for days without sleeping, the body never

changes its function like having no more power over the body to put it to rest. I know that our body can readjust itself in a time of tiredness. This is true regardless of one's work schedule. People work one of three shifts designated by their company: such as first, second, or third shift. One out of those three shifts a person's body can fit to its sleeping time. Our body does not see only nights as our only time for resting. If our system could only detect night we would have only one shift for all business. Since a person's body is capable of changing its slumber behavior, people are able to work one of the three shifts designed by their employer.

Humans have many things that prevent them from sleeping when they should. When the problem is not work related, sometimes it is sickness or other activities. Since we do not have any power in preventing illnesses from overpowering our system, we should not use sickness as going without sleep. When we understand the bodily function, we should fight much harder to make sure we get our rest daily

Not many folks love to take charge of the situation, some leave it to others. When GOD created man, He gave man dominion over all things on this earth. Still we need to see and to understand that we were not given complete control over one's self that we could overpower our self over sleep, food, and all the things our body lusts after. Men have placed many creatures under their domination with the exception of their own body. Sleep has a much greater power with one's body than we have ourselves. Lots of times we lose the fight with our bodies. It is high time for us to stop fighting our bodies. Since we cannot win this fight of stopping the body from sleeping, we should just simply follow the course our system is taking. We should know that it is not a good thing to always fight against the course the body is taking.

As one feeds their body what it seeks, like food and water, the body becomes lax and free of future pain. Freeing the body, of the waste it has no more use for, will remove pain and suffering for years to come. We don't try willfully to keep our urine and feces within our system. Sometime it's the location we are in.

We do all things just about instantaneously to free ourselves of the waste our bodies need to dispose of. I also know that most of the world's population feeds their bodies when the body seeks food. World technology makes this world much smaller than it was say twenty years back. Seeing man's comport we have the same pattern of living globally. We seem to all place food, and other none essential items, over the real essential thing a person's body needs.

There are several ways people do not feed themselves when their bodies are requesting food or something to drink. These are some of the things one encounters that removes eating from a person; (1) Fasting, (2) Famine, (3) Going for medical examination (4) trying to lose weight, (5) some people are afraid they might gain too much weight if they have too much to eat. It's not a diet for losing their weight. It's fear of gaining.

Those are some of the things people encountered; that make them stop eating daily when their bodies are calling for nourishment. Food is not the only thing a person needs as nourishment for their body. Sleep is the outstanding nourishment your body needs. We cannot survive without these vital things daily. After careful evaluation we should all agree that slumber is what our body needs most for existing. Sleep seems to be the one thing most essential out of all the things the body craves for life expectance.

Not every person has the potential to fast and continue physical labor while on a strenuous fasting. It does not seem like everyone can go without eating, or drinking anything while they are fasting. Some do not have the self-will to go on fasting for days without having anything to eat or drink. They simply have a very small portion during their fasting days. Failing to take rest when not eating will drain a lot of one's bodily strength. A person can go forty days and forty nights without eating, and live. I do not think a person can exist forty days and forty nights without sleeping. Looking at sleeping and food, we see that a person does need both of these things. Can we say that one is more important than the other? Should we say they are vital for one's body to remain healthy? And if we continually deny the body daily of its required needs, we are going to kill the body.

Understanding the seriousness of sleep, we should try and find the logic of good slumbering. Should we accept this as the correct teaching or dismiss it as erroneous teaching that we will toss around all night long while we are sleeping. I can recall many years ago, I never knew any better with the doctrine of tossing around while slumbering. I once agreed with those teachings, and then I realized that it is an incorrect statement to the public. I have the answer why men, women, boys, girls and infants toss all the time when sleeping. We can stop being agitated while resting.

At the present I realize that I can sleep with a glass of water on my body. With a glass on my body I will wake in the morning with the glass still filled with water without losing a drop of water. Not knowing right from wrong showed that we are in darkness with healthy sleeping habits. I was flabbergasted seeing a young child resting in a posture most unhealthy. This child's position of sleeping looked like he started to pray at first, then he fell forward as if he never stopped his praying. He crouched forward, until all his body folded together. It was the most awkward posture I have ever seen someone fall asleep in.

Seeing that child, sleeping that way did pain my being very deeply. Do we know that our schools, with all the professors worldwide, including the scientists fail to understand the serious nature of sleeping? In a way we are killing ourselves when we go to bed for our rest. It awakened me to understand that all the wisdom and understanding we claim we have, that makes us feel we are much smarter than early generations, are incorrect. We might develop many new technologies in this era, but we are still ignorant in many things.

Seeing and understanding the error we are making hurts deeply. Do we know that man, who elevates himself to be intelligent, is not so smart after all? The people that teach people that there is no GOD, and that this world did a self creation, are part of our problem. When we leave GOD out of our lives, things will be very difficult; that could be the reason why the correct way to better health is just coming to light. We have been walking in darkness about good health all these years. Look at all the billions of dollars that we have spent over the years, looking for answers about humanity's many kinds of sicknesses. In every way we fail one another.

If man did obtain the knowledge for correct slumbering generations ago, life could have been much more pleasant for people in this era. Failing all these years in our understanding of the seriousness of good resting, we just could not teach others what was hidden from our knowledge. We do not understand the correct way to sleep. We never had the appropriate material for correct sleeping. We just could not teach what we had no knowledge about.

Generation after generation was not able to pass on what was hidden from them. At the present, the way we are sleeping is as one being tortured. Since we do not know better, we have to keep using the things we have. We do not know the deadliness within the materials we encounter daily.

One of these days, I know that you will be awakened and learn that you were only torturing yourself when resting. I have been to places where I see the many torturing devices they had many years ago. They would use them to torture people that were in opposition with their laws or regulations of early barbarous governments in various parts of the world. Seeing those devices makes a person feel great that they never had to live in an era under a regimen so cruel. I do not think we appreciate the freedom there is. People's behavior is like this world is in debt to them.

Yet I find the things we use for resting are as one using a torture chamber for their beds. It very slowly is harming our bodies. Seeing the olden days' torture devices, they would work much more rapidly than the things we use today for our resting and relaxation. Most of the people that under-went some of that torturing might have lasted days or hours. I am very sure that not one person was able to remain alive very long under that inhumane treatment. Yet we sleep daily on a device that slowly works on our system like olden day evil devices. I know that all have been sleeping deadly. It has been withheld from our understanding all these years. Never before did anyone know the deadliness of the things we are using daily to take our rest on.

We should try to be somewhat honest with ourselves. We might just be awakening to the reality that in-spite of all the machinery or technology we have in this era, it only makes us feel we are more superior over other generations. We might just see that we only have a few things that make life a little simpler.

Barbarians and cave dwellers we call early earth dwellers, who occupied the land in the beginning of earth's growth. Remember they are the same people who handed down to us many of the things we have improved on that make life much more pleasant and easier for our daily living today.

Barbaric we address early people to be. In their ignoramus state they are the ones who left many things as a legacy to us, that we apply ourselves like we are above early man. Todays comport of humanity, with technology or without technology, stands about the same or possibly worse. Look back at the early growth of the population, from the only book that has the oldest record of humanity walking this earth, shows that we have not made any better advancement in our behavior. Many people lost their lives in the flood, "Genesee, 7:1-24: Their life was ignoramus. If we believe the teaching of the Bible we can see the same nature in people. Inspite of all the advancements that we have made mechanically we have not improved our behavior.

In what other book written do we find the beginning of humanity and the end of humanity? Since there is no other book we should not completely listen to man's philosophy. The only true GOD: man has not completely heeded his words. We give more time to the one that always hated mankind. We love prevarication more than the truth. We love suffering more than happiness. We just cannot walk away from death. We love death more than life. It's mind-boggling to know that most of the world population is fighting to be very healthy physically.

Millions are being spent yearly on exercise machines, simply because man feels they can lengthen their physical life on this earth. Is it possible we can increase by years, months, or days our life span in the years we occupy this earth? Why are people only living for the time they do? I see in the Bible the life span given to man is only three score and ten. By reason of strength we might make four score. "Psalm 90:10." "In Genesee 6:3 Man's life was shortened to hundred and twenty years". Can man go over the things that GOD placed as a boundary? What powers does man truly have against GOD? What can man do to have things of GOD reversed? What can man truly do for man? Man has been teaching man for a long time about lots of things. Not once have I seen or learned where any man was able on his own to create something that was not on this earth of some likeness.

Look at all the things we use daily as technologies. I see that just about all things that man created come from the surrounding nature. Man studied plants, animals, and other things of nature and turned them into technological equipment. They make our life much more pleasant in some way or another.

On the other hand, it has its draw backs. Many of the items that man created have become very harmful to millions of people all over the world. We have placed our life in man's philosophy so much that it will become our doom in the near future. What we have done is somewhat irreversible. Man keeps looking to man as if to say we have reached a place where we have become super human. Intellectuals behave as if they know all that needs to be known, and very soon with their knowledge, will be able to develop some gadget that we can use to eradicate sickness and death.

Many of the gadgets we use in this era seem to have done more harm in this generation than all previous civilizations. Please do not misunderstand what I am saying here in regards to technology. It's not the gadgets within themselves that are deadly. It's the way we use technology that makes them become dangerous. The thing that makes technology deadly is the way we worship it. I realize that the majority of humans would like to live forever, if possible, in this universe. I am not contemplating suicide. I do not care to live much longer on this earth. I can recall my childhood days. Life was not all that pleasant. The main reason I feel this way was that my life as a child required me to work as a slave. It had nothing to do with my inability to learn. I was not the smartest person in the world. Neither was I the dumbest. We just had very bad procreators that were thinking only for their own welfare and not their children's future.

I know that I was a very foolish child. In my folly I could not think positively. It always seemed that I put my foot into my mouth. As to say, my mouth always puts me into trouble with my dad and others around me. I never knew when to speak and when not to speak. Keeping silent was another matter that was not found in my vocabulary at all.

The reason why my behavior was irrational was that I was an illiterate in many things I did in life. I could not discern right from wrong pertaining to the things that would make others become very angry with me or be pleasant with the things I would reply with. The other thing that I feel made my childhood days unpleasant was I felt my dad only cared for his wife and her children. We were like hired hands. The first seven kids would receive very harsh punishment all the time. The spanking one would receive would be like the way you see slaves being whipped. I personally feel I was not a misbehaving child. All the spankings I received were not called for.

Possibly my dad might have had some serious ill feelings towards me because I was not outstanding educationally as he would have liked me to be. We never really received much from our dad. He was a very hard, selfish person. Even to this date my dad still remains negative towards me. He once related to my sisters "I hated him". That feeling could be his conscience speaking simply because that is what he has in his heart towards me. He does not know how to show me that he never had any love for me. That's the way life goes. I am not the only child whose procreator hates him. Neither will I be the last child their parents despise.

I know that it was a very hard thing for us to starve to death by malnutrition. In each of the two locations we lived, there were always all kinds of different things we could find to eat. Starvation would only come about by a child that meditates cruel evil feelings against their parents. I personally never saw the need to be harsh. I know we all had to work very hard when we lived with my dad and stepmother. Even though they were very brutal towards their children in those days, I am awakened from my slumber in contrast with the days living with my dad and stepmother seeing today's generation's behavior. Sometimes it might take the foolish behavior of others to awaken someone that thinks and feels that their life possibly is the worst that one could ever go through from any home as children and parent.

Comparison of my childhood days and kids these days force me to be happy and very much appreciative of my up bringing. I love my hard up-bringing over the life of young people of this generation. I see an evil, degenerated people today: ones that are very selfish. In their selfishness, love and caring have been driven from their hearts. It's very sad seeing what is transpiring. It's very sad seeing the future if a transition does not take place soon. People are going to be more immoral than those who perished in the days of the flood. As the Bible illustrated about the people before the flood transpired, that within the heart of man was only evil imagination continually. Nothing good was in the heart of humanity. Therefore, the majority were destroyed by flood. Out of the population of millions only eight were saved. All the others perished. "Genesee 6: 5".

I heard someone make a remark that people who are educated do not want anything to do with the Bible and GOD. Only the uneducated people think and feel that there is a GOD. This could be the reason why we have become such a degenerated set of people. We look so much to man and the things we invent as if to say we have out grown the help of GOD. We allow technology to bring us to a state as the early growth of humanity. Man keeps fighting constantly against the Bible. The same book we fight so much against makes us aware that in the closing years of the first resurrection, humans are going to behave and live like the people lived before the flood destroyed them all. "Matthew 24. Mark 13.Luke 21: 5-36 17: 23-37".

This kind of behavior should awaken mankind to accept the Bible much more sincerely than we are doing. We are going to pay dearly for turning our backs on the things that we have rejected all the days of our lives. Our rejection of GOD has brought a lot of suffering to man continually. Who are we to blame for our suffering? Should we cast the blame on the first two that sinned by disobeying the commandment of GOD? Do we find ourselves in the same category as the first two people's transgression? In what way do we examine our lives? Do we exclude ourselves as not equal in transgressing like Adam and Eve? Man! We are paying dearly continually for the immoral lifestyle we live by daily. If we do not think we are paying dearly for the immoral life we are living, just stop and look at all the people of the world that live at doctors' offices and the folks that we find in all the hospitals all over the globe.

It is not only one country in the world population that is undergoing severe depression over the various ailments that are unable to be helped by human treatment. All the health problems that cover the world have had man's life in topsy-turvy for centuries. Scientists in their belief inform us that this earth existed for millions of years.

It should not matter how long or how short this world existed for man and animals and all the vegetation there in. Placing a time span as we are doing with earth being created relates to the atheist and agnostic philosophy, I see no relevance in today's dogma records.

What advantage or disadvantage does man have knowing that we lived on this earth hundreds or thousands of years? It has not awaked us that the devil is controlling our foolish comport. Ancient records comparing early generations with the new millennium population shows that we have not advanced much more over them in some things. I find in the Bible many ailments that always brought man down to nothing, and left us at the mercy of death. They still remain as plagues to man this very day.

Sickness in AD and BC has paralyzed humans for centuries. Our worldwide population might have tripled or quadrupled over early manhood. We have not the knowledge to eradicate one of man's greatest foes. As long as we keep living the way we are, it might just remain until all things end.

Since the population increased immensely, we can find more wealthy individuals today than in early days. It is the same with employees. We also can find more employers in this era than all the other generations in the past.

Perceiving the past and present behavior of man, all these things remain and are possibly worse. We have mass killing of each other. We have not removed envy, strife, hate, bitterness, and jealousy. We look down on others as if to say they are inferior. We fail to see that all the nations of the world came from just two people. We have many beliefs that are different. That does not change the truth to a lie as millions have been doing.

I know for sure that there is a GOD who the Bible ascribed as the Creator of all things in heaven and on earth. If there is anything under the earth they also were created by GOD. Intellectuals teach and believe that there is no GOD that is capable of occupying this universe unseen.

The non belief of man in GOD the Creator, allows man to be irreverent and dishonorable to his GOD. Funny as one might take these words that say there is no GOD, anytime something happens to those who say there is no GOD, they in-turn call out to GOD for help. Why is it we find in many centuries, men spending billions of dollars yearly looking for something in outer space? What is it that man is truly looking for? Is it to discredit the deity of the Supreme Being?

What is it that man wants with space? Are there minerals that surpass all of earth's quality? Time after time I heard the unbelievers speak of their hope of finding people living on one of the many planets in the galaxies.

The other thing that is possible: man has been trying to prove to man that their teaching about this universe is correct and a lot more accurate. They are going to prove someday that there is no GOD as ascribed in a book called The Bible.

Humanity needs to be awakened from their nightmare. It's so simple to eradicate many of the ailments that have people perplexed all their life. Since the answer was always withheld from our understanding, we could not help one another to become healthy or prevent a person from getting sick.

If man was knowledgeable all these years about ailments and was able to restore many to perfect health, we would find more people that would deny the deity of GOD. Since early generations were not knowledgeable pertaining to the bodily function, it was not possible to leave it as a legacy

Therefore, we can only keep on practicing what we know from others who take the time to make us knowledgeable of many things we have and use today. Regardless of all the great items we have in our possession, it has not done much for human suffering health-wise. People spend many hours in their physician's office looking for help. Many end their lives because of the discouragement from knowing that they are unable to get any results from man for their life long agony caused by many kinds of ailments.

Over and over we learn sometimes where a person has more than one thing wrong with them. Some spend all their earnings trying to regain proper health that in-turn cause many to lose their faith, not only in GOD, but also in all things. This has always been man's downfall. People make fools of people because we are creatures that adore prevarication. Deception is our middle name.

Sickness and Death

Chapter (6)

What is sickness? And why is it here? Who is responsible for the origination of sickness and death? Why is sickness making man's life so miserable? Is it possible that man will forever live on this earth with all kinds of aliments? Will this earth remain forever? Will man always occupy this world? Questions, questions, questions: will we ever find the answers for all the questions we ask all the days of our life? When we reach out to mankind to obtain the answers we are looking for, will it make any difference whether we seek the answers from the unlearned or the most intellectual? Man is flesh and blood. As the story goes in the Bible, man came from the dust of the earth: Genesee 2: 7. Each time someone dies, whoever remains alive of the family and close friends, attending the dead person's funeral, they will always hear these words: ashes to ashes, dust to dust, from the place we came, there will we return. Genesee 3: 19

Man's greatest downfall from the first man to the last man, has to do with the way we have lightly esteemed the things that GOD has given to us and shown to us. What man did from the first, and possibly to the last, we have taken the teaching of men, who do not know what the future holds and embrace man's words with greater reverence than that of GOD.

Analyzing the first man's transgression we can find the same behavior that, we can ascribe, is hereditary. Looking at the continual pattern that remains in each generation, we all should agree that we are creatures that are failures. We seem to walk by hindsight and foresight only comes into play after the fact.

In the Bible we find a part that reads this way: "The fool hath said in his heart, there is no GOD" Psalm 14: 1; through men foolish antagonism, we have passed the same rebellious teaching down to man in blindness. Man is a creature made up of flesh and blood. We are not spirits. Therefore we cannot touch the future, nor can we see the next minute. Eve was the person who the serpent convinced that by eating of the tree commanded not to touch nor eat of, Adam and Eve would not surely die, and they would be like gods knowing good and evil, right from wrong. Genesee 2:16&17 3:1-6

Seeing and analyzing GOD and the Devil that spoke to Adam and Eve the first two humans that lived and walked this earth, why did man take the words of the Devil over GOD, and eat the fruit and die? As this question appeared did man within his heart ever ask this question once? We also need to ask why on earth, or in heaven, is the real reason why someone would speak to another person to be in opposition of good to become pernicious. Is it possible, as it was with Eve, so is it with all humans that came after Adam and Eve?

I feel that Eve should have asked the serpent these questions: who are you that you are trying to let me believe that GOD was not completely honest with me in regards to the eating or touching of the tree that was in the middle of the garden? By the way, who ever you are, I know who GOD is. Who are you? Are you more powerful than GOD, who is our Creator? Why are you here? Why do you want me to transgress the commandment that GOD gave to my husband, and I? What is it you want of my husband, and I? Are you telling me that you are much more powerful than GOD? That you know much more than GOD? Do you love us more than GOD? My husband and I have spoken all the time with GOD. We do have a wonderful relationship with our Creator.

What are you offering me that I should partake of the fruit of the forbidden tree? I do not know the truth of what will become of my husband, and I; I know that GOD says we will die by touching or eating. We have to touch before we can eat. It was forbidden to touch and to eat. You I do not know. Give me the reasons I should transgress GOD'S command. Many people have always cast the blame on Eve and Adam for eating of the tree that they should not eat of as commanded by GOD. The thing that we have all overlooked: the serpent is the one that enticed Eve cunningly to eat, and she ate.

The Devil is the same evil creature that keeps working on humanity daily. It is why we have sickness and death lingering with man. I know that death is imminent because of eating. Sickness is another thing. I also know when we might not be able to stop death. I know much better when it comes to sickness. It's appointed unto man to die once. After death is the judgment. If we can't escape death then we somehow will have to face judgment. Hebrew 9:27

Sickness is not compulsory. We can live without being sick. The choice is ours. Eve, like us, saw many things one sided. By not looking to the future or the consequence of eating, she partook of the tree and died. She did not die literally. She then took the fruit to Adam, her husband. He had to die also with Eve so that they might remain equal.

Adam did not ask of GOD what he should do, knowing that Eve was dead. Is it possible it could be something like this? Since Eve was able to still speak with Adam after she ate, which could also make the man look at the tree as Eve did before making the choice to eat. (" We read in the bible when the woman saw that tree was good for food, and that it was pleasant to the eyes, and a tree to be desired to make one wise, she took of the fruit thereof, and did eat, and gave also unto her husband with her; and he did eat.") Genesee 3: 6.

The serpent's words to the woman, "by eating the fruit she would be as gods, knowing good and evil". The cunning deception of the devil got the woman to see blindly by hindsight. She closed her eyes from foresight and lost sight of the things that GOD told them. Not looking beyond the present, the majority of humans will never obtain much out of this life. The life after will be something else.

Adam and Eve might have lived nine hundred years. They did die. The thing that's possible that the death GOD was speaking of by eating of the fruit could have been not just a physical death as when you place someone in the ground. Yet before they ate, death had no power over them. Whether it was physical or spiritual death, they died. If it's both that is very bad.

"GOD would come down and communicate with man in the cool of the day. We can say in the evening possibly when man had accomplished his daily work and was getting ready for rest." Genesee 3: 8. after the eating of the fruit, we have not learned that GOD communicated with man as he did with Adam. Death brought separation.

Since man died when he ate of the tree that GOD commanded them never to eat from: man and GOD could not share as they had before. Remember, it was not GOD that caused separation. It was man. GOD is the one that kept trying to bring us back to the place we once had with him from the beginning. Man is the problem. Once we made the enemy fool us into transgressing the commandments of GOD, he has kept doing the same to us daily. We fail to believe and take GOD at his words.

In the beginning the Devil had to find someone to use as his messenger to infiltrate man's mind and thinking. The devil cannot transform himself into flesh like a human. So, he has to find some kind of vehicle he can use to get man to turn from following the things that GOD placed in front of us, or commanded us.

In the beginning there were only two people living on this earth. The devil and Satan's ambition was to be lord over humanity. In order for the Devil to have the advantage he sought over Adam and Eve, he had to find an intercessor that he could use. If Adam and Eve were always together, the Devil might not have been successful. The possibility the Devil had to study and make some significant maneuver that particular day, to split up these two people that he could work on Eve. Then she could work on her husband.

As we know, if someone wants to be victorious in a battle, they have to plan strategically to win against the enemy. This is only speculation, because nothing was ever written in the beginning about Satan. Possibly, since Adam and Eve had not had any prior understanding or knowledge about the devil; they did not know how to address this person, not knowing that this person once was outstanding in heaven. Being envious of man's status, the Devil gave up heaven. The Devil was once higher than man. Yet within his height and might, he was below man in this matter.

The Devil was a servant to GOD and man. He became envious of humanity and wanted to be GOD over humanity. He was told that he could not rule over man. If he left heaven, to be god over man, he would not be forgiven for his transgression against GOD'S commandment.

In the Bible we find these words "man was made for GOD and woman was made for man". 1Correntians 11:3&7-9. Man would only answer to GOD and no one else. Man had his own kingdom that he should have been god over. The earth was made for man. He was given dominion over all things on this earth. Genesee 2; 26&28 Psalm 8:6.

GOD in the beginning gave great power into man's hand. Man

gave the power away that GOD gave to him. The enviousness of devil over man, made him want the power to rule over man. Therefore he gave up heaven to be ruler over man. We have become the children of Satan; therefore we have to behave like our father the devil.

Man no longer has the power in his hands that GOD once gave to him. We behaved very foolishly and gave away most of what GOD gave to us, to our enemy. We became the servant of Satan. He has become our god. He got most of what he wanted, which is nothing.

Now the devil uses us to do his dirty work. We are killing each other and treating each other without any respect. We show no true compassionate feelings for our own flesh and blood brothers.

Our enemy has robbed from us life, and given us death. He wanted to be much higher than all the angels and man. He became very envious of man. Man has been paying dearly for his transgressions. Our transgressions sure bring a life of topsy-turvy daily to the majority of humanity. It's on the up rising daily globally. It's not just happening in one or two countries or Islands of the world. It's in every corner of the world. We cannot exclude any part of the world, saying, that they are sick free, or pain free. All people can relate about some kind of pain and suffering they are going through.

The Devil knows that GOD is a loving and compassionate GOD. He will forgive our sins when we sin against him. The Devil thinks and feels that GOD would not shut him out of heaven for eternity, if he came down to earth to be god over man. Man's behavior applies in the same category as our enemy. He was outstanding in beauty, and possibly everything in heaven. He must have settled in his heart that he was loved too much by GOD, and therefore GOD would not hold it against him if he should take with him most of the angles to earth to be god over humanity. Ezekiel 28:13-18.

Because all the angels would not leave with him, he created a controversy in heaven until he left. He wanted a kingdom for himself. By obtaining a kingdom as he desired, man became his subjects. We have been paying dearly from that day Eve first ate of the fruit.

Although man was given his own kingdom to be god over he had laws he needed to obey similar to the angels. Angels were always servants. They never received their own domain. Man was lord of his kingdom. Being tricked we gave away ours by disobedience to the command once given to us. Now we are suffering for being foolish.

In heaven GOD had laws that angels needed to obey. If they transgressed they would be cast out of heaven. GOD was not partial with angels. Man was also given similar laws whereby he should walk and live by. If man was able to completely obey the commandments of GOD, man would never die. Neither would there be any kind of sickness that would be able to overtake humanity. 2Peter 2:4

Just say the Devil did not disobey GOD, and he kept the commandments of GOD, death would not apply to him and the angels that left heaven to rule over humanity. GOD would not have created a place known as the lake of fire that will burn for eternity. In this fire both man and the devil will live there for eternity. Revelation 20:14&15

We need to understand that not all men will live in this fire for eternity. Only the people that the devil was able to control their lives during the days they lived on this earth. I am not speaking of controlling man by sickness only. Being sick has nothing to do with sin and death that will cast man in the lake of fire someday. Sickness came into existence because of sin and death.

The cunning deception of the Devil blindfolded Eve's eyes. She could not see the pain and the agony she and all humans would suffer while being alive. We will receive this if we continue living in sin as a servant to the Devil. Transgressing is one thing. Remaining in our transgression is another thing. GOD is not a person who is unforgiving. If we sin and repent and stay away from sin, GOD will not hold our sins against us.

We know that Eve first ate and died. She gave to her husband. He did eat and the both of them died. They still lived over nine hundred years. We have no record of the life they lived after eating the fruit. They were cast out of the garden; all we can do is speculate on their life in just two things: they possibly served GOD or the Devil.

Adam and Eve had two sons. One was envious of the other and took his brother's life. He was the first to die as death. He was more righteous than his brother. Henceforth man has inherited their father's, the devil, trait, knowing that death befell Satan because he was envious of humanity. Man had his own domain. He did not have anyone to serve. GOD was the only one that man would pay homage. Genesee 4: 3-11.

Angels were not given any domain that they should govern as was given to man. Angels had a double service to perform. They would serve GOD and man. Our fearless leader was determined that he was not going to be a servant to humanity. He wanted to be lord over man. He and the angels were not made to be that way.

So he rebelled and split the host of heaven. This guy was able to convince other angels to join him in his conquest as lord of humanity. They took their flight with the devil so that they can steal from man his kingdom. Do we think it would be possible for us to keep fighting this guy and be a winner? Eve should not have given up that easy. This could be the reason why the majority of men serve this guy; the Devil and Satan is a very evil creature. Many just do not care to fight for a better future. They are happy with the nothing that their father the devil keeps them in.

Now that the Devil knows that man does not have much will power and is always quick to jump at everything that is evil presented to him, let's look at the way the Devil continues making fools of people. Over and over the Devil penetrates one's mind. As he enters our mind, he makes sure he feeds us lies and filth about GOD.

All things that are bad he puts the blame on GOD. He takes himself out of the picture, makes himself to be the good guy, and GOD looks like the evil, cruel, bad person.

Look at the way people speak about GOD the Creator of heaven and earth. Everything that happens that is bad in the world we are quick to point our fingers in the face of GOD. We give GOD a bad name that he is cruel and feeling less for humanity. Many become disrespectful to GOD when they lose their loved ones by death. They become very angry sometimes that GOD took away their loved ones. I have not seen nor heard anyone say it's the Devil that causes death to be eminent to humanity.

The other thing that we all seem to overlook is that it was man that chose death and suffering. We should not cast all the blame on the devil; neither should we point at GOD. Humans need to stand on their own two feet for the wrong choice we made. We need to always remember that in the beginning we were like GOD. We were alive. Death had no power over us. We could live forever and never die. We are the ones that see blindly and choose death over life.

In this life of death we should always remember that the fault is always men. The only true GOD is not evil as we all seem to make him to be. We need to always see and to understand that the Devil was not always the Devil. He was the one who also chose to be what he is. In the Bible it tells us of the Devil's status in heaven before he became envious and jealous. GOD never made him cruel and evil as he became. Ezekiel 28:13-18

The devil was the one that was not satisfied being a servant. He wanted much more. In his hunger for power he brought sickness and death to the majority of the human population. Satan too had a choice he could make. He could have stayed a servant and remained in heaven in happiness forever.

Just as man could not see the future and remain alive forever, the Devil likewise lost sight himself. In his belief he felt that GOD would always be very much more understanding towards him, because he was the most outstanding angel of all. He was wrong in his thinking.

The thought in his mind was that he could keep using man. We keep saying and behaving the same way as he is behaving. Folks keep on saying all the days of their life that GOD is love and that he will never cast anyone into the lake of fire as it is stated in the Bible. Man needs to always remember that it is not GOD that is doing the casting here. This place of everlasting punishment was made for the Devil and for all the ones for whom he becomes their god.

We all tend to overlook the reality that all will receive a reward for our service. The reward will be to whom we serve. The recompense one will receive will be as follows. A person who walks in truth and is faithful to GOD will obtain a righteous reward. All that follow and obey the Devil will also be recompensed.

Both the righteous and the non-righteous will obtain life eternal. Both will be alive. There will be the ones that will be with GOD forever in his kingdom. The people that will live forever with Satan will be in death which is the lake of fire. The other thing we should always remember, GOD by Jesus Christ came and died that we might be made free from death.

Each and every person today has the opportunity to correct the wrong choice that was made by Eve and Adam. We need to always remember that Adam and Eve are not going to answer for any person's sins. They are not going to stand before GOD some day and say LORD we are the ones that caused all of mankind to die. It is not going to work like that. "Each tub has to sit on its own bottom". We are not going to be able to have any excuse, to hide, or to have some Attorney represent us as to defend one person. On the Day of Judgment even the Attorneys will have to answer for themselves. The Devil that fills our hearts, minds, and lies, plagues us all the days that we live and walk this earth, will not stand and appeal for any human.

The Devil will be cast into the lake of fire just before the judgment takes place. He will not be able to even plead his own plea; asking for mercy for himself and the sins of all the people that he deceived. It is very sad to see and to understand the foolish way we behave all the time. We should never point our finger at anyone. Each person will have to account for himself before GOD someday.

Analyzing the two rulers, GOD the Creator of all things, and the Devil, the counterfeit of all creation has no love. He knows only hate. Understanding why he hates us so much, to me, makes no sense at all. Man is just flesh and blood, never created as a spirit. We were created to live on this earth forever. All things on this earth were placed here for man's comfort. It was not created for any spiritual creatures. All of earth's substance is only good for man's appetite and enjoyment. This place was created as man's kingdom. Man was supposed to be god over this world. We gave it away for death.

GOD in the beginning gave man great power. The Devil in his jealousy wanted what humanity obtained from GOD. He never had any controlling power over anything that GOD created. He wanted more than what he was created to have. He became the destroyer of the majority of the world's population. He is doing a great job. He did not only steal from us our power and possessions, he keeps using the things that belonged to us, to kill us daily.

Man no longer has the power that was given to him by GOD. We behaved foolishly and gave away most of what GOD gave us to the one that has become our enemy. He caused man to die and to go through a life of topsy-turvy daily. Look at some of the things our enemy has placed in our minds: like we can add more years to our life if we exercise and eat a more balanced diet.

People to this date are being duped immensely by deception. Listen to man's foolish notion that a person can extend their life in good health by eating right and doing a lot of exercise. Man with the wisdom from our enemy lives and behaves just like their father the Devil. The Devil is a liar and the creator of it. Man should understand that GOD is the one that created all things. That we cannot deny. Still we need to understand that the Devil is the one that is responsible for creating death and all things that are bad. St. John 8:44

I know that GOD made the Devil. Yet we always need to remember that in the beginning he was perfect. Men, in the beginning, were perfect too, until we chose imperfection. There is so much deception globally with just about all things in our society; that a person does not know which direction to take daily. Take the food we eat. Analyze it carefully to see if it's possible to ever help a person stay healthy considering the teaching we have to eat all the time.

Following a teaching like that, is it possible for anyone to be healthy? The rapid production of our food, produced in such a large scale, makes it difficult to bring healthy products to the market. The other thing that we have also, that is very unhealthy, is the way we eat. Man's death came through eating the fruit that was forbidden by GOD. We have not learned much about ourselves. By eating we sold our souls to the Devil. We just can't seem to stop eating.

Man was given power to dominate all things on this earth. A very good dominator we have been to the animals and to our vegetation. When it comes down to man, the Devil has man as his slave. We are unrestrained with our own selves. We do not have the power to control our own bodies. We simply gave it away for nothing. Many of us do nothing to regain the power we once had.

Man's Greatest Enemy

Chapter (7)

This is what our enemy keeps on doing to man at all times. We will never see and understand the harm we are doing to ourselves all the days of our lives. We are teaching that if we diet and exercise we can live a much healthier life, with lots less ailments. How can people stay healthy the way we eat and the way we exercise? Our enemy is doing a very good job killing us daily. We just keep on allowing the enemy to have a great advantage over us until the day of our death. At the point of death he knows that there is no more hope to obtain forgiveness from GOD for the wrongs we did all the days of our lives. The Devil, at that stage, will kiss you good-by.

By reaching a point of no return, the Devil will dump you. You may reach a place where life has no more pleasure in it for you, and the Devil has no more use for you. GOD is not going to be sympathetic at this crossroad and embrace you in his arms. The only reason the Devil stops from annoying a person when they reach a place in life where they are of no use to either GOD or the Devil.

I see many old folks that are dying. They behave very despicably. They speak ill-mannerly with all kind of vulgar languages. They are very much impatient with the staff in the old folk's homes or their family members if they are still at home. Frequently I hear people say that not one person ever came back from the grave, or death, to relate to them what death is all about. The thing that all seem to overlook is that each time someone die's, they are technically speaking of death without words.

Because we do not hear them speaking by literal words, we claim that death does not speak. They remain in the ground being dead. The dead will remain in the ground until the day GOD resurrects them. Still, they speak inexpressibly. Not much escapes this guy's tricks. It matters not to our enemy who we are, intelligent or illiterate. He works hard to keep us from thinking of being true to the One that loves and cares for us.

What most of us are failing to see, and to understand; it is the intellects that the devil uses to keep the illiterates in ignorance until their death. Not discerning the game we are playing with the Devil, we feel that we can defy death by believing a lie. Billions of humans serve this guy for nothing all the days of their lives.

The one we serve faithfully has nothing to give us; even death that now belongs to all that are born of flesh and blood parents. It does not belong to him that he can give it to anyone. Someday in the near future he will be cast into the lake of fire with all the people that heed his words. This place is called the second death according to the Bible. Revelation 20: 14&15 "And whosoever was not found written in the book of life was cast in the lake of fire."

Seeing what the Devil is doing to humanity is very painful, knowing that we can shut down this guy forever if we work together in truth. The cunning maneuver of the enemy does counterfeit just about all things there are on this earth that man thinks are great. The things we love to enjoy, that we call pleasure and happiness, we need to reexamine.

After careful evaluation we might just find that in the end it will only bring death. The devil is the author of torment. He does not know how to give true happiness to man. His only ambition is to annihilate man from off the face of the earth. He still can't see and understand that man is the only reason why he is still walking this earth. The day all things end for mankind on this earth, is the day it will end for the Devil and the angels he persuaded to abandon heaven with him.

What we should try to see and to understand is that the Devil, at this point in time, is unable to make a change to stop his destiny. He can't maintain his reign in this universe after man ceases to exist. The Devil's reign will come to an abrupt end little before the second resurrection? The second resurrection, known as the judgment day, is when all will have to stand before GOD to be judged. The Devil is not going to be judged like humanity. His judgment is the thousand years of being shut up unable to cause man to sin. Why should man remain on the losing team?

I also know that if man was able to completely resist this guy in the beginning, he and his followers would have had to repent and ask GOD to grant them remission for their sins. Because man did not heed the commandment of GOD, the Devil was able to continue to occupy this earth. He made life very unpleasant all these years.

Not once in the life of mankind did we unite to fight against our enemy. I do not think many of us have come to the realization of the things he has done to us. He makes people behave ignorantly one towards another. The Devil keeps us in ignorance in such a way that we cannot differentiate between right and wrong, good or bad, and from our right hand or our left.

Just as he enslaves humanity all their life, we treat others in the same manner. We are flesh and blood. Humans are the only creatures that are created in the image of GOD. It should not matter the color of one's skin, or the appearance of any. All people came through the only two that were created in the beginning. GOD never created any more humans after He made Adam and Eve. There is no need for anymore creation to be done as in the beginning. The exception is the thousands years, known as the millennium. That epoch GOD is going to create new things. Man needs to regroup and have one common goal. The goal should be to reclaim what was taken from us in the beginning; man is too lax with death.

Man, being controlled by the Devil, behaves as he commands. We hate each other. We kill each other. We enslave each other. We are envious one towards another for no good reason. All the things we kill each other over belong to us in the first place. Man has become a very despicable creature. The only reason we are the way we are is that the One that loves us, and cares for us, we keep failing to heed His words.

The one that keeps us continually at each others throat, we enjoy intercourse with daily. The people that keep trying to disassociate with this guy, we call them stupid. It's not the ones that are trying to completely separate themselves from this person we should call foolish. All the people that love to fellowship with their enemy should be the ones called stupid.

Man to man, we do not allow anyone that we feel is in opposition to our well-being to ever get the upper hand easily. All the ones we think and feel are our enemies, we keep them at a distance. The way most of us behave, we love to be alive. To many, it matters not how difficult life is we would all like to live healthily forever. Many will not accept the reason we all visit doctors and hospitals. We want to live much longer. People will go through a lot to extend their life on this earth. Death is something we all are afraid of. Why are we afraid of death; is it because it hurts to leave what we know, and that we are going to a place that we are not sure of what is going to take place?

I know that it's no secret that death is eminent. Daily we see and learn of people dying all over the world. Many books have been written about the past life of great men. The great and wonderful things they accomplished during their life on this earth. Only a legacy remains of their greatness.

Not one person lives on this earth for a thousand years. In all our great accomplishments death is still eminent to all. It matters not whether we are poor or rich, illiterate or intelligent, death is disrespectful. It never postpones its date when it's your time. It always takes its victims. The only one that death respects is GOD. He is the only One that has complete power over death and the grave. He is the only one that can postpone death eternally. No other person can. GOD can. GOD is the only true super power.

The one that's responsible for death to humanity knows nothing else. He cannot do anything else. His only goal is to keep people in death. He despised mankind in the beginning by being envious of us. In his envy, he wants total control of all men who enter this life. He plagues every person that remains alive that came from their procreator. Not one escapes this person and the other evil spirits with him. Remember this guy and his associates are called evil. We should always try to remember evil stands for bad and not good. He can only govern with sickness, cruelty, and it ends in death.

As long as we are having intercourse with the Devil, we are under his control. He is one guy that does not want to let go of any person. I am not saying I know what the lake of fire will be like, or what will be the full reaction of people when they are in that place of torment. This I know: all the ones whose names are not written in the book of life will wind up in the lake of fire. They are going to look upon Satan that weakened the nations. Isaiah 14:12-17

Knowledgeable of the future, Satan will be visible forever in the lake of fire. This is also known as the second death. Can we scrutinize that it might be possible all the people, that will be inheriting the second death, will be able to see Satan and his confederates and know that they were our tormentors when we lived and walked the earth?

Living in the lake of fire is hard to comprehend. Using earthly knowledge, a person cannot endure tremendous heat for long on this earth. Can we imagine a person having a body capable of being alive forever and cannot die. The place where those people will be living, the heat will be tremendously hot. All the people that will inherit the lake of fire will have no food, no water, or anything to cool one's thirst. Are they going to be hungry? What is it going to be like being tormented forever?

The possibility is that all that inherit the second death will in some way plague the Devil and his host. Man will be angry with their deceiver, who they allowed to play tricks with them all the days of their lives. They are going to be very angry with themselves. Because man did not take GOD at his words, we allow the Devil and his evil spirits to play tricks with our mind and thoughts. We need to keep reminding ourselves each waking hour, anyone who ends up in the lake of fire, they are the one who made the choice to be there.

The Devil became envious of humanity because men had their own world for self- government. He never wanted to be second fiddle in man's kingdom. He was displeased with man. He was lower in rank, yet higher in power. Man is flesh and blood. He is made to be an earthly creature in the beginning, and only an earth dweller. He was never given the power to transform himself to a spiritual being and ascend into the heavens.

Over and over we read in the Bible where spirit beings called angels are seen talking with men. Not once have we learned of man transforming himself into a spiritual being. The Devil at first was an angelic being. He was able to change as he was permitted. He would be able to communicate with man. He never wanted that servant like job. To him that was below his beauty and grace. He felt that he should be lord over a lower creature than himself. So he disobeyed GOD to be lord over humans.

His disobedience brought death to man. He would not have had any ruling power over humanity if man did not heed his deception. Just as it was for Eve that day it seems to be the same way for billions of people daily. Man just simply down right can't take the words of

GOD very seriously. We keep living, as though GOD is just the figment of a person's imagination.

Many confess with their hearts and lips that there is no GOD. The things that are hard to understand, I have never heard these individuals who confess that there is no GOD, also confess that there is no Devil. Any person with any kind of honesty, by now, should not need anyone to tell them that there is a devil. When someone thinks, or feels, that there is no such thing as the Devil, just look around you. Ask yourself a question. Why is there death and evil?

Why do people behave so despicably one to another? Why do we hate one another so much? Why are we so greedy and selfish for food, money, and all the substances of this world? Why can't we wake up and analyze our lives in a way that will be beneficial after death? We need to see and to understand that all things in this world benefit the occupant only. In death nothing in this world is of any use to the one that is departed.

Let us analyze the Devil and his confederates. They have no use for any of the substances we need to live with daily. Money, food, clothes, water, air, homes, cars, or any other substances that people use for their comfort and relaxation are of no value to any spiritual being.

What is it the enemy wants of humanity? Why is he so forceful and so demanding in oppressing us into living a sinful, wretched life? He seems to want death for all, since he lost his life because of man. The envy of the Devil caused him to reject GOD as his GOD. He wanted to be lord over man. Man would only answer to GOD and no one else. The hate he now has in his heart for humanity is because he is envious of man. He became very bitter against us because he lost the status he had in heaven.

At one time he was able to enjoy all the beauty and pleasures of heaven. Now he knows that the place known as the lake of fire awaits him. Is it possible for him to ever correct the wrong he has done? Can we see and understand the pain this fellow must be undergoing continually?

Many of us do the same thing to ourselves all the time. Envy and greed allow us to behave the same way as our father the Devil behaves. Do we think this person has a right to be the way he is? He gave up a beautiful place for a corruptible place that he made. He cannot reverse his corruptible place he made for himself. Still the people that live in the corrupt place have the opportunity to occupy the wonderful place that this person gave up. All because: the Devil wanted to be lord and master of humanity.

The Devil possibly will never humble himself and beg GOD to grant him forgiveness. Since this guy cannot make heaven his home anymore, he is going to keep working on man to prevent us all from going to occupy the wonderful and very beautiful place he gave up for nothing.

He gave up heaven for nothing. He does not want us to give up our nothing for something. He wants us to remain with our nothing forever and ever. There is a question we need to ask ourselves. Is life ever going to be pleasant on this earth while the Devil occupies it with man? He is very much disrespectful to each and every person that is born in this world. We need to know that even before we are born he starts to work on us that we never make it alive on this earth.

It's a constant battle we are having with the enemy. In some of the ways he opposes us, we are not aware. We need to understand that this guy, even when you are true and faithful to him, keeps you under his full control, and in torment all the days of your life.

We should understand that nothing good is in this person's vocabulary. The only thing he knows is evil continually. As long as we allow this person to be our lord and master, we are always going to have lots of pain and sorrow all the days of our life and in the end, death. Genesee 11: 1-9.

I also know that all the people that walk with GOD still have things very difficult all the days of their lives. Still, we need to remember that the opposing one still walks this earth. As he tricked Eve to believe a lie, he will forever keep doing the same to us all the time. It will be worse for those who keep opposing him in trying to walk pleasing with GOD.

All the people who are being very faithful to GOD have life much more difficult than the ones who have nothing to do with GOD. The other thing we all fail to see and understand is that the people who are faithful to the Devil will wind up with him in the lake of fire that is the second death. There will be weeping and gnashing of teeth for everyone who ends up in the lake of fire. In heaven, where GOD is, there will be happiness and rejoicing for everyone who makes heaven their home. The other thing we might ignore, or has not entered into the heart of many people, is that we are not knowledgeable of the devil being the one that made the choice to live in the lake of fire forever. The same goes for all that will wind up in that place of torment.

At this stage Lucifer has no other choice to make possible. I am not GOD, and I am not the one that forgives sins. At the same token, I have not created anything. I am just a man like everyone else. I am powerless. The reason I am what I am is that too many of us were not molded correctly when we were younger.

Our Bible teaches that we should bring up a child the way they should go and when they grow up they will not depart from it. Proverbs 22: 6 Men allow the enemy to teach us only ungodly things that profit nothing. As long as we remain faithful to the enemy we will never have a pleasant life in this world and in the world to come.

Today we can find millions of people globally who keep saying they are walking with GOD, and they know that they will someday make heaven their home. Yet the same person fails to see and understand that they are only walking with GOD with their lips.

Man, by the craftiness of our enemy, takes the words of GOD and makes us believe a lie. As we believe a lie, we remain as a servant to our enemy. Many will profess they are the servant of the true and living GOD. They feel the Devil is their oppressor. Through his oppressions they are claiming GOD as their LORD and master.

If that was the case the majority can claim the same. The reason I say that is look at all the people that have a very hard time making ends meet in this cruel world. We should not look upon worldly possessions as blessings or curses. Man looks at the things a person obtains in life as either blessings or curses. We should never apply wealth or poverty as blessings or curses.

Man's life does not only exist by the things a person obtains after birth. Several times I hear people say what a blessing that person has obtained by the skill they have in playing all kinds of instruments.

It is not only instruments that people address as a blessing from GOD, but other things we would be addressing as blessings from GOD. The thing that is very hard to comprehend with men is this: the things that we address as GOD sent blessings; we use the so-called blessing to exalt the Devil.

Man is a failure to himself. We find it difficult to truly lift up the One that really loves and cares for us. In my opinion I feel that it's overdue that man ties to recapture the life that was once taken from us. Once in history we see where man united with one common interest in building a tower that would reach into the heavens.

In the day when man was determined to construct a city with a tower whose top might reach heaven, man only spoke one language. The tower was being built just in case GOD would change his mind and once more plan to eradicate man from off the earth with water. Genesee 11:1-9

GOD shut down man's plan by changing one language to several, whereby dividing man and the earth. With all that GOD has done, we cannot find it within man to work together in unity for our own good. We just keep separating farther from GOD. We keep embracing the one that only keeps hurting us all the days of our life. 1Chronicles 1:19.

By understanding modern technology, and the things we have created, we behave as if we are responsible for creating man and all things on this earth. Man keeps spending billions going out into outer space looking for other humans. We have not taken the things in the Bible as GOD stated. The heaven and the earth were created by GOD for man's dwelling place, known for man as our kingdom. We need to remember we have given our subduing and dominion power to the devil.

Now we have become his slaves. We do all his bidding for him. We behave irreverently to GOD; as our master the Devil commands us. Our neighbors are hungry and naked before us continually. Yet, we spend billions all the time being destructive to our neighbors.

When are we going to develop feelings for our neighbors? Is it possible we are not in love with ourselves? We have no feelings for the folks we are in contact with. Being selfish, we are unable to touch each other spiritually.

Man has a love hate nature within his being. We all claim that we are in love with ourselves. At the same time we hate ourselves. When a person is in love with himself, he would shun the Devil and turn to walk with GOD will all his might.

Analyzing the way most of us behave, all of us know that if we do not eat, sleep and drink something we will die. Because we are somewhat in love with ourselves, we eat, sleep, and always have something to drink. Many listen to men who they think have the answers to good long healthy living. They then guide their lives upon those teachings, hoping that they will extend their life in good health. We walk in man's teachings because we love life. We do not want to die or go through pain and suffering.

We hate ourselves. GOD offers us real life if we live a sin free life while we live and walk this earth. We find it so hard to heed the words of GOD for our own benefit. Yet, at the same time we seek earthly physicians to extend our lives. Man might help in some ways to extend one's life in many categories. Yet in truth, they are not extending our life. The day death really knocks at our door, it's the day man will have to take a back seat. Man is unable to stop death. The end of this life does not eradicate man's existence forever.

Man has placed many humans on life saving machines that he has invented. People would lie there being kept alive; yet being dead. They never know if anything is there or not, because their functional understanding fails to consciously acknowledge their surroundings. At that stage they are dead. It's the machine that's working. A machine hooked up to a man cannot detect what the person needs to regain consciousness.

Man is a creature that is very difficult to understand. I do not think that we are ever going to change. I see we are becoming more and more despicable daily. If there is a change being made it looks like it's only for the worse and not for the better.

Man made the Devil place a blindfold over our eyes. I personally am bewildered why we can't try much harder to boot this guy so that he does not keep harassing us daily. Look at the use of drugs, alcohol, and all the various things that the Devil uses to keep us as his slaves.

Take all the sicknesses that have had man's life in topsy-turvy.

They are not from GOD. We should never point our fingers in the face of GOD that He created these sicknesses as a method of keeping man in check. I know that GOD always wants man to call on Him for help. That is not the case with GOD. He does not ill-treat the man he loves so much. All things cruel, with evil treatments, come from the enemy.

All sickness comes from the one who desires to continually oppress man. Sickness is a way of enslaving man. We love and enjoy being treated shamefully. GOD made a promise to the children of Israel. If they would faithfully obey him, and keep all his commandments and his statues, neither sickness nor any plagues would over take them and their children forever. He would make sure that the plagues that were placed upon the Egyptians would never over-take Israel. Exodus 15:26. Deuteronomy 7:15

When they reached the Promised Land they were commanded to completely annihilate the entire inhabitants they were commanded to destroy. They should never make an agreement with any nation in that area. They were supposed to be completely separated from them and never live or behave in corrupting themselves in the evil ways the others did. Deuteronomy 7:1&2, 20:17

Israel's lifestyle should have been according to the standard set by GOD. Look at man's continual behavior. It matters not the year or time. From the day of Eve and Adam, to this present era, we can see we are just as guilty as the first two that rejected GOD'S words and heeded the words of the Devil. The thing is this; we have not stopped heeding the words of the Devil.

Man, all these years, has nothing good to show that Satan has done for anyone. GOD is the one who is responsible for all the things we love so much and enjoy. Our food, homes, and cars, or whatever our souls lust after, we are able to still receive them by what GOD did in the beginning. There is never a time when GOD needed to be envious of man or behave the way man behaves.

The day GOD holds a grudge against man will be the day GOD becomes vile. Man needs to understand that GOD can never become a vile and evil person. That is why he cannot associate Himself with evil. It is one of the many reasons why He has required all the ones that serve Him to separate themselves from all the ones that walk in an ungodly way of life.

Just as GOD cannot have a double standard in his kingdom, he would like man to behave as he behaves. Man cannot serve two masters at the same time. We need to choose GOD or the devil. There is no neutral ground here. One has to serve either of the two. One of these two masters is a counterfeit. One is very sweet and compassionate. He will not hold us in sin if we go to him seeking for him to forgive us of our sins and trespasses.

Look at life in general as a very broad picture. Not in a pattern as we have been doing for centuries. People have been behaving on a small scale with their minds. We have not learned to be thankful to the One who has been there all the time for us, even when we keep turning our backs on him.

If GOD was not there for us all the time, by now man could have been completely annihilated by the Devil. To me the Devil does not think positive. Just as man thinks and behaves ignominiously, the Devil behaves the same way. He is very much disrespectful to man. He hates us with a passion. I do not think the Devil recognizes he only has a kingdom because of humanity. The day he should completely annihilate his enemy, which is man, he will have no subjects for him to govern anymore.

Looking at how he behaves, we can apply man's behavior to his. Despite similar behavior like the Devil, we are not as completely ruthless as he. Man to man might be unjust, yet in all our unjustness the pattern of behavior is not really man. Men in truth really have many good attributes still embedded within their being.

A man is never completely ruthless to all people. Even in the hottest battle with our enemies man to man, we find time to have compassion. That is where one has taken prisoners of war. Prisoners of war, in many countries, get somewhat good treatment. They do not kill the prisoners of war; only the ones that remained in battle lose their lives. When we go to war with any country or Island, if they should surrender before the beginning of the battle, the battle would be over before it starts. The party that is the victor would be the controller of that people that seek peace. Man's greatest foe would never be compassionate in his battle with humanity. He does not want man to be in heaven with GOD.

Man was not the one that forced this guy to leave his home in heaven. Men were not knowledgeable about angelic beings before sin infiltrated them. Communication was with GOD and man. When man sinned, angels were placed to protect the tree of life that man would not eat and live forever in sin, and never would die. Genesee 3:24

When are we going to wake from the sleep of ignorance the Devil has over us? We have not tried to understand how cruel this guy really is. All he does care for is to completely eradicate humanity from off this earth. He did know that if man ate of the tree forbidden by GOD man would die. What about the tree that would prevent man from dying? Why did he not show man they would never die by eating from the tree that would remove death?

Understanding the truth about this guy, we should learn by now we need to try to unite to fight against our enemy. The Devil is man's only true enemy. He fools us to think man's enemy is one another. We should love and care for one another, knowing that we are humans, flesh and blood alike. We need the same things as one another. It matters not whether a person is a king or a peasant, all need to eat, sleep, or work, take a bath, and use some things to smell pleasant.

Take from a person all the things above, and they are unable to survive in this world. The majority have not seen, or understood that it is not only sickness the Devil uses to plague man all the days of our lives. I wonder how many see and understand that sickness seems to play a very large part in the life of people globally? It removes millions from this life yearly. In this era the enemy is having a field day with sickness to control man as he pleases. We just can't see the need of doing something to get this monkey off our backs.

The majority of humans behave like they are very happy with this guy being a very cruel master to them. We are not doing much to dispose of this guy. He keeps plaguing us all the time. Night and day, even in our sleep this guy does not even give us rest. Many times the dreams we have make us go and do the things we dream about. That becomes sinful for many people all over the world.

When our enemy feels that we are not dying fast enough by the sicknesses he plagues us with, we become angry with others because they do not do the things we feel are according to what we like. If they break the law we simply remove them from this earth because the enemy placed bitterness in our hearts towards our brothers and sisters.

When, humans are not the ones who take the lives of their brothers and sisters, the enemy finds many other ways to annihilate more humans. There are floods, fires, tornadoes, hurricanes, earthquakes, tidal waves, and volcanoes. Don't exclude cars, trucks, buses, trains, airplanes, ships, and submarines. We can think of many other ways that our enemy uses to annihilate man from the face of the earth. Don't forget he uses man to keep killing man.

Humans are not willing to fight this guy; he just keeps beating us up. The thing that might be possible, because so many do not believe in GOD, or do not accept that there are devils, they might feel nothing is wrong with killing another person. It is just reducing the population because people are unable to live forever. The world would become over populated if people do not die one way or another.

Man, from the day they first transgressed, started to die. In this era man no longer lives as long as the very first people that occupied this planet. Looking at the death rate, I feel man has much more death daily than people say a hundred years back in time. If they had cars and much of modern transportation a hundred and fifty years in the past, men and women would not die with as many accidents as we have these days. We have more immoral people living today than just eighty years in the past, and it seems like it was just yesterday. Look at the kids that are having kids, and all the men that have been going to men, for sexual pleasures. It's because man refuses to unite in one common bond to stop the enemy from overpowering us.

Many people believe that there is a GOD. Likewise, they accept that there is also a Devil. We can resist him and all his confederates so that they will be powerless in all their effort in trying to destroy man. We have no power to look upon this demon and knock him around a few times. Even though we cannot see this person, or spiritual being, we can still be successful in shutting down the power he has over us.

We need to understand that if we do not allow the Devil to access our minds and our thoughts, he will not be able to have any power over us. The Devil can only beat upon us if we allow him to infiltrate our thoughts and mind. If we should analyze the counterfeit maneuver that our enemy used against us, we would be ashamed to realize what foolish creatures we are.

I am not saying that the devil is powerless and that he is only a figment of our imagination. This guy is a spirit. He is not visible to man. We can only see things that do appear. Since this person is a spirit, he has to put on a body that will be visible to man's eyes.

How sweet it is to know that Satan, the Devil, is unable to change himself to human as so many angels have done. If this being was able to change himself to human and walk this earth the way many angels have done, what a despicable world it would be.

He would constantly keep changing himself to keep man even farther from walking with GOD. I would like many to know that people would not be happy seeing the Devil and his confederates. They are such hideous creatures. We have seen many movies man made with some ugly looking beasts. These creatures are awful looking, but the Devil and his companions are much more terrifying than we can ever imagine.

The Devil knows how to bring many evil plagues upon man. Still he cannot harm anyone if we stand strong in unity. There is not much he can do with all the power he has. All the power of the enemy relies on the weakness of humanity. In the day when man becomes as one in unity to defeat the enemy, we will find out that the enemy has no power over man. We are going to feel very small because we did not fight harder in this race.

Shame will not be necessary anymore. I cannot speak of what hell will be like. I have to believe what the Bible teaches. I know that the good book indoctrinates us that there will be weeping and gnashing of teeth {Matthew 13: 41&42} for all people whose names are not written in the lamb's book of life. Revelation 21: 27. We need to remember the fault is not GOD'S if a person does not make heaven their home.

Looking at this life, and the various things that befall many people in this life, we cannot cast the blame on others. For many years we find various types of people that are rich. Also you can find many who are very satisfied with their poverty. Many just do not care to be their own boss. We can find many who are very unhappy if they do not get the opportunity to be the employer. Many just care for some alcohol, some women and they are very happy. All the people that live on benches, I do not feel they are happy with their life. I know that the Devil has total control over their lives. That is the reason they are living the way they are. Total control of the enemy, over their lives, removes from them the feelings of caring for themselves and others.

If people could go without eating and drinking, or even sleeping, they would go without, but because of the power the enemy has over man we are unrestraint. The reasons so many people comport that way, is that these evil spirits cannot die, and they go from humans to humans. They were never cast out by the power of GOD. They love to keep man from consciousness so that man will continue to be servants to his master the Devil.

The other thing many of us have overlooked is the reason so many angels turned from heaven to serve under the Devil for nothing; it's the same reason we reject GOD. Man's heart should ache seeing the suffering of many that are unable to be set free. We set up places for many so they can have things natural like clean clothes, and somewhere to lay their heads. Still the greatest relief they need we are unable to give. We are still under the control of the Devil, even though we do not behave as the ones who sleep on park benches.

Because we refuse to care for ourselves we keep listening to people that are the instruments of the Devil. We truly cannot help one another. What we fail to understand, the Devil does not have the power to possess each and every person as he does the ones who live on the streets. What can he do? He can infiltrate the mind of humanity and use it as he pleases. What is needed to be done to wake up humanity from a life of sin and death? Millions are suffering and dieing yearly without mercy from the Devil.

He has done this to millions globally. When he has people that way, they become his ministers to do his dirty work for him. This is how he works. That is how he gets his power. Will man ever be awakened from his slumber to realize that he is the servant of Satan and that he obeys his every command? It might just help us to go to GOD for the first time in truth, to band together to bind this guy, and to cast him from this earth forever and ever.

We need to remember all things can be possible if we can unite as one. We should be awakened to the fact that nothing that man has been doing all his life, on his own, has worked to bring harmony to the population of the world. The longer we keep doing evil sinful things as we are doing we are not going to help one another. Not able to help each other, we are going to remain a cripple forever.

The thing we fail to see and understand, because we are not physically crippled and handicapped, is that the reason why we behave as if all things are normal? It's our faculties that the enemy has crippled. The way he has done it is so subtle that we never know where we are and what we are doing until it is too late. When we part this life we know nothing. The day we are awakened to know anything then it will be over. There won't be anything anyone can do for us.

The person who is so subtle in his deception over our lives will be on the pleading side begging for mercy. The thing we should ask ourselves, who will be merciful to this guy after he was so unmerciful to us all our lives? I do not think any person who obtains the lake of fire will have any feelings of forgiveness towards this person. He crippled the majority of people's reasoning and judgment and faculties that they could not see the truth and put their trust in GOD. When we do not trust GOD, we will end up in the lake of fire with the Devil and his confederates.

Believe the things stated in the words of GOD concerning damnation to all those who are obedient to the Devil. Many would not have allowed the devil to condemn them. Looking at man's life on this earth, I see constant agony for all. Many might address their lives as great and pleasant. They think and feel they are not undergoing any agony in their life. I would like for you to take stock of your life. Think if you have ever encountered any colds, flu, or any kinds of problems from your childhood days with your parents and teachers, or had any kind of accidents whatever they may be. That should show that you will never walk this earth trouble free. If you have never encountered any kind of illness or any problem in this life, then you should be able to say that you are above GOD.

When Jesus walked this earth as a man, the Devil was disrespectful to Him. He gave Him a very hard time. Many times He was displeased with men's behavior because of the hardness of their hearts in accepting who He was. To the day of his death, the Devil was working on Him so that he would sin. If the Devil did cause Jesus to sin at anytime while He walked this earth, He would have been a very poor example to us. His coming to die for our sins would not have worked because He sinned.

We should always remember it was the people that GOD showed great things unto all their life, such as the deliverance from Egypt, and the land that flow with milk and honey. Israel was the chosen people that Jesus should come into the world and die for all sinners of the world. The Devil used the people that knew more about GOD than any other nation. They treated Him oftentimes with no respect as He was nothing in-spite of all the miracles He did in their presence.

We need to ask ourselves this question. The devil that treated us so disrespectfully all the days of our lives, what has he done that a person can think of, that is pleasant that we can thank him for? I personally have not seen anything pleasant this guy did for anyone worthy of thanks.

I feel man should be so angry with this person, and we should all try immensely to wipe out this person once and for all eternity. I heard these words from when I was a child, and they have not left the lips of humanity, "playing with fire one will get burned." We are playing with fire. I know that we are going to be burned with the one that we are playing with.

I will always have this to say. The majority of humanity is in love with the life they have. We might not look at loving our life because we seek a physician when we are sick or we eat, drink, and sleep to live a long time. Because we do not know what death is all about we do what is necessary to stay alive. Do we know the real reason why we fight so much to occupy this earth? Is it because it's a natural thing built within the human bodies that make us automatically take care of our bodies? What is the real reason why man lives on this earth? At the present time man seems to only do what is insignificant and valueless all the days of their lives.

What is there in life that causes man to say they are in love with life? We would travel to the end of the earth to get help when we are in need of help. People who have lots of money would spend a tidy sum for a physician who they think would be of great service in eradicating their problems. As a rule, they would go because their colleague made the recommendation. It's not necessary that a person's colleague visit that physician as patient.

Having feelings and consideration for others, people will tell someone about a good physician if they know someone is sick and not getting help from the present doctor they are seeing. Man is not all that bad of a creature. If we were ruthless as the Devil, we would not care what happens to anyone.

Many of us might just go along being selfish, not thinking about others. Yet, if there should be some catastrophe, the same person that has been walking with their head up in the sky, would become compassionate to the ones that encountered the accident. In-spite of the ruthless nature of the Devil over humanity, the Devil to this date still is not able to have complete control over humanity. He has been trying very hard from the first time he gave up heaven to be god over humanity. Man, in all the opposition he encounters, still manages to remain with compassion.

Since we are capable of rejecting many things that our enemy casts at us, we should be strong enough to resist him in everything he throws at us. Man, in many things, is a weak creature. He fails in many cases to understand what is best for man. I realize that people have a very hard time believing that they are controlled by the Devil.

As I travel daily and converse with people of all walks of life, I learn of many different views. I have not seen a lot of people that think and feel the Devil is their lord and master. Many claim they are not walking with either GOD or the devil. The Devil is not their master; at the same time, they are living a life that is very sinful to the laws of man and GOD.

How do we apply man's laws when men break the laws of man? Are man's laws counted as sin, or is sin only counted by GOD when we break the laws of GOD? I do not think we have analyzed the three governing bodies of this universe. We have GOD, then man, and then the Devil.

Two of the three have laws that govern. One has no laws or

government. The devil is just an outlaw. He keeps humanity lawless all the days of their lives. The laws of man keep man in check, so that we do not live like savages all the days of our lives to one another.

By being honorable to man's laws we have a very pleasant place to live. Harmony brings happiness. Being honorable also to the laws of GOD makes life much more pleasant for all of humanity. When man keeps man's laws, there is no need for them to stand before a judge. They do not need anyone to defend them in the court of law. Only a lawless person needs an attorney to represent him when he is caught breaking the laws of the land.

When man breaks the laws of GOD, there is no one he can find to be his defender before GOD. The only reason we break the laws of GOD is the Devil has us in his power and under his control. The Devil is the one out of the three that has no laws and no real government. He is the only one out of the three that never tried anyone and sentenced them to punishment.

We need to understand that this person is a counterfeit. He has nothing and nowhere to place anyone. All the ones that are in the grave are not his to have. The grave is not a place of any kind of punishment. The grave is a place where no one thinks, feels, or is in need of anything. People that lie silent in the graves never need food, clothes, or anything. They never fuss or fight with anyone. Their love and hatred lie with them in the grave. Taking a person from this life in a sense is favorable to the ones who die, if they are in love with GOD and obey his every command. One is much worse off when they die being a lawbreaker of the commandments of GOD.

Life might be unpleasant many times. The only reason why life is not always harmonious is because we have a lawless person that forces humanity to be lawless.

All that the Devil or Satan has done is to keep man in torment all the time on this earth, we cannot awaken to his control. Instead, we acknowledge that there is no lawless demon and that the Devil is only one's imagination.

I feel it's overdue for humanity to wake from their slumber. Then we may see that there has to be a ruling evil force over humanity. If there were no evil force controlling man's existence, we all would be able to live our lives without anyone breaking the laws that man made for governing man.

If Satan was just a self made entity, man should be able to govern this earth without all this evil standing in our face. Looking at Satan's behavior and man in the same order with the Devil, we should agree that the same nature is in man. We do have continual hate, killing, stealing, fuss, fighting, and almost all the ruthless nature of the Devil. We should never forget sickness and death still reign with humanity.

Look at the evil things that the Devil keeps giving us and we keep being harmonious with him. This shows that we are not willing to let this guy go that we might have life much more pleasant than the way we are living.

Man can do much better than we are doing. We only need to stop, look, and listen to our own laws and rules to know what we need to understand. We do know and understand that man can't live without some kind of government. We should also understand that there has to be a much greater power than man that teaches us laws and government that we can work in a manner that's pleasant.

Just as in every country or Island we can find opposition that makes things unpleasant. One of the parties just wants to look good to their subjects. This takes us back to the Devil and his opposition to man. The Devil has become our opposition because he wants to rule when he should have always remained a servant. This could be the reason why most of the world's governments are the way they are today. The people that are running the world today possibly should be in the back seats, not in the driver seat. Many of the world leaders are the Devil's henchmen. They are destroyers of their citizens.

The reason why countries and Islands have so many lawless citizens is that they are sons and daughters of the devil. He is the only ruler that has no laws. He is the lawless one. All his servants are lawless as he himself is.

The Silent Killer

Chapter (8)

Life seems to be a waste if we look at the way we all take things for granted. We live like there is no tomorrow. The world's population today behaves as if man's only purpose on this earth is to eat, drink, and have lots of pleasure, and then die.

Is it possible man is unable to see the real truth of good and bad, life and death? Until someone who knows better can show good and bad, right from wrong, and what will happen to all the people who live without planning for life after death. I am not saying that I know all things. I was once in the boat of ignorance just as millions are still in that same ship. I was not able to see the evil I was doing to my body; just as millions are unable to see all the danger they are encountering daily.

The opening of my eyes showed me many things that are very devastating to man. It makes my whole being ache. I realize that man needs a teacher: someone, who is a very good educator with love and understanding, and that is something difficult to find in man. People are creatures that are very easily persuaded to turn from caring for their fellowmen.

The things we place over one another are of little value. Man is the true value of all. Man has been placed on earth above all things. Yet, we find it so difficult to do what is right and to care as we should. What is it about man? Why do we behave disrespectfully and place vanity above each other?

More than once I have heard this saying, that before his death, a man requested that he would like for those left alive of his family to place some of his money in his casket with him. The day of his death, several members of his family placed cash into his casket. I heard that one of the members of his family came along and took out all the cash, and for the cash he placed a check in the casket. He then addressed the deceased, that the check was good, and he could cash it anytime he so desired. This should show us that one of the family members realized that it was a waste to place cash in the casket. So he exchanged the cash with a check, knowing that a dead person will never use money anymore. Yet we all crave wealth so much. So many are in love with money even in death; they would like to carry it with them.

I know that we have created a society that requires a lot of money to live these days. If we do not have any money, we are going to have a very difficult time living, especially when we live in a society where we fight so hard not to be criticized.

Man, through our enemy, has become very greedy for power and wealth. We kill one another to become wealthy and to stop criticism. If we do not become rich, we envy the rich and point only at them saying they are thoughtless and greedy for themselves with their riches. The poorer people have not noticed that they too are greedy. In our greediness we behave foolishly. Fighting for equality, to be in the same category with rich people, makes life unpleasant for millions.

Today's generation does not have this word in their vocabulary: "contentment". It is not found in the heart of people that live in rich countries and Islands. In parts of the world where we find people living where it is still undeveloped, where technology is not available, one might find contentment in those people's vocabulary.

Living in vast developed countries and Islands makes people behave outrageous and dissatisfied. Man has to keep developing all kinds of gadgets so as to make people feel content. What would man be like, having such a large population as we have globally, with nothing to do all day but just hunt, fish, or be a farmer?

Living as farmers in ancient civilization made composure much stronger in man's existence than today's much faster pace of life. Looking at man's conduct, living in countries and Islands that have modern technologies, I see a life of misery that's full of unhappiness. Because our eyes are blinded with the facts of realities, we live as if this type of life is much more pleasant than those of the undeveloped nations.

The question we have facing us is: out of the two types of lifestyles, which one do we think has it better? Can we find comparison in any form of equidistant with life in the developed nations and the undeveloped nations?

In my opinion, I feel that we have not educated ourselves

correctly as we have developed. We have cast behind us a healthy lifestyle for a very unhealthy one. We do not know the road back. We have become so advanced that we will never return to a lifestyle that makes a person's life much healthier. Despite people being forced to change, folks are still controlled by man's philosophy.

Man is so much in love with this kind of living, even though it is a killer. We are not going to give it up for better health. People are somewhat half way happy with their unhealthy outrageous life. Some people will never give up their despicable life for all the happiness and better health a person can obtain.

I am not saying that modern conveniences do not have great values. Yet, in the pleasures of today's advancements we can find great danger. Because of poor education from our educators, we live in places that make life hazardous. We feel this type of living is far better than those that have a lifestyle as ancient people.

Ancient populations never had the luxurious living conditions as today's people have. Even the poorest in many parts of the world have some of the luxuries of today. The majority might not accept that lots of modern day technologies are the cause of man's down fall. They are very deadly. Man's fast pace in this era makes folks unaware of the danger we are encountering daily. Because we love comfort so much, no one ever thinks of harm when making many of today's mechanization.

Advancement is a very wonderful thing. But failing to be knowledgeable of people's shortcomings with today's technology, it can be harmful to the users and very deadly. That is where we find the silent killer.

Our scientists and our educators with all their teaching might have overlooked the silent killer. The reasons why the knowledge was never found, the first amount of machinery built was less in quantity, and we lost sight of the hidden dangers to the users of these mechanical devices. They were not able to make us aware of the dangers there are with them. The other thing that might be possible, man has become so greedy for money that he is just downright selfish, and does not care for any person. He may think that as long as he can make, or get, the amount of wealth he desires for himself while he is alive, he does not care.

What is the reason why humanity fights so hard to become rich and will do whatever it takes to become wealthy? Why do we also weigh success by the amount of money or the abundance of things we possess in this life? All the wealth we fight so hard to obtain, has not removed death from either rich or poor. Sickness and death still plague humanity.

People have become very complacent in this epoch, that these words are a common phrase in today's society. "The learning of anyone coming back from the dead, or from the grave, to address what dying is like." People tend to close their eyes to the reality of death. The Bible tells us that after death is the judgment; death does speak. Despite the apathetic behavior in people, people still keep dying daily and sickness is on the increase. Even with modern technologies, we have not slowed down death or reduced illness.

Analyzing the increase in sickness, being knowledgeable with nescience within humanity you can see many things which are being overlooked. Because we have been using these devices for many years, and have not seen physical injuries, we just let them keep bringing harm to the users. It's not the users fault. Man has to have an educator. When we do not have anyone to indoctrinate us, we are going to remain in our ignorance all the days of our lives. I see lots of ignorance prevailing as I travel this earth.

Let us for a short time analyze the life of the people that we call barbaric or uncivilized. The people of the modern world live in homes that are beautiful. They can walk-over to a switch and instantly the darkness is extinguished. That is very pleasant. A person has no need to grope in the darkness to find the toilet, or to get something to eat or to drink. At that time each person can satisfy their craving. They do not have to go back to their bed if they are hungry and would have to wait until the morning to get something to eat. Electricity is a very pleasant thing. People who do not have electric live with lots of restraint.

Life with electric is wonderful if we are able to not let it govern our lives. Those who have modern day technology should be the ones that should have a much better, healthier life than those who do not have the use of electricity.

That is where men have failed one another all the years we have had electricity. Think about what has transpired since the creation of lights with a switch. People have become very careless in their living. Man thinks that life in the dark years must have been barbarous. Now that man developed a thing by the name of electricity, that allows us to get light by pushing a switch, all life in the dark years has been placed in the trash bin. Electric development keeps humanity busy all these years making all kinds of gadgets powered by electric that enable time and space to be much shorter.

Looking at all the various things we have in our world that run by electric, what would man do if someday we find ourselves without any means of generating electricity? What if we have to go back to the dark ages when man had to use candles and other methods for lighting? Although we have the power of extinguishing many areas of darkness in our world, and have so many commodities at our fingertips, we simply use many of them as our toys. This gives great pleasure to man in this era, but man still behaves barbaric.

Fascinating as it may be, technology is somewhat hazardous to our health. Since we are not knowledgeable with the unseen dangers with technologies, we live as if we are going to remain on this earth forever.

By the power of electricity man developed many types of transportation. Each type of vehicle made by man snuffs out many lives yearly. When it does not take one's life, one can remain a quadriplegic or paraplegic, and suffer in many ways the rest of your life.

It is very hard for millions to imagine a life without the flick of a switch to eradicate darkness. I feel that this generation would hurt one another if by chance something would happen that would cause electricity on this earth to fail forever.

I know that electric has its advantages and disadvantages. It also takes many lives yearly. Man developed many great things that are powered by electric. They likewise take a lot of lives because men still have a difficult time understanding the principles of electricity.

Electricity is very dangerous. Men created it. It has been giving men a very difficult time to understand its property. Regardless of the deadliness of electricity, it will never be deadly to humans if we use caution being in the pathway of electric current.

We might be able to correlate money with electricity, but money might be a little different in the use of it. Money never moves itself. Wherever you place money is where it will remain until someone moves it. Electric is a current that moves rapidly. It does not move slowly under any circumstances. The flick of a switch and current will move from one location miles ahead with no hesitation. Even when there is a short in the system, it does not stop the flowing of electricity. It will go to the ground and snuff out a person's life, if they don't take the proper precautions.

Most places where we see high voltage signs, we will always see barriers in place as a precautionary measure. As long as a person does not behave ignorantly with electric, it will not hurt you. Behaving unwisely with electric current spells death as it is with many things man has created. Money in itself is not deadly. It becomes very deadly when we are in love with money and place money before humans. That is to say, we are in love with filthy lucre more than people. Many humans place filthy lucre, at a great value over the life of man, and many will take even their procreator's life to obtain lots of money.

Money is similar to guns. Man is responsible for creating guns. It is not guns that do the killing. Remember, just as electric does not have the power on it's own to move as it pleases and take the life of whom it desires, it is the same thing with all things that man has created. All the things that are created for man's benefits, they were not created deliberately to be destructive.

Man with his poor loving and uncontrollable desire has lost sight of his brother's children, or whatever category we place humans under. Knowledge was not given to man by GOD to create technology for the purpose of destruction. Wisdom, understanding, and knowledge were imparted to man for a much better living with great understanding for one another. It was not to be selfish and greedy for obtaining more filthy lucre than your brothers. Man by the influence of the Devil sees only one side of the coin. Seeing one side, we lose respect for our own flesh and blood. Humans place more love and care for items that cannot feel or think.

I know that we have lots of people who have developed more love and consideration for animals than people. I know that many people behave unlawfully all over the world. Many feel they don't have to be respectful to the laws of the land. Many behave dishonorably to their countries or Island's laws because the sovereign heads of state themselves are dishonorable to the laws they make.

Their behavior is like this saying that I keep hearing all the time about preachers. "Do as I say; and not as I do". People's self-government in rebellion will forever lead to self destruction. I know that we all have to have self control in all things otherwise we are going to live barbarously one to another. That's where we can find a form of self-government.

The kind of self-government that is outrageous is when a person behaves like they are above the laws. There are a minority who refuse to obey the laws of the land, because they see their leaders are breaking the laws they made.

All sovereign heads of state should always remember what manner of people they should always be. People that choose to be leaders should remember they are also responsible for all people of their country or Island; not only their citizens, but other nations that visit their country or Island as well.

All cannot be leaders in the governing body. There is only a small space in each country or Island for a governing body. The governing body should always remember their responsibility to their subjects.

They were not only elected to make sure that their citizens have jobs, homes, and all the commodities needed for daily living. They need to understand that they should be held responsible for many of the crimes committed by people that become disrespectful to their homeland. Due to inconsiderate leaders of the people many occupants become criminals.

Before we proceed any farther, we need to realize that in-spite of all the wisdom, knowledge, and understanding imparted to humanity by GOD, all the deadly things we created are not of GOD. GOD would never develop within man the feelings of killing one another. There is where the Devil once more steps into things that GOD gave man, and uses it for his own selfish well-being. His only goal is to do all he can within his power to annihilate humanity from off this earth. Daily we surrender to this person. Look at all the weapons of mass destruction so many governing bodies have all over the world.

They were created to kill one another, because we allow the Devil to have full control over us.

Man hates the oppression that other countries do to theirs. They will try to protect what they have with their lives from outside predators. Man's foolish comport brings more harm to one another than we can imagine. We should stop pointing our fingers at other people and look to ourselves for our own shortcomings. The failure is not always on the ones that are leading. We have some responsibility for our own sins.

I know that all were not chosen to be a pastor or an overseer. Yet all have to think of their lives and what they want out of life. That is why we need to understand that anything created by humanity that has become evil in its use should not be addressed to GOD as the one who imparted such knowledge to man.

I believe the Bible is the written words of GOD to humanity, to make man behave respectfully to GOD and man. Man, in his ignorance, behaves as if he is much mightier that his Creator. We have become irreverent to our Creator. The one that is the counterfeit, we honor with more reverence.

In our Bible we find these words. In the book of Isaiah 2:4 and Micah 4:3 "He shall judge among the nations, and shall rebuke many people: and they shall beat their swords into plowshares, and their spears into pruning hooks: nation shall not lift up swords against nation, neither shall they learn war anymore".

GOD'S promises to man are not as man makes theirs. Man is a creature who will never be able to keep ninety nine percent of his promises. We cannot guarantee the next moment, because man is just a vapor or similar to the grass. In the morning the grass is beautiful. Cutting the lawn and the grass loses its beauty. Man is the same. This minute one speaks highly and the next minute one is dead. This should show that we should never rely on man's promises because humans are creatures that are powerless. This minute we are alive, and the next minute we can die.

Man should never express any evil thing we invented as obtaining the knowledge from GOD. Death to humanity was not in the plan of GOD. We are the ones that hate life and show more love and care for death. GOD is the one that keeps showing us a much better way, and we are the ones that seem to keep saying to GOD why not just leave us alone.

Looking at GOD and man, we can find many similarities that we have all overlooked. Man has the ability to create many things. All the things we have created are not alive as human's are. Neither can they remain forever. Man was able many years ago to make cars and trucks, likewise other automobiles as transportation.

Things that man has created cannot become procreator. Man has to keep manufacturing his inventions. The day when GOD completed His work, He never needed to keep making anything that he made. Humans are able to keep multiplying forever until the time that GOD designated as the end of man and all things on this earth.

Analyzing man's workmanship, I realize that man needs spare parts for their creations. They never last very long. That is why we have to keep manufacturing to keep enough supply for the vast demand. All things created by GOD were able to maintain the same course of nature from the first day they came into existence. I wonder what life would be if man had never fallen into sin. All I think we can do at this junction is speculate on the possibilities and leave it there.

GOD was not selfish when He first made man and all the angels in heaven with Him. He gave them a choice and many sinned against Him. Man likewise had the same choice. Man sinned like the devil. Both will be cast into the lake of fire, if?

When the devil will be shut up in the bottomless pit, I see in the Bible that man will never learn war anymore because the tempter will not occupy this earth for a thousand years. Not having any tempter to make man behave irreverent unto their Creator what will man's comport be like? All man can do at the present is speculate on what life will be like without opposition from one's enemy.

Understand that man will not do anymore fighting because our Bible makes it plain enough that man will turn their swords into plowshares and their spears into pruning hooks. Living in a place where there is no need for weapons, it will be possible for men to live for the first time in harmony. "Isaiah 2:4. Mic.4:3"

Instead of weapons you will find equipment for farming. Instead of killing we might find embracing. Instead of an argument you might just find sharing. In those days it will be the first time man will ever truly live loving one towards another with real honest caring. I am only speculating because the force of evil will not be present. We should not wait for those years. Many might not make it to that day. We have the opportunity to be true now, please do not wait. Today is yours; do not put it off.

Since man has been inventing major machinery for today's industries, we have manufactured them without proper education. The reason why man might overlook the dangers we have facing us daily is that we just think only of the labor time shortened in manpower and the money there is to be made. Man just keeps looking on one side of the coin we have in our hands. We do not use foresight over hindsight. Wealth is the game. People are second place or second nature in life. Man's interest seems to point more to wealth than health. We only think of our health when we start to get sick frequently.

Because we are not knowledgeable with all the things we encounter, that can work as a silent killer as we live without caution. The day our eyes are opened to many things that we do daily that work in favor of death, it's the day many will change many things they are doing that are unhealthy.

I know that the vast population will not care. Man just loves to do their own thing without someone else telling them what to do. Rebellion is buried deep within the soul of humanity. It is a very hard thing to remove from the majority of the world population. Most people today behave as if life is indebted to them. Since life owes them gratitude, they live as if there is no tomorrow.

The other thing that might be possible with mankind is that it's not in every man's ability to self govern. Most need the guiding hands of the ones who have the ability to lead themselves and others at the same time. Misleading the ones who need someone to hold their hands, they are going to be lost forever. This could be the reason why so many of us live, eat, and breathe things that are killing us daily as the silent killer. There are many things we have in our society that are killing us silently. Yet, there is one that is much more dangerous than all the others.

Let us look at some of the things that man publishes that works on man's structure and very slowly shortens one's life. They make a person develop many ailments as they journey through this earth. What are the things that man credits as the causes of many illnesses? Should we all take their teaching as correct or simply prevarication? Since the vast population can't afford medical school, to learn about the body for personal satisfaction, it places medicine at a height much greater in value. I know that there are many types of occupations where a person has obtained more than a profession. Many years of study for the medical profession weeds out the ones that are slow in grasping the things they have been taught.

If a person cannot reach an advanced stage in their schooling, they need to find an occupation that is most suitable for their educational background. Many times money is the factor why lots of individuals never reach an advanced stage in life. Being poor can be harmful to people in many ways.

Riches have their drawbacks likewise. In this life a happy medium is very hard to find, especially the way man behaves in this era. Men, with their advancement in technology, place themselves in a much greater category of intelligence than all the generations that lacked the knowledge of today's industrial advancements.

In my estimation, today's advancement in life has not given us any kind of longevity or any better health. We have lots of people today joining all kinds of fitness centers fighting to be healthier. The question one should ask: is it working and are people getting healthy because of what we have been taught? Is there another motive behind the fitness promotion? Money is a vital part of our daily needs. Many behave superficially only to increase their wealth through people who are vulnerable.

People are creatures who easily fall into deception. The truth is a very difficult thing for a person to accept. Lies go over much more pleasantly than the truth. I have seen over and over where lies find a place of comfort in man more than the truth. I see many would kill people when they speak the truth. I know the days when the truth of physical exercise reaches the public that it is very much unhealthy, people are not going to accept the truth. People listen to their educators for health tips. We have taught for years that a person needs lots of physical exercise to keep them healthy and to burn off calories. One day man will find out he can get rid of many things that man once taught could only be gotten rid of by exercise, without any physical labor. "Mr. Silent killer is on the prowl."

Man sure has a great time misunderstanding things that he says are killing us. But, what about the silent killer that has man fooled and playing a bigot? : Which is right? The silent killer has man blindfolded, and keeping man downright lying, or the truth is man does not have the answer.

Oftentimes I hear people say that man is very much knowledgeable about many diseases: that have been plaguing man for centuries and the reason people keep getting sicker. People invest in companies that make drugs for the sick and afflicted that will never give the sick folks the correct medication to help them become better. It would reduce large profits from investors or reduce employment.

It's a very sad thing if that's the truth. Then we have placed wealth over man's well being. I personally have this feeling and will hold them as long as I keep seeing the rich and the poor die. Businessmen that invest in the large corporations that manufacture drugs die of the same illnesses that the poor and middle class people die of. People that own the drug manufacturing companies die also with incurable diseases.

Scientists and the researchers are dying with the same ailments without any help. Why would someone behave so foolishly because of filthy lucre? If I personally worked in a lab where medication is developed or manufactured that's capable of eradicating many ailments, I am sorry, I am going to get some for myself. Then I can die of old age without sicknesses.

I am not being selfish. I am just trying to relate the truth about myself. If I was working in a place where I could obtain medication to remove illness from my body, I would help myself first. Why would someone find a cure for sickness, and the company they work for have them conceal the matter? It is very difficult to understand that even the owner of the company and /or the workers would not have access to the drugs? I know that man is very devious, and the love of money makes us behave despicably.

When I was a child, I remember my granddad saying these words once to my dad "money is king, it can give you almost everything".

The other thing I learned about money when I was small, "money makes friends, money breaks friends, and money will make you take the life of your procreator, your friends, and your neighbors".

When it comes to obtaining money, many lose their feelings for others. Most of us think first for ourselves. Not many put others before themselves. So the question we all need to ask ourselves, is it possible that man has always known and understood the cause of all the ailments that are responsible for millions of people's death yearly? Is it possible we are going to learn the truth about man's knowledge in connection with man's health enigma?

Possibly the fire is going to get very hot in the kitchen. All who cannot stand the heat should resign from the activities of the kitchen. If man has been playing games with the lives of men for filthy lucre, I know that we need a change in the course we have been taking all these years.

What I have learned and understood is that man has been teaching us many things to use in our daily life: are these the culprits that cause many of the various illnesses we have in the world? They have been a nuisance to man for centuries. Yet, there is still a question I hear all the time, "my mom never smoked, or my son, my daughter, or my dad, but they died of the same kind of cancer that people died of that smoke."

I also learned that people who are obese drink coca cola or a lot of pop. I have learned about diabetes being caused by eating too much starchy food that removes the insulin from one's body. I learned of many people who are upset with the teachings that if a person watches what they are eating they can avoid many of the various ailments that are plagues to people, like parasites, all the days of their lives on this earth.

Which one of these teachings do we find correct? Which one would we address as incorrect? Is it possible that both are incorrect? Where are we going to go to find the correct answer? Man's behavior is like this: in this era, if you are not a graduate from one of the many universities you are a no-body. You stand to be rejected by just about every person who has obtained their ticket. People should be flabbergasted with man's doctrine for this generation. Please do not think that I am against higher education. I have always encouraged children to get as much education as they possibly can, because this world has become very technological. A person needs to be educated to maintain a half way decent life.

The controversy one hears daily makes life full of unanswered questions. This only brings to mind that theory seems to be a guessing game that leaves humanity in perplexity. As we travel this life daily, we learn many things about the past. But we only take the things of the past for granted.

We have bookstores, libraries, and many other facilities where you can find all kinds of books that relate to us the past, present, and the future. All the knowledge they have stored up within the pages of the books that are read by millions of people of all walks of life has not truly done much for the vast population of the world.

The thing we have not done is to read between the lines to get the full understanding: what each book has to offer to its readers. Many just read because they love to read. Some read because they would like to find a special answer they are looking for. People seem to read for various reasons. Yet we all seem to miss the main objective in the writing of books.

I know that not all authors write for making a lot of money. Many write to express their inner acquisitions. We can find many that just simply write to become wealthy. All the books written showing the behavior of humanity have not made man behave any more or any less moral than any other generation in the past. People, as they were in the beginning, have remained the same today.

What we have overlooked is that early people never had any examples after which they could pattern their lives. They were unable to walk soberly continually. In their misfortune, we have a pathway paved for us that we should not follow in their pathway of life. We should be able to escape the agony they have been through in their lives. What is the benefit for all the books written, if we never adopt our life to be much more sober in everything? Then the same evil would never befall us as it did past generations that went through all kinds of pain and agony.

I also see that many things that should have been written a long time ago, have not reached the pages of our books as yet. There are possible reasons why all the necessary things have not reached the pages of our books as yet. Either we lack the knowledge, or we might just only care for money, or we are willing to keep people in ignorance.

Is There a Real Killer?

Chapter (9)

Is it possible we always had a silent killer in the life of humanity; from the day we found out we were naked? Or is it possible it is within the eighteenth to the twenty-first centuries that we can only find the silent killer? Let us backtrack a few years before the twentieth century. We know that most of modern technologies came within the last three hundred years of civilization.

Things like automobiles, ships with engines, planes, and other forms of transportation, that were invented in the eighteenth and nineteenth centuries, changed man's way of living three hundred and sixty degrees. They make us live a life completely different from past generations.

The advancements in living, with modern day technology, we should all agree, help us to make life simpler in many ways. On the other side of the coin, it has some hidden dangers that we have not put into perspective because we do not see the need for alteration.

Man behaves like he woke up one morning and all things appeared on their own. For example, the teaching there is about evolution, where the universe is self-created. The understanding I obtained through the theory of evolution is that things started through a massive explosion with the interaction of the various gases that collided in the atmosphere.

The massive explosion created a chain reaction that made things start to develop. This produced all the things there are in the world that man now inhabits. We seem to live our lives with industrial affairs like they were here before men. I feel like our educators leave out the best part of their teaching to humanity. We just sit back and allow them to indoctrinate us with anything they feel like telling us. We easily fall into error. The majority holds to erroneous teachings because blindness is imparted.

We have in our society, in all the countries and Islands of the world, various teachings on man's beginning. One teaches this, others teach that, and a few say so what. We have many kinds of teachings: good, bad, and indifferent. Our perplexing teaching is very much unhealthy. I feel that it is time that we should start to behave much wiser.

Our form of educational philosophy can use some changes. There are too many variations in the dogmas used today. Most humans in this era apply themselves as though they are superb. With our educational background we think we are it. Being overbearing in our daily walk, we overlook some of life's greatest values. This keeps us in ignorance until the day we stand to be judged for being puffed up with pride.

Taking stock as I walk through life, I was one of the many individuals that always took things as they were handed down in existence. Poor nations are not fortunate to purchase for themselves the luxury that wealthy people have in the beginning. The more I traveled, the more areas of the world I learned of that are not developed in every country or Island. We can find areas that people live in that are far from popular; areas where you find a smaller population that cannot afford the convenience of developing towns and cities.

The areas where you find larger populations you find more activities in everything. Looking at the undeveloped areas, one does not find hospitals, police stations, fire stations, or movie houses. You will find churches and stores for food, clothes, or other more important items for one's daily need. People that live in the poorer undeveloped areas seem to have a lot less need for many of the things big cities and towns have.

What is the reason why in every area of every country or Island one can't find the same things as the large cities and towns have? Is it because not much money is in the area where few people live? Living with fewer people tends to show more caring and more neighborliness in all things they do.

Looking at the way people live their lives, in the undeveloped areas of the world, should be the way we all live. Living in an area where we do not find electric, we can find a completely different way of life that we do not accept in large, developed areas of the world. When people move to large, developed parts of the world, many people do not like to return to their poorer homes. The majority can adapt to pleasure very easily.

As the saying goes "When you are in Rome, do as the Romans". Should we accept that saying when we live in large, developed areas of the world? Can things be much better for people if we always live by the golden rule? Is there a law that is golden or is it a saying? I learned these words when I was a child that if you should train a child in the way he should go; when he is old he will not depart from it. Proverbs 22:6.

Can we accept that teaching in this era, since we think we are so advanced? We simply ignore the proper procedure for bringing up kids. Do we just enjoy killing ourselves? I read in the Bible where GOD spoke to the children of Israel when they still occupied the wilderness. He warned them to be careful when they reached the Promised Land. There they never planted any fruit trees or any vegetation, as GOD described the land as flowing with milk and honey. Reaching that place, they should at all times be very careful not to make eating control their behavior that they would sin against their GOD. Deuteronomy 8:7-14.

It had to be a very good reason why they were instructed to control their life of eating, drinking, and gaining wealth. Just as Israel rejected the warning of GOD and ate in rebellion to their deaths, I see the same pattern in humanity today. When people from poor countries or Islands visit places that are developed with all of life's pleasures, a person soon forgets where they came from. If there was a correct teaching they had, it would be a thing of the past.

A person becomes overwhelmed with all the abundance of things they behold in a large, developed area that they have never seen before. One becomes lost in a dream or wonderland. All the teaching one had from their childhood days never was there. The reason why so many behave the way they do is because it was not much of a doctrine to a person when they lived in poverty. It was the only way they knew. That is where we have made many mistakes in our lives.

Living in poverty has many advantages. We have overlooked the good there is in areas where people live in poverty. Being poor, is not a crime. Living in poverty is not sinful any more than living in wealth. I feel poverty has greater advantages than wealth.

I say that for this reason. In the countries, or any parts of the globe, where there is poverty, we can find that most of the people are more content in their lifestyle. It's only when people travel among them that are from wealthy countries or Islands that make some of the people, that are poor, crave the things these travelers carry with them.

When the travelers speak of their lifestyles, it makes many of the poor start to hunger for the life the traveler impresses them with. What nobody seems to think about is what makes the people from the rich luxurious countries, travel and visit poverty stricken places? If one's place of occupancy is so great, and you have things so wonderful, why does a person of such caliber want to visit people in their poverty? Are we in truth having consideration for these people's feelings and to really help in improving their living condition? We possibly need a sense of composure in our own life. So many people travel to other countries daily.

Being somewhat unhappy in a rich environment, you then make the lives of the people in their poverty as unhappy as you are. Because we do not look at our traveling in that aspect, we keep making the life of people unhappy all over the world. People that travel from one country to another shows some kind of fatigue and that they seek rest for their exhaustion.

One's selfishness hurts many in the long run. I am not saying that we should not travel to other parts of the world. We need to think and feel for others as we travel. I know that millions of people, from all walks of life, would give up a part of their lives if the door was open to America. People from America live very extravagantly. When they visit other countries, they make the people yearn to come to America thinking they too can have a life like the visitors.

I constantly hear many people say living in America is much better than any other place on this earth? Is it only because many feel it is so wealthy and it is so easy to become rich? I am not lying, when I lived in Jamaica before my migration, I felt that I would not need to work as long to get something out of life in America as I needed to do in Jamaica. I wanted to move to America very much. I used to say that it is very hard for a person to ever walk with GOD in spirit and truth in Jamaica.

What I found out, since living in America, is that this place, is the most difficult place on earth for anyone to walk with GOD in spirit and in truth. I see people behave like GOD is not very serious and his words are just simple jokes he is playing with humanity.

I have a lot to give thanks for. When I came to this country I did not adapt to the very fast moving pace of this place. This could be the reason why I see and understand who and what is the silent killer.

When I immigrated to America, I was a stranger to the people and their way of life. I was not any better than they, neither was I any worse; I was not inferior, nor was I superior. The only thing that's different with America over Jamaica is that it has more opportunity in all things pertaining to living on this earth.

On the other hand, I see many evil, deadly things that are much more devastating to humanity's health than when I was living in Jamaica. Today, as I visit my birth country, I see the same ugliness overshadow that place. It's not because of the growth in the population. It is caused by the many travelers from many parts of the world that seek a place to relax.

No one truly ever thinks of being destructive to the place they vacated. Most seek relief for their fatigues. This in turn becomes harmful to others. I know that people think what they are doing will, in the end, make others have a better living than they had before vacating to these places.

Because we have not noticed our bad habits, we take them with us everywhere. People pick up our bad habits. Because as a child we lived that way, and because our parents and their parents did the same, none knew any better. So generation after generation walks the same pathway.

Looking at some of the things that we have done unto ourselves, since we have electricity, folks changed the way they eat and drink. Years before we had electric, man would behave completely different in many things. The way we are living, now that we have electricity, makes us unhealthy in this generation.

It might not make much sense to many people living today to correlate Israel's behavior after they reached the promise land. They completely forgot the instruction of GOD that they should not make the milk and honey cause them to sin. We should not make the advancements of life cause us to eat ourselves to obliteration. Israel was forewarned that they should always remember not to over indulge in eating without restraints.

This universe is being destroyed rapidly, not only by erosion, but by one of the greatest destroying agents there is: humanity. We look at life one sided only with hindsight. Man is only after the fact. Being simple, we fail to heed perfect instruction. We constantly keep behaving repugnantly with one another. We are much more rebellious to GOD. GOD is always being patient with humanity, until time will be no more. GOD set a date and time when all things on this earth will come to an abruptness.

The most outrageous phenomenon there is has to do with humanity living the way they do. We create lots of things, and allow the things we made to more or less run our lives. Many might disagree with what I am saying. We are unrestrained with ourselves so much that non speaking items are making human life shorter than intended for it to be from the very beginning.

GOD created all the things that exist, seen and unseen. We touch and handle them, and they also touch our lives daily. The understanding I have obtained is that nothing created by GOD is able to control him in anyway that will hurt him in anyway. We are instructed in the Bible that if GOD is hungry, he does not need to relate his hunger to man. People cannot give GOD any physical food to eat because we are unable to bring ourselves in the presence of GOD. GOD can be standing right in front of us, or even holding our hands, and we will not know that He is. Psalm 50:12.

Right there holding our hand. In what way can man do anything that we will be able to control GOD? We allow the things we create to weaken us and eventually obliterate us from this life.

We are the ones that created electricity by the knowledge given to us by GOD. We also created many other kinds of gadgets to make electric more efficient in its source. Electric by itself would not be of much value. Electric, with all the machinery there is, makes electric come alive. Remove all the appliances we have in our society today and the entire wonderful power one receive from electric companies would be useless.

It might be hard to accept where we made the wrong turn as

we move forward to the future. The wrong turn could be one of the causes we have a killer that works very silently. Our scientists and researchers keep looking for an answer to help eradicate the ailments that have been a thorn in our side all the days of our lives.

The thing we might not see and understand is that we have not studied past generations living habits as eating, working, or last but not least sleeping. When we developed refrigerators we felt we did something wonderful. We can keep food fresher much longer than it was before the fridge came into existence. Man also developed several types of stoves for much better and easier cooking in cleanliness and in many convenient ways.

Open fires make it very difficult to clean cooking utensils. It takes a much longer time to prepare breakfast, lunch, and dinner when cooking the ancient way. Cooking with stoves that just take the turn of a knob to get their cooking started, works wonders. Cooking with natural gas, kerosene, or propane in many cases can also make one's cooking utensils black on the outside. Cooking with electric is one of the cleanest and safest ways of cooking today. Today's cooking sure makes it much more pleasant. Yet, it still has its drawbacks.

When I was a child, I remember we had an open fire in our kitchen. The wood we boys had to gather daily made the fire. The fire would take time to make. One has to start the fire with small pieces of wood first. Then, as the fire started to gradually burn, one would place the larger pieces piece by piece, on the fire. When we felt that the fire was burning correctly we would place the pot on the fire.

In my childhood days cleaning cooking utensils was no fun at first. We never had any scouring pads or any cleansing compound that we could use to help clean our pots and pans. We would get a coconut. From its outer covering we would make straw that we would use with the ashes from the fire as our scouring agent. It was not easy cleaning one's cooking utensils.

As time marched on we developed a better method for our pots and pans. This is what we would do to our cooking utensils. First, before we started to do the cooking, we would get some ashes from the fireplace, wet pots, and place ashes all over the outside of the vessel before putting it on the fire. After you completely covered the outside, including the bottom, you placed it on the fire. After the completion of cooking, it would be very easy to clean the vessel you just took off the fire. Even after hours of cooking, you just placed the vessel in water and the ashes would wash off without any effort when cleaning the pots. Modern technology does make life in every way much more pleasant. By the flick of a switch or the turning of a knob, a person can reduce lots of their time, and danger.

Open fire as it was in my childhood days was harmful in many ways when putting on and taking off vessels from the fire. The fireplace in our kitchen was higher than normal. Removing hot cooking utensils while the fire was burning high was very dangerous. A person had to use caution a lot to prevent an accident.

The one who was responsible for cooking would breathe in lots of smoke. Do not misunderstand what I am saying. The kitchen was not covered with smoke. Open fires always have smoke, especially when you have an open fire that's not contained in an area where the smoke exhausts through the chimney. When there is no chimney, the smoke will travel within the confines of the building. You always find soot on the ceiling.

There was another problem with an open wood fire like the one we had in St. Ann's Bay. When a person had high heat, with somewhat high blaze, you would place the food in the pots. Many of the ingredients would be placed in the pots when the pots started to boil.

Shuffling pots on the fire where you cannot turn up and down the heat can be very dangerous, especially when it's in a building where access is only on one side.

In those days we never had a refrigerator. I know two ways my dad and my stepmother would keep their meat lasting longer. One-way was by smoke, the other way was by salt. Placing a wire mesh in the ceiling of the kitchen did the smoke procedure. The smoke from the fire would preserve the meat placed in the mesh. The other one was done by salt. It was properly covered with salt and pimento, and then placed in an earthen vessel; the cover was made from a piece of board. Using a stone as weight for slowly removing the blood from the meat, that would melt the salt.

As the salt slowly dissolved, it worked to preserve the meat.

Sometimes flies laid their eggs on the meat, which, in turn, spoiled the meat. When the meat is contaminated with larva, it will be good for nothing.

These days a person can place their meats and vegetables in their freezer for a long time. Your meats and veggies do not spoil very easily as they would without an icebox. They would not be contaminated with larva, other insects, or dust, or any other contamination.

By not having a refrigerator a person would not have cool liquid to drink. A person would always try and buy some ice to cool their liquid they would have to drink. In those days one would find many ways of keeping their drinks somewhat cool, especially when you were at locations where there was no ice.

Although the weather was hot all the time, we managed to keep things very cool. Things were great then. The kids never knew about fridges. My dad was knowledgeable with electrical appliances. Since he was working on his plan, he never saw the need of purchasing an icebox or any other home appliances. Dad's employer at the home they provided for the operators furnished all the necessary appliances.

It is mind boggling thinking of one way we would keep our water cool all day. My dad had a farm where we would reap pimento yearly. In those days there was no running water at our farm. We had a large container we would call a kerosene pan. It would contain about five gallons of water. We had one we would use for cooking when we were harvesting pimento. We had two for water.

The water containers did not have any lids. We always filled the kerosene pan with water, and placed several branches with leaves in the pan with the water. We had to walk more than a mile with the water on our heads. We would get wet with the water splashing while walking with the water on our heads. When we reached our destination, we would not remove the leaves. We would leave the branches with the leaves in the water until the water was completely empty. The water would remain cool all day long. It was a lot cooler than the ambient temperature.

I could not to this date understand the reason why these containers were called kerosene pans. They were not containers for kerosene oil. They were receptacles for cooking oil that were shipped to

Jamaica from overseas. I have not learned to this date the reason for the name of this receptacle as kerosene pan. I know when I was living in Jamaica, in the area we call country; those containers were plentiful. In other countries, one would call the undeveloped areas rural areas.

Emigrating opened my eyes to many things different in culture. Should I say behavior or culture? Humans are the same in every country or Island. The difference I see with each place or country I visited is this: there is great wealth, and there is poverty. There are rich countries and poor Islands, there are well developed and under-developed at the same time. In life we have good, bad, and indifference.

I think this has to be more mental than cultural. The reason for my analogy is the unrestrained attitude. Possibly all this mentality could stem from the abundance that a person has exuberantly. Through the vast great wealth and great advancement, people behave as if they are super and that people that live in poorer countries are beneath them. Because a person comes from another nation, where their birthplace is undeveloped, does not make them a lesser person.

Some of the things that we might have overlooked, is that people from poorer nations, might feel inferior. Not thinking about the people that live in a country that is developed with the modern technology, although that country is more advanced, you can find poor, poorer, and the poorest living in that country. I often hear people say in each country that there are always three standards, or classes of people, like rich, middle, and poor. We have never spoken of the people that have nowhere to live. They live on the streets. Some organizations take the responsibility to cater to these people who are the poorest of the poor.

I know that not every one in each nation is capable of becoming wealthy or even in the bracket of the middle class. I realize that there are more poor people in every nation of the world than the two other classes. As I was saying about the poor, they have somewhat a better life in this category, because they do not have the means to have the abundance of food as the wealthy or middle class. They are forced to go without sometimes.

Because the real poor do not have things superfluous, they have to go without things to eat sometimes. They often go without a meal here and there. As the poor go without a meal here and there, their bodies can rest. Because we cannot understand the body, we feel when a person goes without a meal here and there they are going to have more health enigmas than those that have four or five meals daily.

We live in a society today that teaches us that we need to constantly keep eating all the time when we are awake. What I am actually driving at is this: years before we had electric, mankind never had a place where they could keep their food as fresh and as long as we can today. By the power of electricity man made lots of devices that cause us to overwork our bodies that become very destructive health-wise.

Having refrigerators and modern day devices for indoor cooking, does make one part of our life a lot simpler. On the other side it is more deadly. Take the years when there was no electricity. Man would have to close up shop much earlier. All of one's activities would cease when it became dark. Not much could one do when it became dark. The lighting system in the days when electric was not developed was poor. The children who had homework had to try and do as much as they could while it was still daylight.

With electricity today, man's behavior is yet to be desired. Man has become an unrestrained creature that seems to live to eat, sit up late, and keeps eating to obliteration. I cannot point my finger at the vast population for such a gluttonous behavior, because most people have to be educated by the educators. When our educators lack the knowledge, one has to live in ignorance. I feel that is why we have too many sick people today. Our educators need to be educated with the proper procedure of dieting first before they should teach others.

When a person lacks the knowledge in the correct procedures, how can they teach others something they themselves need to know? This is where we have been going wrong since this generation has known electric. In early days of electricity, man might have behaved in a similar way when there was no electric.

In the days when there was no electric man's eating lifestyle was completely different from these days. Look at our conduct in comparison with the folks that were using candles, kerosene lamps, or other sources as their lighting. They did not have a place within their facility where they could sit up until one, two, three, or four in the morning. The only reason why they would need to be up that late was if they woke up and were unable to fall back to sleep for the rest of the night.

In the days when there was no electricity, when a person woke up, and they could not go back to sleep, they had to have a very difficult time. They had no proper lighting, no fridge, or stove, where they could make themselves something to eat. They were unable to read a book, watch TV, or go for a drive. There were no forms of medication they could take to help them fall back to sleep.

In the days of no electricity, was it better health-wise? Did the days of no electricity give people more sleeping hours of the night? What was life like not having electricity?

Are we better off these days having electricity than the years when there was no voltaic current? What are the changes in people's lives that make it different than the people that never knew anything about electrical current?

Should man try and learn if there are any advantages, or disadvantages, with the two types of living that we have learned about? One is the one that man calls the dark ages. The other is the one we know today, the age we should call the age of light and power.

I personally like this age. I am glad I was born in this age: a stage in life where one can turn a switch and get to find what they are looking for. I am not the greatest lover of the cold weather. When I think of an outhouse in the winter, it sends a chill to my body. I don't mind urinating in the winter cold outside, but excretion from one's bowels in the cold, that is hard to swallow. I cover my body correctly in the winter, because I hate to feel the cold air hitting any part of my body.

When I think of people using outhouses in the winter, I ache all over. The reason I might feel that way about an outhouse in the winter could be because I am from a tropical climate. I might feel and think completely different if I was born in the winter climate. Humans at first never knew winter, because in the beginning there was no cold weather. It was years later that the four seasons came into existence.

Man's body was made perfect. We are the ones that are unrestrained in just about all walks of life. I know that our greatest foe truly makes life very perplexing; that causes many over the years to end their lives. It does not give anyone the right to end their life because things are not going the way they would like them to go. If a person's life did end at the grave, it would not matter the time one lives on this earth, or if someone takes their own life.

Living on this earth from generation to generation, all seem to have their own lifestyle related to technologies. This takes us to the light and power age. For people without electricity, life was completely different in the Dark Ages compared to this age where we get our lighting with the flick of a switch. People today, with all the gadgets there are, should be able to be much healthier than the people born in the age when there was no electricity.

Oftentimes, I hear words like these: people who live in the age that has light and power are much healthier and live much longer than Dark Age people. Are those statements really speaking the truth? Can we find only subterfuge in those words concerning long living and better health? Looking at people's appetites today, and the way they eat, one has to say that people that live without electricity should be able to live much healthier lives. Understanding what we are doing wrong with our being, I can only say that people who are born in the age of electricity have more unhealthy gadgets to encounter. We just keep going like life owes us a favor.

People of the dark ages were restrained, like it or not. They did not have the source of keeping food fresh as this era can. Not being able to maintain wholesome foods, one was kept from eating all the time as this generation does. Not living in the dark ages, many have to speculate on the behavior of the people living in that era. Since there was no electricity, no icebox, no gas or electric stoves, all cooking was done with an open fire that made lots of smoke.

In the time of no electricity, there was no icebox where one could keep their food from intruders such as roaches, ants, rats, or the various insects that would invade people's food. A person would not have the convenience at hand where they were able to have foods and drinks to partake of when awakened in the night to alleviate their body waste. In this dispensation people eat all the time, day and night. Some would step in the kitchen for a quick snack when they arise to use the bathroom.

Dark Age dwellers never had it as good or as unhealthy as it is today. Back then, they never had any kind of night jobs other than people that would be guards to watch other people's properties from those who would seek to steal what was not theirs. Life was much simpler. I do not think this saying was being used "that time is money, punctuality is essential, and one needs to move much faster than they are". Since there was no clock to punch, people were much more composed. Today's businesses keep people under great stresses all the time.

Man has not looked back to the time when people were much happier than now. The thing I can't understand is the teaching that people are much healthier and living much longer than the people of the Dark Ages. The people that lived in those days were able to go all night after eating at sunset, knowing that their next meal would have to be in the morning. The other thing we have to always remember is that all their liquid would be more or less room temperature. There was no ice or icebox, otherwise known as the refrigerator.

In that generation people were able to obtain lots more rest by sleeping. Less eating and smoking were done. In this era, when people get up, the first thing they do when they turn on the lights is smoke. They would first turn to their cigarettes and start smoking. Then, they would head for the bathroom or the kitchen. Since there was no switch to push or turn then, a person could not overeat or over smoke themselves to death as they do today.

The other thing we need to keep in our mind is that they never had indoor plumbing as we have today. They had out-houses. I can remember as a child a container was available that we would use at night for our urine. In the morning we would dispose of the waste and clean the container for the next night. This we would do when we lived at the place where we had outside plumbing.

Man has become so impatient and greedy. We have overlooked the more pleasant life once lived when man had not yet developed all the industrial equipment there is today. We have allowed greed and selfishness for filthy lucre to blind our eyes to the real facts that are destroying humanity.

I am not pointing my fingers at any one person. Unconsciously we have taken many things for granted. Most of our educators have overlooked man's shortcomings. It's not necessary to say that neglect is the culprit. What we have done, through fast growth and development, is make the most important part of our lifestyle slip right through our own hands. We have become so busy with all the opportunities that are knocking, that we simply dive head long into the advancement of progress. We never foresee the danger that lies ahead.

Now that we are so deeply involved in working for one's daily, weekly, or yearly ration, we keep killing ourselves ignorantly. We do not think of the changes that would affect us in the near future. I am not saying that change is impossible. I know that it is possible that some will try to alter their lifestyle. They care somewhat for their health. Millions are irresponsible, and they will not care one way or another. We need to stop being selfish, and care more for one another if we want this world to be a better place.

I spoke with several individuals, who are still alive, who once lived in the days when electricity was not as common as it is today. In all corners of the earth you might find some kind of plant or some kind of gadget used to generate electric. In the unpopular day of electric, I know and hear the old timers say their lives were completely different in many things than they are today. Food was not as plentiful. There were no restaurants and snack counters where a person could have something to eat at their fingertips.

I stated before that they would have a lot less to eat all the time. The people who lived when life was much more difficult never had any electric lights or any appliances. Therefore, they had a very hard time surviving.

I came from a very poor country. I also have experienced a place where there was no electric. When I was a child, in the country where I was born, a tropical area of the world, it got cold in some areas of the Island: still not as cold as countries where snow falls in the wintertime. To get warm was not as difficult as those places where it's like living in an icebox.

Imagine living in the cold where there is no central heating, no proper windows, or a correct barrier for reducing the pressure of the wind blowing through your home. The only thing people had to help stop the cold from freezing them was their blanket.

The Un-recorded Danger

As a child living in Jamaica, I had a very difficult childhood. I lost my mother when I was a baby. I could have been one of the most backward children growing up. I had a very strict father who saw one sided. I know that I was slow grasping what was taught in school. I think my dad was not pleased with his children's educational background, especially me. My stepmother was something to be desired. All she cared for was her children. My dad's kids, in her eyes, were beneath her children, and we were treated like that.

I know that my sisters and I were not the only children in the world that had either a stepfather or a stepmother with either stepbrothers or stepsisters that obtained partial treatment from either procreator.

What I have learned over the years about unrecorded dangers will follow in this chapter.

I always felt that my dad was selfish and inconsiderate in his treatment towards us. He always had the best for himself. Not once did he put any of his kids first. His wife's behavior was similar to his. As the saying goes, "two peas in a pod".

When my mother died, I was not capable of understanding what happened to my mother. For instance, if my mother emigrated at the age I was, and returned years later, I would never be able to recognize her. Babies do not have their faculties developed enough to correctly understand lots of what is in their environment. As a child develops, so does their understanding.

As a child, I was very slow in developing. I just could not grasp what I was being taught. Being my dad's first son, my dad behaved shamefully on my behalf. It could be, as I always hear when I was living in Jamaica; "a child is the pension for their parents that when they become old, their children can be their financial institution".

I personally do not see anything wrong with a child caring for their parents after all they have done for their children. It is the way many go about cultivating their children's lives. Many become very bitter.

The things that I have seen, slips through many of our hands and minds, make many behave very despicably. If we did recognize the hidden dangers as we progress so many evils would not befall us. As I said before, I know what it was to go without a fridge and many more electrical appliances. Not having many of today's modern conveniences did, in a way, make a person behave unconsciously healthier. Not thinking of what they were doing, when there were longer hours in making preparation for whatever a person was doing, it would take a longer time to go from one place to the other; unlike today's traveling where with modern day technology, a person can travel from one country to another in hours.

Years before man created all the traveling machines, a person would take months or weeks to go from one point to another. Lighting was very poor then. When electric was invented, that was a very great thing. The thing I see we have overlooked makes us live a life that has become unhealthy to the majority of humanity all over the world.

The power people have at their fingertips to push a lever up and down, allows man to have power to remove darkness for the time they so desire. It also produces all kinds of gadgets that shorten time and traveling. Yet, we have not used all this technology wisely so that we all might enjoy a much happier and pleasant life. Instead of longevity and better health, we have more unhappiness and more death.

I know that man keeps relating all the time that we are living much longer in this era than previous generations. One thing we need to remind ourselves about is that all the nations that existed before the creation of electricity had to work much harder than people today.

In the days when tilling the soil was done by animals or man power, cultivation was much more difficult than it is today. Reaping and separating grains took more time and effort. In this era there is a lot less pain and effort. Today's people is eating more and doing less physical labor. In all the great advancements we made, with luxury and comfort, we are not awakened to the danger we left ourselves open to.

In the years of hard labor the population was a lot smaller. I don't think it was done willfully as in many nations of the world today. Trying to stop over population, we create a very unhealthy society. Daily in the world people keep aborting their babies for various reasons. We also can find many women that are too busy to have a family. They are looking after wealth and other things that people feel are more important than a good family life.

This generation sold out a good healthy family life for an unhealthy, deadly, lonely life. There is lots of misery in old age today as soon as one's procreator reaches a certain age. The children become as busy as their parents, parents' were, when their children were smaller. They would always leave their children to a babysitter.

Illogical as it might seem, yet it is the fact, the ongoing behavior is passed on in this era since man has all the technology in the time we like to call modern days. Man loves to speak of this era as if all the people before these days were barbarians. Man feels they are so advanced. Even the houses of worship, known as churches, change their style in their worship services.

In every way, and in all things today, we can see all the changes man has made. All the changes I see only keep bringing out the ignorance of humanity. I feel that as we speak about all the improvements we have made over the years, we should also learn to make adjustments in our lifestyle just the same. The pattern that I see keeps going around is like this: when both parents work very hard, they normally send their kids to daycare. When the parents get old, the kids shove them to the old folk's home or give them a cold shoulder. This is similar to what their parents did to their kids when their kids were younger. Because of the law, they could not leave their children at home at their age alone.

What we have done as we move up technologically, we have not moved with foresight. We move with hindsight, as if we are blindfolded. It shows that man always needs a helping hand to guide us so that people can always make the right decision.

Even the men and women who say they are chosen by GOD to be the shepherds of the fold have not truly walked as they should. They too have allowed the blindfold of the enemy to overpower them. They are not of GOD anymore. If they once were of GOD, now they are of the Devil.

I am not a super human. I am a man just like everyone else. I have been through a very hard life, possibly more than most. My dad and my stepmother were not very compassionate. They made the lives of their children unnecessarily unhappy. One, because they where selfish. Two, they were bad procreators. Three, they were greedy for money. They wanted to have a lot in the bank, just in case their children turned their backs on them. If they did not get help in their old age, they would be worse off in their old age. Fighting for some independence can be more devastating than it has to be.

The lack of compassion by my stepmother towards us, turned out healthier. In her ill –treatment, she did us a great favor. When we lived at St. Ann's Bay, I can recall we had very hard childhood days. My stepbrothers and I would have to go and gather wood for cooking. We would do that say six or five days a week. Oftentimes when we returned from wood gathering, we had to look about going to school. I always hear people say that a person should have something warm to drink in the morning to break your fast.

In the days of our life living at my stepmother's home, we would have cold things to drink. We would get water and sugar with lime and mix them together. We would go to the bakery shop and buy day old bread. The bakery was right across the street. We would have that mixture with a piece of bread as our breakfast. Sometimes it would be the same for lunch. Sometimes it was porridge. Even at dinnertime we would get porridge. Life in Jamaica was poor then, and we would use all kinds of things to make porridge.

The way our eating would work when we got home from school was that our dinner would be ready for us. When we ate dinner it would be our last meal of the day from dad's food supply. If you wanted anything more to eat for the day, you had to find another method of getting something for yourself.

The great thing about Jamaica, when I lived there, there were all kinds of fruits and other eating products one could find to eat. Many times on our way home from school, we would stop in various places and get things to eat before we got home. There were always people's gardens planted near by. We would always help ourselves.

The day we moved to the location where my dad worked, things were somewhat different. Moving to the area where my dad worked, the company furnished a stove and a refrigerator. It was an electric stove, and electric refrigerator. Years later I learned about a kerosene refrigerator. Now we had a stove that only took turning a knob to do cooking. We could now have something warm each morning before we left for school.

When we lived at our stepmother's home, there was a wood burning fireplace for cooking. She would possibly make sure there was no fire for us to have anything hot in the morning. If we were to have anything hot we would have to be the ones that made the fire ourselves.

At the location where we had an electric stove, we were able to always have something hot. We were not allowed to have coffee or tea purchased from the store, at the location where dad worked. We could always get all kinds of leaves for making herbal tea. We had all kinds of plants that we used daily to make the things we loved to drink without costing my dad one penny.

The other thing at this location was that there was more than enough land. That enabled us to plant the majority of the food a person would need. We had sugar cane and fruits in abundance that we could eat as our snacks. After dinner a person had nothing more to get from our dad's food stock.

My dad would give us a spanking if he knew that we took any food and ate it without his permission. He called that stealing, because he never gave us permission to take the things we took to eat. The only reason I feel my dad always did that was he never wanted to keep spending all the time to make sure we had an ample supply needed in the home. He would go to the market Fridays and Saturdays for the weekly supply. He was determined that what he use to purchase as the weekly supply was not wasted in a few days.

This is my view of my father's action when we lived with him. I could be right, as well as being wrong. Our dad could have been looking at the picture from a completely different angle. We always looked at the picture as to say our dad was cruel and selfish, and only thought one way to save his money. He knew that he was limiting our eating.

Our dad and stepmother never sat down with us and reasoned one to one. They didn't show us the better way of coping with things to come.

I got into big trouble once with my dad. We used to keep company with one of my dad's coworkers, because someone tried to break into his house one night. He would go out on nights when he is not working and drink. He would always give us his supper when he would return home from his drinking. One night he asked my stepbrother and me if we had our supper already. I, being slow in understanding, replied we had not had supper at our home.

My stepbrother, always being the stool pigeon, ran back and told my dad that I told his coworker that we never ever had supper at our home. My dad was very mad with me. When he was angry you got a whipping that hurt for days. My dad was not a person to accept his fault. It would not bother him if I lied like my stepbrother did.

I was the one that got into trouble for speaking the truth. My stepbrother was the one they thought was good and caring. I was the illiterate. I know the Bible teaches us that the truth will offend. It is not sinful to always speak the truth, no matter the pain it might bring. Because I was not the wise one in the family, I did not know how to keep the family lifestyle in the home.

I say all those things for a reason. My dad was not showing us the good or the bad in the way he brought us up. We thought evil of his ways. Likewise, the way my stepmother was treating us was so cruel. In ignorance, we speak bitterly of others only because we see things one sided and make even the good evil as we did.

I once heard a tail being told. It was like this. "There was a stepmother to a stepson. She had a son, and she disliked her husband's child. She gave her stepson all the pot liquor. Her son was given the food that was more pleasing to her. She then noticed her son was not as healthy as her stepson. Visiting the doctor, she learned that in her ill feelings toward her stepson, she was looking or thinking that she was being cruel to the child that was not hers by giving him the thing she thought was bad". It turned out to be the best. Her evil became good to her stepson.

It is the same with my stepmother and my dad. It was a good thing they were doing for us. Even though they never knew it was a very good thing that they were doing for their children.

We, as kids, saw only evil in their treatment. We felt it was cruel. Not knowing better, we only saw it as cruel and injustice. I know

185

that we were not the only family members in the world that had a procreator that was inhumane in their treatment.

Let me show you what I see now I should have been doing all my life. We always got things that were cold in the morning going to school. The bread was not that fresh. Lunch was not a lot. Dinner was not all that great either. We would always have one little piece of meat in our dinner. We always called it the watchman. We would always leave it for the last to eat with the dumpling. The only time we would have a lot of meat would be fish. My dad once had a partner, and he was fisherman. When he caught a lot of fish we would have fish for days. We did not have a fridge in those days. We had to fry them and eat them up quickly.

I found out that one of the best diets anyone could live by was the way we were treated by our stepmother. It might have been evil intended, because they never treated themselves the way they treated us. If they were treating themselves as they were treating us, then one would have to say no evil was intended. Doing the opposite, a person will see the opposite of good. The behavior of most humans at first is to always think evil. Many change their minds later in life when they realize that no evil was intended.

Understand that the keeping of a person's body temperature at normal is much better health-wise for you. A person should know what to drink and how to drink it. That was what they were teaching us even though they did not know what they were doing. Today, they still drink very hot liquid every morning.

I saw my dad and stepmother, morning, night, or midday, with their tea so hot that their body temperatures increased so much that their bodies began to perspire to cool their systems down.

I have been hearing that perspiration is very good for a person because it's one of the body's methods of ejecting toxins from the body. Conflicting as this might be, perspiration has two purposes for the body function. Man says one is to remove the bodily toxins and the other is that perspiration cools the body down when it begins to overheat. The question one has to ask our philosophers is at what time does our perspiration eject the toxin and why only fewer than three circumstances that the body perspires?

If ejecting toxin from the body is done by perspiration, why only when someone drinks hot liquid, or does physical exertion, or fright, or nervousness causes a person's body temperature to change, and thus produces perspiration? If a person never does anything by physical exertion, or drinks hot liquid, or becomes frightful and nervous so as to eject their bodily toxin, what will happen to the person's bodily toxin? If it is important for all waste matter to leave the body, where will it go when it is not being disposed of? Will it be destructive to the body when it does not release perspiration?

The truth of the matter is this; perspiration only serves the purpose of reducing the body temperature. It's not a toxin-releasing agent. When a person's body temperature, within and without, rises above normal, the body quickly sends out a signal to do something to reduces the excess heat. Perspiration is the body mechanism of keeping the body cool. It places water on the outside of the body that works as a covering for the body that reduces it's overheating.

That was a great thing our parents were doing for us when we were not getting hot liquid to drink all the time. I know when I drink hot things sometimes I will perspire. When I labor with great exertion for a while I also perspire. In the winter having on lots of clothes, when I begin to exert myself it increases my body temperature and I begin to perspire a lot. Sometimes I get so wet that all the clothes I have on get wet all the way through. If I never exert much in the winter I never perspire.

In the summer I also know how to keep my body temperature cool so that I do not get as hot as people I hear complaining. See, the malicious behavior of my both so-called parents was doing me justice, even though I never knew better. I used to always say they were cruel and devilish.

They fed us very early in the evening. Not giving us supper was not unhealthy. That is a very healthy method for all people of the world. A person should always try their best to make their last meal, in their system, digest before going to bed.

We always had a lot of fruit to eat after dinner. Meats, like chicken, beef, and pork take more than ten hours to digest. One should try their very best to avoid large portions of meat when it is getting closer to bedtime.

Look at the way people are killing themselves, and they are

not aware of it. Our educators are in the same ignorant ship as the uneducated ones. We continue behaving that way until death.

TV is one of the most deadly silent killers. We are not willing to give it up. Man over the years has become malicious to cigarettes. They keep trying to completely eradicate the use of tobacco in the market place globally. They keep saying it is a very unhealthy substance.

We now have another product on the market that our educators are making the public aware is also unhealthy. This product is known as pop. They are beginning to develop a malicious name against pop as they did cigarettes. They hope that people will heed their messages and withdraw from the use of pop.

The thing that man overlooked all these years is that because we look only to the scientist and medical researchers, we just relax and leave the driving to them without a lot of objection. Their answers, they claim, are correct because of many years of research.

What I found out is their research is on a one sided basis. The reason it is that way is because they do not know the proper procedure in research for the answer.

The malicious activity, against the cigarette manufacturers, is forcing manufacturers to make cigarettes that it will stop burning when the smoker quits inhaling the cigarettes.

A question stands out forcefully in each daily publication of the charges made over and over on the various items that are the causes for many illnesses. Are they correct or incorrect? Is it possible for us to find the answer elsewhere? The organizations that have taken the responsibility all these years trying to find the answers to the many ailments, they are only making people's lives topsy-turvy?

Comparing TV, cigarettes, pop, and other industrial items that are blamed for health enigmas, which one can we place as more harmful? I have not broken down each substance's name that is blamed for illness enigmas. Yet, if I should describe each item by name they still would not correct the malicious name given to the products. There is a product on the market, that no one has written or made any comments about, that is very deadly. This product is the deadliest of all, and still remains silent.

What of TV? Is there any flaw within the contents of this complex device? Is the problem with the device or is the flaw with humanity? Are we looking at the coin at the wrong angle? Is it possible we have crushed the coin and only imagine that there is nothing wrong with the coin? Should we point our fingers now at television that silently is the deadliest object on the market that man has overlooked?

The influence of television in the life of humanity is as in the days of sorcery when people would use evil omens to keep people under demonic control.

I understand that women who others thought and felt were witches, were tied to a stake and burned alive. The person's life was not first taken then burned. They were yet alive when they were set on fire.

These people were burned alive because others were fearful of them. Knowing the evil they indulged in, if someone did not like that person, the malicious feelings could cost the person their life, same as we have thousands incarcerated all over the world that are innocent.

With lots of misunderstanding and experimentation we keep making lots of mistakes. We set the guilty free and send the innocent to prison. It is possible we are making the same mistake with many products we designated as unhealthy?

Looking at the undetected behavior of humanity with their televisions, we can find a more harmful enigma than cigarettes. I am not a smoker. I do not promote smoking. It's the malicious name that needs removing from the public. It's the injustice that needs to be removed from these companies. I am not only addressing cigarettes. I am also speaking about pop, asbestos, and all the other food products that man says contributes to illnesses.

Television's sorcery power seems to put man into a trance that makes him hurt himself unconsciously, unbeknown to the person. Oftentimes I see and hear people say they are in severe pain because they slept on their sofa watching TV. When a person sits up late watching TV, they eat and drink a lot. This is to say that TV makes you hungry a lot faster. When a person smokes, they smoke more watching TV.

Sleeping on your sofa does all kinds of harm to a person's body. This takes us back to people not knowing the importance of sleeping correctly. Failing to know the importance of sleep, we live, eat, and sleep carelessly.

All people do not have great will power to restrain themselves. Since our educators are guilty of the same unrestrained living, their students will also behave as their teachers. A few behave differently.

I find it hard to understand the reason why it has taken this long a time to give humanity the answer for the way we have been living unhealthy all these years. I was not aware of the healthy treatment we had when we lived at St. Ann's Bay. We took the unhealthy pathway when we moved to the location where dad worked.

Before we moved to Roaring River, the location where our dad worked, we never had hot substances in the morning when going to school. At home when there was no school we had the same cold drinks in the morning. We had hot tea in the morning when we worked harvesting dad's pimento. When we moved, we had an electric stove. Preparation of food was simply, turn a knob. We could have a hot cup of tea morning, noon, and night.

When I moved to America, I never got into the habit of drinking tea, morning, noon, and night. I never had coffee when I lived in Jamaica, although we grew coffee. Coffee was at our home all the time. Upon my emigration, I never liked what was available at first, so I never drank hot liquids in the morning. I love soup, and I love it very hot. I know better; I changed many of the bad habits I had.

The Unrestrained Behavior of Man

Chapter (11)

In this era we can find hundreds of people all over the world who are very disrespectful to their own bodies. The way we live and behave, it has to be mind boggling looking at people's actions today. It is as if their bodies are on climate control.

Today's dressing is inadequate. We have four seasons: winter, spring, summer, and fall. The way we dress in these four seasons is as if we are hurting the weather. The most deadly of the four seasons is winter. I see where we are very disrespectful to winter.

Can we cast the blame on our educators in this matter? If the fault is not on our educators, whose fault is it then? Should we, from this moment, point our fingers at anyone for our many problems?

Humans always act as if they have never done anything wrong. When we are caught, we always try to cast the blame on others because we hate criticism. In hating censorship we should all try harder to walk the pathway of morality.

Each season has its advantages and disadvantages. In many parts of the world, where the temperature drops below freezing, a person will find snow. Snow is a very beautiful thing. Yet, in its beauty, it is the deadliest of all. The reason why it is the deadliest of all is it can be subzero in its temperature. A person needs to adorn him or herself much more appropriately, so as not to suffer frostbite or other complications.

In the winter a person's blood changes its property. This makes us incur more sickness in the cold season. In this century people are outrageous. Our dressing is insufficient. Why? I am not too sure why we dress inadequately today in the four seasons.

The question is, is it the fashion of the day? Is it because of the growth in the population why apparels are made with less material to be sold cheaper? The other thing that it might be is that this generation feels they are more advanced, and they do not need to dress with as much clothes as the people did when technology was not yet developed. Now we can live in the four seasons with less clothing, being modern, and it will have no effect on a person's body.

The other reason why people of today dress inadequately, could be because sin always is the controller ever since man transgressed. Since we are not controlling ourselves, we do not know how to behave correctly.

Back in the beginning of humanity, I read in the Bible that man was naked at one time. They were not knowledgeable with their nakedness, until they transgressed. At that time they realized that they were naked. They made coverings from leaves for their nakedness. I see where GOD made clothing from skin and gave unto them, because that was much better than the leaves to cover their nakedness. Genesee 3:21

I also realize that there was one season also in the beginning. They never knew rain. Much of the devastation in the weather today, early people had no knowledge about. It was after the flood that four seasons came into existence. The first rainfall was the destruction of the majority of the population. Genesee 2:5&6. GOD created the four seasons after He wiped-out early civilizations. Genesee 8:22.

I do not know if the majority of humans see and understand that it was sin that caused the four seasons to be on this earth. It is man's disobedience to GOD that caused man to be clothed with clothes. The creation of four seasons came also by man's transgressions.

All the hardships that we go through daily have not wakened us up, or taught us to respect our own body, soul, life, or simply care for ourselves. Each day we behave more and more disrespectful to GOD. As we live our lives daily we all dishonor His words. We walk just about naked because sin has blindfolded our eyes.

Sin blinds men's eyes and leaves us in pain and suffering all the days of their lives on this earth. It is sad to see that so many people believe this earth is self- created. Who then is responsible for the creation of suffering and death, knowing that life is not a pleasant thing? This minute we feel great and wonderful. When we think we are having fun, with lots of pleasure, we are cut off forever with no hope for better in the future.

The other question we should always ask ourselves is if this earth is self created, how did it create four seasons? Are all the trees and vegetation able to adapt on their own if there is no one responsible like the Creator?

The other question that needs to be asked relates to the theory of evolution. If all things are self-created, why do people die if it was not pronounced by GOD? To me it is very difficult to ever acknowledge the theory of evolution. The regeneration of humans and all species is too perfect to be credited as self-creation.

In this era we find the world population dresses with little or no pride. The fashions of today show poor morals. The enemy of humanity has so much control over us that we are dishonorable to our own bodies.

Is it possible our educators lost their backbones and joined the system so as to not rock the boat? Over and over, I see negligence in the lives of thousands of people as I travel this pathway of life. Is it possible that many cannot stand the hassle of dressing or undressing? What is it? Why do people tend to walk inappropriately in their clothing?

Are we trying to disprove a point? Are we showing the world that we are not going to respect anything that GOD commanded us? Are we going to make the devil be our lord and master in our daily dress code?

The majority of the population seems to behave like they are telling GOD that He needs to repent and come down from his standard of right to people's likes. If GOD does not like the way man is behaving, too bad. It is not GOD we are hurting in this game we are playing. Man is the one who is going to be sorry in the end. Look at the ones who are having all kinds of health problems. We might think and feel that we are getting away with murder now, not realizing as we journey through this life, we will inherit all kinds of ailments.

We are not receiving a just compensation for being disrespectful in our dress code. Most only receive a little sickness here and there, because their bodies are exposed too long to the various climates. Many humans that have no regard for the cold weather dress like it is still summer. I have seen many that say they are too hot even when it is very cold. I live to see many of the people, who once said they were ok with dressing inappropriately in the winter, whose life has ended at a very early age.

Pleasure might be great for a season. It is not forever. Sooner than we expect we are going to be awakened to our ignorance. Many die without the opportunity to correct the erroneous way they did dress.

A person should not need another person to educate him/her to be clothed correctly. It should be automatic within each individual. It is so easy to fallow evil and join the devilish system, where you find that the majorities are not determined to separate themselves from immorality to a life of morals.

A person needs to cover their body properly in all of the four seasons. Each one can have a profound effect on a person's body. When a person is young and strong, they feel they can move mountains. As soon as we begin to climb up in age, we start to regret our past behavior. When a person reaches that stage, it has become too late. We cannot reverse the damage done to our bodies. At that stage we seek medical help, to no avail, for any further damages.

At that crossroad in life we become very unhappy because our life savings begin to dwindle away. It hurts when all a person works for in their life will be gone forever without any comfort or hope in regaining the life one disregarded many years before.

Continually, I see and hear people compare their life with nature. We even have our scientists and researches using small animals for experimentation to obtain the answers they are looking for. They want to eradicate ailment that makes men's lives topsy-turvy.

The study of nature by men makes men teach us that people are a higher class of animals. Thus, to find an answer, it might be more appropriate to use the lower class of species because they are of less value than humanity. They suffer casualties through man's ignorance. They do not have to be judged someday in the near future.

Man is the creature that will be cast into the lake of fire for being dishonorable to his Creator. All other creatures are in complete subjection to GOD. Man is the only creature where we find a statement that we were made after the likeness of GOD and in the image of GOD. Man is the only creation of GOD that gives him the most trouble. All things suffer immensely through human disobedience. Genesee 1: 26&27

Let us study for a short time the four seasons with plants and animals. Let's see if we can understand how we behaved very foolishly. Take the trees with spring, summer, fall, and winter. Each year we have four changes. Not all countries are able to see the four seasons as they change yearly. People that live in the tropical climates also have the four changes take place. Because they do not have snow, it is not as noticeable as the locations that have snow when it becomes very cold.

I came from one of the Caribbean Islands. I can remember a tree in our yard would always shed its leaves completely in the fall. The trees that are in the tropical climate never fall asleep as those that grow in the cold climate. Not all the trees would do that all the time in that abundance.

I realize that all trees renew themselves by changing their leaves yearly. That's the way they rejuvenate themselves all the time. Trees' leaves are their covering as men's clothes are theirs. In the winter the trees don't need leaves because they are sleeping. If they should maintain their leaves, and they refuse to work according to the plan of nature, working in opposition will bring death to the trees. Over and over we see many trees that are dead. We might not know all the reasons why these trees died. We have to cut them down. Trees do not answer for themselves to GOD or anyone. Man likewise does not see the need for finding the cause of trees that are dying especially if it does not relate to food supply or other important factors.

I know that man today is trying much harder to preserve trees globally. The preservation of trees is not necessarily an accounting for what they are doing. The purpose of preserving trees has to do with man's well-being on this earth. Man is not capable of existing alone without plants and animals.

Consider all plants and animals that occupy this earth. They need nutrients just like humanity to survive. Just about all plants and creatures need water. All things on this earth that fight against nature always suffer in the end. It matters not what they may be; opposition only brings pain and death to the opposing ones.

Plants and animals all seem to behave wisely, not like mankind. In spring, the trees put out their buds. They are making preparation for the hot days of summer that is ahead. Not making preparation for the hot weather ahead, when the hot season comes around, the trees that refuse to wake up will remain asleep forever. The survival of each plant depends on their leaves. Having no covering, death will be imminent.

Each of the four different climates allows the trees to make preparation to meet the next climate or weather pattern that is on the way. Take spring for instance. The trees get ready by putting on their protective covering to combat the hot weather so that it will not kill them. In the fall, the trees make the necessary alteration for the winter weather or climate that they are not wasted away by the cold climate. A tree cannot survive in the cold winter that has leaves. Pine trees have no leaves and they can remain alive all year in all kinds of weather without shedding their pine needles.

The survival of trees depends on the quality of their leaves. Unhealthy leaves show that something is drastically wrong with the trees. The development of insects depends on eating the leaves of a tree. That is the reason tree surgeons keep a very close eye on the leaves of a tree to see if they are being affected by insects. If they see signs of moths' intrusion, they get the plant medication. If the plant has parasite invaders, they eject the moths from the tree so they do not kill the trees.

Plants and animals all have a covering to protect them from the environment. Not all trees lose their beauty in the winter. The trees that shed their leaves in the winter do that to retain their life. It matters not whether it's a tree or an animal they all have a built-in mechanism that is able to preserve life. Bears are animals that hibernate in the winter, something like the trees. They eat a lot in the summer so they can sleep all the days of winter. The animals that do not hibernate are able to change their body's properties different for the winter than the summer, fall, and spring so that they do not die.

All the animals, that stay awake in the winter, maintain their correct body temperature in-spite of the cold weather. They never need to make a fire to warm themselves or cover up to help from freezing.

A human, on the other hand, needs an outer layer as a covering and a fire to help maintain their body temperature. Mankind's body does not have the built-in mechanism that changes its outer layer to combat the cold weather. Most animal fur, which is their outer layer, increases to maintain the body temperature. Then, the cold weather does not have much effect on them so that they would freeze easily like people.

The other thing with animals is they do not need to outfit themselves in the cold weather with any kind of clothing. As long as they can get the necessary food that they required to be healthy and strong, they will not freeze that easily. Take a rat, or other rodents one would see running up and down in snow, you will never see them all over the place dead. When you see many of these creatures lying dead, they must have eaten something that affected them. Sometimes they run up against a shortage of their daily ration. Insects are not prevalent in the winter climate. Summer brings out the best in all things. Take the little ants, how busy they are in the summer gathering for themselves their winter supply. They are unable to find their food in the winter.

We need to study the ants. These creatures do not have any master or lord over them that they need to follow the laws their governor forms. People are suppose to behave with lots more intelligence than all the other species that live and walk this earth. Man is the creature that gives the most trouble in just about everything.

I do not think people know and understand what is good for them. I have a very hard time accepting man's behavior, especially addressing animals. I know that birds and animals do not have use for man made light. Even when we domesticate these creatures, it does not change their life much.

Birds, animals, and creatures eat to maintain their living. Their eating habits are more controllable than humans. Most of the domesticated creatures' man treats healthier than himself. These species do not have the power to get their meals as man does. Many cannot obtain their meals when it becomes dark. They just remain without until the next day.

Even when people have them as pets, they still eat wisely. Their owner shows more love and caring for their animals than for other humans. Man's love for money keeps him doing great injustice to himself, without understanding what he is doing.

Man is the intelligent creature over all other species of the world. Because humans are like GOD, man should have been the controlling power in this world. We gave it away for foolishness.

This in-turn brings great sorrow to our hearts, because we failed to properly control ourselves from the beginning.

As I say, people with their pets, treat them better than themselves when it comes to their diet. Continually I see animals are kept on strict diets. I have a friend that has horses. I was at his home out in an undeveloped area. He had several types of feed that he gave to his horses. This included the fresh grass they ate daily and the hay they fed them in the winter. He related to me that if you do not restrict the horses' eating, they would keep on eating to their death. I personally find that very hard to believe because horses in the wild do not have a master they are subject to. How come they never eat themselves to death?

Man addresses himself to be the higher class of animal. We have been studying the lower classes of animals for many years in laboratories looking to find cures for various ailments in humanity. One of the greatest things we might have overlooked in our research is the way these animals eat and their total behavior.

The eating behavior of birds and animals might not be important in the eyes of our educators, and our medical researchers. We are educated with what they were educated with. They are unable to go beyond their educational level. If we are pleased with the doctrine of those who are teaching, we accept their teaching. When we are displeased with what they are lecturing us about, we just disregard their teaching.

I often see birds, animals, and insects stop eating sometime before night falls. The only time we find insects, birds, or animals eating in the night hours, has to do with man controlling them. They pick up man's bad eating habits being unrestrained.

Animals are uneducated. They do not need electric or any of man's technology for survival in this world. They get sick and die similar to man. We eat their flesh as part of our diet. It has been taught that we need meats as a source of great vitamins and protein.

Man's diet is separated completely from all other species in the world. Man is the only one that changed their eating habits since the creation of electricity. In the days when there was no electricity, man would not have the hours of the day as we do these days. Man has twenty-four seven, three hundred and sixty five days yearly to eat and to drink as he pleases. The day mister and mistress are overpowered by some ailment: at that cross road, we regret our past in the way we diet.

We need to not only use the lower class of animals for laboratory experimentation for illnesses, but look at our own weakness as the example to the animals that we are commanded to be over. Their restricted life shows much better discipline than humans. Man's behavior looks like people live to eat, instead of eat to live. Man just keeps pigging out.

People walk this earth, in a manner of speaking, as if they do not care for tomorrow, like today is forever. Yesterday is gone and tomorrow addresses tomorrow. So, man only knows today. The past is gone. The future is yet to be seen. Man thinks he does not need to make preparation for tomorrow.

What would it be like if the animal kingdom's eating behavior was in the same category as man? I understand that chicken farming is something like this. They never stop eating from birth to death. They stay awake all the time. They have lighting all the time, making the chicken think it is always daytime. To me, that is a very hard thing to accept. I have not been to a chicken farm to confirm the story if it's true or false.

Animals, like humans, need rest. It is not only at night that chickens rest. I was one that raised chickens when I was a little boy living with my dad and stepmother. I saw our chickens all the time in the daylight take a nap. Man and animals have to sleep. Vegetation, they say, needs rest too. I understand that all creatures need to sleep. Cats, dogs, and birds do not only slumber at night. We have animals that are domesticated that sleep much more than animals that live in the wild.

Domesticated animals do not have to fend for their daily meals. They have their masters that tend to them morning, noon, and night. Man does things for his domesticated animals that they have as their pets. People are so involved with pets these days that they will incarcerate you if they feel you ill-treat any animals. That includes domesticated and the ones that live in the wild.

I am not a person that hates animals. Neither am I a person that abuses animals. I just think we should be much more attached with our own specie and show much more affection for one another. We have not shown real affection for one another. Oftentimes we put this world substance over humans. Not one object of this world is capable of helping humans when something happens to them, when there a need to be moved or transported for some necessary purposes.

I hear people say all the time that dogs are man's best friend. I am not saying that dogs cannot seek help when you are in trouble. I know that they cannot call for help on the phone. They cannot cook or clean anything for you. There might be a few little things they might be able to accomplish for you. That's not enough for anyone to say that a dog is man's best friend. Do we ever wonder how GOD reacts when humanity keeps on saying that dogs are man's best friends?

Each species serves its specific purpose on this earth. The animal's purpose we might not see and understand. Since they are with us, we best try to make life pleasant for all. We are all in the same world together. We should just make it pleasant as best as we can for all.

Man in his search for better things in life studies plants and animals. This is a determination to obtain an answer that has man perplexed most of his life. The perplexity of many, especially in this era, confesses that there is no GOD. These people are trying to prove that their theory is accurate, even more accurate than the people who are content, with the words of the Bible, that there is a GOD. And they are happy that GOD created the heavens and the earth.

What has the study of animals truly given to man since he has been using them for experimentation to find the answers to cure many aliments? Is it possible that he will find what he is looking for?

Man is his worst enemy. We are looking elsewhere for an answer when we should be looking at ourselves for the answer we need.

Looking at many of the things we created, we need to see where we made the wrong turn as we push forward into the future. Technology is great. Not one thing is wrong with being advanced. The problem is what we have allowed ourselves to become. We are killing ourselves for no reason at all. The pain we go through daily is not necessary. All the pleasure we crave so much day after day keeps us continually in unhappiness.

Look at our foolish behavior as we walk this earth. We love to eat and do what our bodies crave. We never try to think if what we are doing is necessary and what are the things we can do without in this life. Most people do not see the need to give up anything they are doing, even if it will cost them their lives.

Take the bewitching power of the most watched or listened to device created by humanity. TV! It makes the watcher eat more, waste more time of his life, and sleep in a very unhealthy posture that is killing more people than cigarettes and pop.

I can bring to light another item that we use daily that takes millions of people's lives. To this present moment, the men and women of the world who dedicated their lives trying to finding the answers needed to make millions healthier are having a very difficult time. Regardless of the difficulties researches are having, they are persistent in their effort with the hope that one day they will find what they are looking for.

There are many things we need to study that we are not studying. Finding out that many things that we have, and we are using incorrectly, might open our eyes to a much broader or wider avenue of greatness, which might just make us change our unhealthy lifestyle.

Because humanity has placed GOD, the Creator of this universe in man's imagination, and being irreverence Him in all things what we should have learned hundreds or thousands of years in the past are still has remain a mystery. This is because we think and feel we are very intelligent. And the reason we might feel that way, is because over the years we have developed so many gadgets.

I have to agree that people of today have things more pleasant than all the generations that were before us. On one hand, we have some things that are much more unpleasant. Regardless of the pleasant, and the unpleasant features there are in our society, we can remove difficulties for most people of the world if we stand united as one. We are so involved in today's advancements that we could never live if many of the gadgets should disappear.

People in this era are so spoiled that they are controlled by the many power companies. They dictate to us. They are demanding. They threaten us monthly if we fail to pay our utilities. They never use their consideration in correct judgment. A person has to rely on the government system for help. The reason things are this way is that we are spoiled and set in our ways.

I often say that this era is great. We turn a knob or push a switch and we can get heat or cold temperature. It has to do with the type of weather we have. When it is cold we turn a knob to get heat. When it is hot, we do the same. We get cool air that keeps us cool. Man is a creature in this century that loves a lot of comfort. I find most complain about the weather all the time. There is no happy medium for some. One day it's too hot and the next it's too cold. I wish the rain would stop.

When there is a power outage, especially when it is in the winter, it sure makes a person's life very cantankerous. Many homes are built with wood burning fireplaces. This does help a little in heating a person's home in the winter. Central heat is great. It gives us much more time to goof off. It reduces us using our body for physical labor producing wood as needed back in the days when there was no central heating system. It reduces the physical labor that was a help to us in so many ways. It kept the people in past generations healthier than we are today with modern technology.

Physical labor by men and women in the days when there was no electricity was very beneficial health-wise to that generation. As they worked, they kept themselves very healthy. They were exercising unconsciously. Yet they were being kept healthier than this generation. When a person does their exercise these days, they are hurting themselves with all the exertion they are putting on their joints and nerves. Someday it will make your body hurt horrendously.

In today's push for healthiness, it brings great disappointment in later years. It is not giving people longevity as taught. If anything, it is reducing a person's life span. You are going to be angry with yourself in your older years. What I would like for all to know and to understand is this. When I speak of people labor during the years when there was none electricity, and say they would be exercising differently that is the truth.

We do not look on a laboring person and dresses their daily routine as exercises. What I am trying to bring to people understanding, is the life of the people in the years when there was no electricity man had make provision for their comfort, and it put great restrained on them compare to the stage we are in this century.

Man had to eat less, get more rest, and had a lot less time to goof off. With today's gadgets man become more destructive to themselves. Was their foods that they cultivated was much healthier than ours that is produces by our farmers? That is the question we need to find the answer for. I know the answer as you read this book you see if you know the answer also.

It is very sad to see what is being transpiring in the world these days. Man in truth does hate himself. We are not in love with ourselves; if we did we would behaving as we are doing.

The Unanswered Answers

Chapter (12)

What is man? Where did man come from? Is man a creature that evolved? The real question is: is GOD truly responsible for man's existence? Why did GOD create man? GOD'S angels are spirits like Him and occupied His habitat with Him. Man was created, as the Bible teaches in the image of GOD. Genesee 1: 26&27

Man was never at anytime created as a spirit. Man was always flesh and blood, a much lower creature than all the angels. Man's habitat was always this earth, because he is human.

Angels are spirits. They do not need to have the spirit of GOD dwell within their being, because they are spirits. Man is not a spirit. Therefore GOD can dwell in man only because we are flesh and blood. Man can die, because we are the ones that choose death. Angels are spirits. They were not made like man. They were created to serve GOD and man. Man was made only to serve GOD.

Man's rejection of GOD brings man to serve angels. The devil is an angel. He is known as the god of this world and he is doing a number on humanity. He also is responsible for the many unanswered answers. 2Corinthians 4: 4 and St. John 12: 31

Does it seem correct to have such a chapter as the unanswered answers? I would say yes. Many might disagree, while many will agree. It is hard to understand the things that are over one's head and in a person's mind. Man is a creature that cannot see the depth of a person's heart.

Man is flesh and blood. That is what we need to remember. Man keeps trying to exalt himself above others. That could be the reason why man strives so much to be kings, governors, presidents, prime ministers, or one of the many government members. Man is a creature that loves to be seen and to be heard.

I am not being mulish with humanity. I realize that someone has to be the leader, and that all cannot lead. Yet, in this era, we find too many who are fighting for leadership who do not have leadership quality. When we have leaders, who are of such caliber, they are going to be detrimental to the population of their country.

The minority of people, who crave for power in many areas of life, bring others to misery and to a place where many hate being alive. Some end their lives, because of the pressure placed on them by men. They seek to have complete control over other people's lives. It is very sad to see what humans brought on themselves. All because they constantly give heed to the words of men, and not GOD'S words. Man cannot see tomorrow or the next moment. We need to stop, look, and listen for our own good.

The answers many are looking for they are not reaching. They keep being unanswered all the time. Many just give up with both GOD and man. They feel life is unfair having constant problems all the time.

I also realize that some people feel within themselves, they fail in many things in their life as they walk this earth. This takes us to another unanswered answer to many people who are perplexed with life in general. Why is man undergoing such a horrendous life? Why did GOD make the devil and why did he allow him to ruin his perfect creation?

{"I will give you the answer that was shown to me, why GOD made things to continue with the Devil and man being in opposition with his laws, in the next book."}

Man's quest for answers fails to answer his own questions. Because man fails to see his own shortcomings, he points fingers at other people; this includes GOD and the devil because we overlook our own selves.

Take our researchers: they are looking for ways to help man with their many health enigmas. What have they given to the people that are going through many kinds of ailments: more unanswered answers? If we never behaved irreverently to GOD, we certainly would have fewer problems today.

I do realize that man needs help from some other source, whether from GOD, as the loving and caring one, or from man. The majority are aware of the evil creature that the Devil is. He and his confederates force man to be evil like him all the days of their lives.

Despite how cruel this person is, we find a minority of people who knowingly serve him faithfully daily. These people who serve the Devil faithfully ask help of him. Man is a creature who is helpless in many areas of life. Therefore, we seek help from wherever it is available.

It might seem outrageous to say that man seeks help from the Devil. Remember, there are many individuals that pray to the Devil and serve him faithfully. The majority of humans unconsciously are serving Satan. The true reason the majority are serving Satan unaware, is because they confess with their lips that they are not a servant of the Devil. By deception they serve Satan unconsciously. They keep confessing they are the servants of the Creator and pray to none other but GOD. Yet they are irreverent to the words of GOD. Who then are they serving but Satan?

Remember, when we go to men and women who are agnostics and atheists for help, we are going to the Devil for help. The same with people who say they are fortune-tellers. We can find many other things in our society that are of Satan that the majority seek help from.

By man's thinking and behavior, he keeps giving deceptive answers to the seekers who are having trouble in many things on this earth. Various ailments, or other problems, confront us daily. It can be all our faults. Still we are censured continually for man's many problems we encounter daily as if it's not our fault. Living a life that is not restrained in the way we eat and sleep helps to contribute to our health problems.

We should not get angry with our physicians, our researchers, or anyone that has anything to do with producing any means of help to the sick and afflicted people globally. We need to stop suing these people. They are not GOD, just man. Remember humans are subject to all kinds of errors.

The lack of patience, that's imbedded in people, makes many lives very unhappy. Since man is powerless in changing people into much better individuals, we cannot help in anyway. We can't make that impatient person change from their intolerance, especially if he refuses to heed what's been shown to him.

We should, in some way, learn to be thankful for the smallest of help men give to one another, even if we think that all doctors, scientists, or researchers are only there for a job. A job is so that they can have some of life's commodities without having to steal or obtain by killing others for their daily ration.

Man has to survive on this earth. We keep making mistake after mistake; all the mistakes that we keep making, has not removed man from the face of this earth. When one dies, hundreds are born daily. The thing we might overlook is that all things cannot continue as they are going these days. Something is about to give way. It is not going to be very pleasant.

People in general do not like unpleasantness. We love to be pampered. When things are not going the way we would like for them to go we become angry with man, like man has any power to make things any better for us. We should stop, and contemplate on all the things that man has been trying to do for man since development of electricity and all the other gadgets. We should be somewhat thankful, AND NEVER FORGET TO BE THANKFUL TO GOD.

Since the development of voltaic current, man tends to have many more ailments. We have acquired all kinds of occupations to cope with all the jobs that opened since we found voltage. Take all the jobs that were found because of electricity. Some of the jobs are great. While we have many that are deadly, at the same time, lots of people love to make a lot of malicious remarks. Could be because they are unfortunate being poor. Poverty has become commonplace in today's living. Mankind will never be able to totally understand man's problems.

Researchers, and all the research that has been done all these years, have been looking to find answers for all the ailments that have had man perplexed. Do not be negative with our men and women who dedicate their lives seeking answers for the people that are going through many ailments.

We need to remember that our scientists, who dedicate their lives in search of cures, run into the same problem themselves. Because they seek answers, does not exclude them from sickness. They are not looking for the solution only for the people that are undergoing the problem. They are in some ways trying to prevent future health problems for themselves and others.

They are thinking that they can, in the near future, find the answer for diseases. That will help the men and women, who dedicate their lives in many hazardous ways in their search for cures to the various types of diseases there are in the world. Remember, these diseases are not in just one country of the globe. They are all over. They have been plaguing humanity all their lives.

All the years that these men and women have spent in medical research, they are still hitting their heads against the wall looking for answers. They cannot come up with what they are looking for. We still have unanswered answers daily with us without any in the near future from the people that give up their lives seeking to help eradicate man's greatest fear.

We have hundreds of diseases that keep men and women perplexed. Since we developed electricity we are able to do greater things than all the generations that ever lived before us. I am very sure that if they had all the ailments we have in this generation, they had to be very unhappy with their lives.

I know that sickness is not a new thing only in this era. Sickness has been with man possibly from the day we began to multiply and started to live ignorantly. Is sickness a method of keeping humanity in bondage all the days of our lives? What is the real answer for man's aliments? Is it because death is eminent to humans that it seems that sickness has always been around?

Answers, questions unanswered, as we go on our journey through life. Many have become perplexed with life, especially with diseases and the pain it leaves us with. Death hurts a lot, still not like sickness. Over and over, I see and hear many people speak of their loved ones suffering before they die. They lose weight because of what the disease does to their loved one before parting this life.

Many times you would hear them say it was much better for their loved ones to die then to keep suffering as they were doing. When a person dies, many feel it for a while. Many keep speaking about their loved ones even after death. They miss them. The ones that suffer the most are the ones that feel inappropriate to talk about it.

Men, with human wisdom and understanding, are trying their best to eradicate all the various diseases that shorten millions of mankind's lives yearly. I feel that if we truly want to obtain the answers for all the diseases there are, we need to show much more respect to GOD. I am not speaking about the devil. He is the author of confusion. He feels that as long as men live and walk this earth he has to make us speak irreverently about the One who really does love us.

In our ill feelings towards GOD, we fail to come up with the answer needed to stop sickness. Men's behavior tends to ignore GOD, as if to say, we can solve our enigmas without the help of GOD. Not realizing the wrong path we have taken, we blindly continue the same pathway hundreds of years.

Many answers given by man in connection with diseases are still unanswered in every detail. The reason our dedicated men and women have not found the answer they have been looking for is they allow the piece of paper they receive from one of the many institutions for learning to blindfold their eyes. They cannot behold good from bad or right over the wrong.

For instance, we can bring to light several answers that are unanswered in the medical philosophy. We have several types of cancer. It does not only affect one area of a person's body. Not all people are affected with cancer. Some are more affected than others. Some are wasted early in life. Some reach a good old age. Many lingering diseases continue to overpower the human body when the body fails in its operational strength.

One of the many teachings we have, also shows us an answer that truly is unanswered. It is a statement in this regard. All humans are born with cancer cells. We have to eat or drink something that triggers the cancer cells into growth. Once again we have to say a statement like that seems far-fetched if eating and drink was the culprit that ignites one's cells into growth. We then would have each and every human all over the world, develop cancer within their body. Is eating then the correct answer or is that another unanswered answer known to man? The truth is cancer does not develop by eating, just as cigarettes and other products are not the cause of cancer. I will give the answer in the next book how cancer and other sicknesses develop in the human body.

Man loves to teach the unlearned. We think in this era everyone should be educated. Thinking that we can make this world a much better place, most are illiterate in the profession of medicine. We have to go along with their teaching because there is no one else we can seek any answer from. That could be the reason why so many organizations jump on the bandwagon about the various foods and drinks that contribute to the development of cancer.

Knowing correct from incorrect, many refuse to associate themselves with an illiterate. They say that a person that is an illiterate is not book wise. When a person cannot read or write, they are the misfortunate ones of society. These people, who lack knowledge in-conjunction with the human body, are in the same category as the people that we look upon as illiterates. One has a little more understanding in some things than others.

The other thing we might overlook is our educators are teaching us about the human body, but they still lack knowledge in many things about the body. I have been hearing, for a very long time, that cigarettes cause cancer in the lungs and in the throat. Likewise cigarettes do harm to a person's heart. What is it a person gets from a cigarette, just smoke? Is smoke really deadly? There are thousands of people that die yearly as a result of lung cancer. Our researching organizations are connecting cigarettes as the culprit. Millions have been trying to free themselves from the use of tobacco. They hope to extend their lives for many more years.

Let us say that cigarettes are the culprits that truly cause cancer of the lungs and throat. What other substance do we take orally, away from cigarettes that contribute to cell growth in one's body? Knowing that there are breast, liver, colon, prostrate, and many more cancers, why are only two types of cancer pointed to that cigarettes trigger?

I am not saying that there is no answer for the cause of other cancer growth. I have not learned of a lot more products that man says causes cancer than chemicals and asbestos. I have not heard or read what type of cancer other products develop. I understand that asbestos are being removed from the population.

Should we go along with the teaching of cancer as it is today? All the time, in many doctors' offices and other businesses, a person can find all kinds of magazines. They are trying to encourage old and young people to never start or just stop smoking because it is so deadly. Restaurants, businesses and other public facilities ban smoking. Millions join in a malicious maneuver against the use of cigarettes. Is it correct or incorrect in the answer given to the population of the world in connection with cancer development in all humans that have their cells growing within their bodies?

It's within the era of electric that we have found many diseases that develop in humans. In the age when there was no electric, there where fewer ailments. The thing that might be possible was that there were less people in the population, the earth had better quality soil, and the abundance of products was not necessary in those days. People were a lot more content with life. There was no need for a great supply of food globally.

The other possibility is that man was not able to keep correct data in his daily living. Not able to work correctly, because of improper lighting, it would take a longer time to record all things that happened. Therefore only the necessary things they felt were vitally important would be recorded. The other thing that might be possible, there was a shortage of doctors. The other possibility was that there was no electricity and man was unable to x ray people's bodies. They might not have had proper microscopes, as there are today, that are used to analyze blood.

Men, in their quest for knowledge, desire life to be much simpler. In our search for making our labor easier, we develop all kinds of machines. All that were created are pleasant in man's sight. They made us more and more cantankerous in our daily lives. We created many great things. They would be wonderful, if we had not created envy, lust, and greed in the process. Through the creation of electricity, man was able also to create better optical lens. This enables men to divide cells and bring greater understanding of the body better than ancient civilization.

The advancement in technology brings other complications in man's life, because we feel we have outgrown the usefulness of GOD. We feel that we have surpassed all the other generations before us in knowledge. We have not noticed we also surpassed them in diseases. We have not noticed that we behave much more despicably in everything we do daily.

Take the increase in crimes and the use of drugs, likewise the up-swing in immorality. Something is going to happen to keep men in check, whether we like it or not. I know that many people are unbelievers. We have lots of skeptics, including atheists and agnostics that inhabit this world. I am not excluding atheists and agnostics in the writing of this book. Having placed GOD so much in this writing might make you feel you are not wanted. I personally cannot do any better. I know that there is a GOD. All the knowledge I am imparting now GOD is the one who gave it to me. Man is not my educator. So I have to bring to light the hidden things that were not knowledgeable to man. This is not a put down of any sect, color, or creed.

Life is not pleasant when a person even catches a cold or the flu. It matters not who you are, black or white, male or female, Christian or none Christian, atheist or agnostic. Let's not forget the skeptics. All are in the same boat when colds or flu occupy one's body. Because diseases are disrespectful and impartial, all suffer that are alive and in it's part when they move in man's habitat.

The only thing is this: people fail as they grow in knowledge, population, and everything else that comes along.

I made the statement that men have been studying animals for sometime. They are trying to obtain an answer for man's many ailments. To this date they are only coming up with unanswered answers. Why is it so hard to find the answer to alleviate many of man's diseases? Man can invent so many gadgets to make a person's life more lax. What is the problem? Why is man's health getting out of hand?

Thousands are employed globally in trying to aid the people that suffer daily with all kinds of illnesses. Billions are spent yearly in research all over the world. In every country, and Island, one can find just about every sickness one is knowledgeable with. Not one nation or country is excluded. We cannot find one nation where people can stand up and proclaim that their nation, country, or Island is uncontaminated with sickness.

Take the simple common cold that makes man's life very miserable. You can find it in every nook and cranny in every part of the world that man inhabits. I keep hearing that there is no cure for the simple common cold that has been plaguing humanity all their lives. Man keeps getting a beating with an answer for the common cold. Since they keep coming up with an unanswered answer, they tell us that it's incurable. We keep buying the answer they give us. This takes us back to the fact that all cannot go to medical school to know more about the body.

Man's body is a very complex, unparalleled beauty, perfect in many ways. Yet in its perfection it suffers great traumas. It is a very difficult thing to understand man's philosophy, because people are creatures that love self-will. They take punishments like prisons that are man made. They have been incarcerating all the lawbreakers for thousands of years.

Man would love to live and walk this earth without any problems, free of normal everyday enigmas. Man would love it if from this very moment all problems one encounters would cease forever, never to return.

Life, with its atrocities, has not forced many to eradicate themselves from pain and suffering. I know that a few people who could not face the atrocities end their lives. We have hundreds in this era with all kinds of incurable diseases as stated by man. People with ailments such as theirs end their lives because they are unable to endure the pains that they are undergoing.

I know many people that gave up on life, because of their suffering. They would not have requested help to annihilate themselves, if someone was able to show them there is hope for their suffering.

Millions have cancer or diseases that have our researchers knocking their heads against the wall. They are looking for an answer that they might give the people who are suffering with various illnesses.

The unavailable, immediate assistance to the ones that are encountering problems, they simply lose sight of their life. The ending of this life is not the ending of a person's existence. It would be great if it was over when death snatches us out of this life, like the animals or all other creatures that die. There has to be more to death with man than the other species on this earth. Man is the only being that governs all the other species on this earth. The other thing is this: man should be the governor for himself.

When man fails the responsibility that was handed to him, he casts it away, and chooses death and destruction over life. We never see the need to maintain correctly what was handed down to us. Over and over I hear other people cast the blame at Eve and Adam because they were the ones that first disobeyed GOD'S commandments. In their disobedience death passed down to all. Should I agree with those words even though we read them in the Bible? Is it possible we might just get the wrong understanding or answer in the words that say all die through Eve and Adam?

Is it addressing a physical death? Or, is it speaking of death as separation from GOD? Because of sin we became evil and vile in our nature from birth to death. Knowing we came into this world through the transgression of the first two people that occupied this earth, should we live as we came? I learned that a few escaped death. If a few were able to escape death we all could, if everyone was able to live like the ones that escaped.

If man was able to take the words of GOD very seriously, even in this era with all the technology that we have in our society, there would be no need for a medical doctor or anyone having any ailments. Man's disobedience is the cause of all the problems he encounters all the days of his life.

What a wonderful life man can have walking this earth, "If" we could only just stop, look, and listen, so that things would be better. Why can't we make the right choice? Why can't we wake from our slumber? The evil force does have the greater grip on humanity. We can't deny it, if we are honest with ourselves.

We can change the future if we try. If we refuse to try, things are only going to get worse. Do we have enough of life's agony? Are we glutinous for punishment from birth to death? Can we answer our own questions? Are we always going to look to someone else for an answer? The power is in the hands of everyone. It is up to the individuals what they do with what they have.

Death Brings Pain and Suffering

The uncontrolled nature of humanity brings all kinds of diseases on people. Once more we address man's creations. Look at electricity and the other appliances that were developed with the use of voltage.

Don't be negative completely with your thinking about man's inventions. We need to be our own judges in these issues. I know that man always looks to man for the direction to take in just about everything that pertains to this life. Not many look for anything good in the life to come. If we were looking honestly with a pure heart to the life that is yet to come, no matter what man creates that would cause distraction, we would not be distracted. Diversion comes when we are not properly grounded.

When we are determining to maintain positive thinking, nothing can move us out of the pathway we step into. When we are not shown the correct path to take, we remain walking and doing the things that are not convenient for anyone to do. There is a saying that goes this way where there is no vision the people perish. Proverbs 29:18. 1Samuel 3:1.

We do not need for someone to make a proclamation to show the population that we are suffering. In every direction people look they can see lots of unpleasantness. Because of the lack of vision in the indoctrinators of people, there are heartaches and pain. The pain is very much unbearable to millions all over the world. At the present time there seems to be no hope for millions. I am very sorry to know so many people have to take their lives because they feel all hope is gone. They spend their lives in agony and every direction they take only disappointments continually.

In this chapter you will find out why so many people contract many diseases in a very early stage of their lives and even cause death to many. This might be something man has overlooked or possibly never has seen the need to pursue investigation in the matter. The way research is being done, it was passed down from other researchers who thought the way they did research was right.

The continuation in the same pathway that started, maintains the erroneous beginning.

Medical researchers throughout all generations had no knowledge that a woman's monthly is not something to be taken lightly, especially the way we are involved in this century sexually; it's outrageous. We behave barbarously sexually both male and female. It is not only men, who are the fault of sexual misconduct. Today's women seem to be much more aggressive in everything in life than men. They are much more business oriented than men. Women are the ones who are doing the proposing to men to get married. Men keep on running away and seem to fear commitment. I have seen many men that are unhappy with the way marriages end up. They say it's better to remain single. On the other hand, many would love to have hundreds of women that they can call their own. Most are not content with one woman. Why are human so unhappy and not contented? We covet one another and kill one another for what they accomplish in life. We do not think that everyone cannot be educated and become wealthy.

Having sexual intercourse with a beautiful woman is outstanding. Still we need to understand that beauty is in the eyes of the beholder. All things that glitter are not gold. We have men and women who behave despicably today. Both are uncontrollable in sex. This possibly has to do with machines made to view all kinds of sexual materials?

Once again we can point our fingers at the creation of voltaic current, not that within the confines of electricity should we converse dangers. Man's deadliness is unrestrained. It takes away a full life of living from us and places us in a constant battle all the days of our lives. The reason we live as we do is that man's attitude is outrageous. This could be one of man's downfalls. The other can be that we seek a life of nothing. It's possible that a majority of humanity does not believe or have any regard for the Bible. They live disrespectful to the things that GOD shows us to come.

A person can read in the Bible where GOD shows humanity that a woman is unclean fourteen days in each month because of their menstruation. It was commanded that if a man should uncover a woman's fountain, both parties should be killed. It was not the man alone they should kill. It was the man and the woman that they should take their lives. Judgment should not rest if any man uncovered woman's nakedness during the days of her uncleanness. Leviticus 15: 19-3. 18: 19, 20: 18.

All my days, from childhood to this present day, I personally have not seen or heard anyone teach that GOD required death to humanity for uncovering a woman's fountain during her days of separation. Especially in this era, with all the available sexual paraphernalia there is, men and women live unclean daily.

It is not all the fault of the individuals who are involved in a sexual act of being unclean we call barbarous for what they did. We place a greater value on making lots of money, so as to become wealthy. In our craving for wealth, we place our brothers and sisters in the background.

Once more we see technology play a significant part in the immoral life of today's population. With all the available gadgets people have at their fingertips, they see things only one sided.

Considering man's misconduct, is there a nation we should hold guilty because they never taught the rest of the world what GOD requires of all humans?

I realize that it is very important for a person to have money to live an honest life today. Nothing is evil with money. I say that electric is not evil or other gadgets created by humanity. Nothing man makes is capable of self propelling, speaking or living as man does. Man's creations require man to operate them at all times or constantly oversee them. Nothing has the power within itself to maintain its operation. Man has to keep on providing the source of energy required to keep their gadgets fully operational. And don't ever forget making spear parts to repair the various gadgets made by man.

Having to keep supplying the required source to all things created by man, we should agree that within the contents, there is no evil at all. Look at guns that man uses to take other people's lives. It's not the guns that are the killer, it is man. Remember not one of the guns can load themselves or can they fire themselves. Wherever man places their guns, there will they remain forever.

Money is no different than any other creation of man. Money in itself is not evil. Wherever it's placed, there will it remain forever. It is evil just as the Bible said it; it's the love of money that makes it become evil. Over and over, I hear many people keep saying that money is evil. They keep using it out of its context, and change the proper meaning. A person should place things in its right order that all might understand the general purpose.

The love of money especially, in this dispensation, makes humanity behave barbarous and inhumane. Man, in his behavior today, sees things one sided because we are not in love with one another. It is quite easy to speak with one's lips; the heart behaves another way. Both have a very hard time working together as one. Not able to have an honest and true heart towards another person, we place wealth in front of people.

The other problem can be this: mankind in general in this era tends to look at the Bible in a manner of speaking that a person should not take the Bible literally. People often say that man tampered so much with the Bible, that he no longer knows what is correct. Others claim that it is too hard to understand. We find another group saying that it's a contradictory book, because it contradicts itself all the time. Others made the statement that the 'these' and the 'those' in the Bible should be removed. All the things one keeps hearing daily shows that humanity is a creature whose hearts and lips cannot coordinate even though their life depends on coordination.

I personally feel and think that all the commandments of GOD are not taken very seriously by humanity. There are only ten that man tends to place a greater emphasis on. All the others we place in a vault as if to say they have no value to man. Because the fingers of GOD wrote the ten does not give more propriety over all the others. All stand the same with GOD. GOD is the One who gave them to man in the wilderness even before he wrote the ten on the table of stone. He first spoke them to the congregation. There were a lot more than ten spoken. All that the men of GOD did was write them all in the book we now call the Bible. Exodus 20:1-26

Today in our modern day society globally, only ten are presented. All the others that possibly amount to hundreds are locked up in a vault never to be used. We feel they do not have any significant value in this dispensation. Even the ten are still disregarded.

If that's the case, because they are from the Old Testament, then we should not use anything from the Old Testament. According to the words that say, "All scriptures are given by GOD'S inspiration and they are profitable for doctrine and correction to reprove to instruct that the man of GOD might be perfect thoroughly furnished unto all good works". We should also disregard these words that are found in the second book of 2Timothy 3: 16&17. They should not be used in this era simply because we leave out so many other commandments. The possible reason why we are ignoring many of the laws written in the Bible, we are interpreting the words, instead of understanding the words.

I do not think the things that once were given to humanity for our welfare were done to keep mankind as a slave to GOD at all. When this earth was created for humans to inhabit, they were given the power to rule and have total control. Man was supposed to answer to none other but GOD. Since man never fully understood all the laws to properly govern their world, someone needs to enlighten man as to teach them the proper self government.

Man, is not self created. Neither is there in truth any such thing as the great explosion that caused a cosmic chain reaction that ignited things to come into existence. Things are too perfect to believe that an explosion would likely be that powerful to make plants, and animals, and all creatures in the globe come alive.

I am not trying to put down any person in their theory in connection with earth's development. I accept the teaching of the Bible and all things therein. I also take all the words of the Bible literally. I think when someone accepts the 'theses' and 'those' in the Bible, they do a wonderful thing. I do not have any interest in adding or taking anything from the Bible. Man loves to add and take away from the Bible, trying to make the Bible please them in their sinful life. This I know: GOD is not going to accept all the changes made by man to satisfy his own rebellions.

The uncleanness of a woman's monthly cycle requires her to be separated from other people each time her fountain starts. She has seven days where she menstruates. At the end of the first seven, she is required another seven for purification. During the fourteen days of her separation she is counted to be unclean. Not one person should touch anything or lie on anything she touches or handles. The individuals who touch anything of the person who is separated for her uncleanness, they too would be counted to be unclean.

Our Bible teachers today do not teach men and women about separation when a woman's blood is being issued. I was not taught that it's unhealthy for a man and a woman to be sexually involved this time of the month. I did commit a sin worthy of death. I know that millions all over the world are in the same category as me. When I learned the truth, I gave up that sinful act.

When I lived in Jamaica, I was a person that did chase the women all over the Island. Sometimes I would drive sixty miles or more to look for a girl. When I got there, and her fountain was flowing, I just could not see driving that far for nothing. I had to get me a little piece.

I was a person that loved having sex. I was not thinking of self control or sin. I never knew any better, because I was not taught. Now that I know better, I do better. It's not because I am much older why I do not behave as I was when I lived in Jamaica. Now that I know right from wrong, it is pleasant to always do what is right. I have learned that it pays to serve the LORD. Sin is a reproach to a nation. [Proverbs 14:13] Man should serve GOD in spirit and in truth. [St. John 4:23-24]

The other thing that possibly made me change my behavior sexually is I spend a life in fasting   and praying since I emigrated. I made a promise to GOD if He should open the door for me to move to America, I would serve Him forever. Upon my arrival He reminded me of my vow and from that day to now, I keep trying to completely obey Him. The years I spent in fasting and prayer reduced my sexual craving.

I see people, especially today, do not have any true feelings for themselves and GOD. They just keep going along with the crowd. Such as when in Rome, we do as the Romans. This is a very poor example for people who teach greater advancement over other nations. We should be completely separate in all our teachings since we are so advanced.

Why does GOD place such strict punishment on humanity's involvement in women's uncleanness? Looking at the harsh punishment; it is death, it's got to have a very significant meaning to it that we have overlooked. We have not taught one another to fight hard to withhold ourselves from menstruation of a woman.

Because man was not instructed of the danger in sexual intercourse while a female is having their monthly cycle, we often in this era have sex without allowing the female to complete her uncleanness, and make sure she purified herself before we are involved sexually.

Adam and Eve were told not to eat of the tree in the middle of the garden. The day in which they touched or ate thereof they would die. Not seeing the danger in touching and eating, they partook of the fruit and many died because of their disobedience to GOD. All my life, as I journey, I am awakened and made aware that we were not completely shown all the dangers in things created by man. Failing to see the danger within man's creation, many people over the years die because of the oversight.

It is the same thing with man and many things given to us by GOD. Because He has not given us all things with complete instructions, we head into many things that bring pain, death, and unhappiness to millions yearly. We need to understand that man sometimes just simply needs to take things as they were given to him without great details.

Obedience goes a very long way. It speaks not only of things pertaining only to GOD, but also man's behavior with man's laws. Yearly we find hundreds or thousands of men and women all over the world who suffer incarceration. It is not the law that is unfair to the individuals when they are incarcerated. It's their disobedience they are being punished for.

In every country or Island, one can find laws given to control the occupants therein. Whether a visitor or citizen, it matters not. All need to heed the laws of the land. Being lawless will bring punishment either by death or incarceration. Justice in the laws of a country should never have partiality, for the rich, poor, or the middle class.

Disobedience is not only found in the poor and the middle class. We can find the same in rich or poor, black or white. Whatever race or color there is, we can find the same sinful behavior everywhere. A person that constantly disregards the laws of GOD will also disregard

221

the laws of men. Not being brought up in the fear and knowledge of GOD, man just keeps being lawless forever.

In the beginning, just as GOD did not show Adam and Eve the sin of death was the consequence for disobeying GOD'S commandments, it is the same we find with sexual involvement with a woman when she is on the rag, as many people call her uncleanness these days. All they knew was only the expression of words; they never fully understood death not seeing anyone die physically. All we know is not to have sexual intercourse with a woman when she is unclean. We were not taught the danger or deadliness.

The unchaste behavior found in humanity today, in the world we call advanced, has become profligate and preposterous. Looking at many parts of the world, we call uncivilized or undeveloped, we can find a better restraint in their lifestyle. People that live in the developed countries and Islands have all kinds of unrestrained people that live with bitterness, envy, and anger all the time.

All the ones that remain in the undeveloped world, even though they live naked, they have not over populated their areas. Crime is less and rape is not found in their communities. Their lives seem to be much more harmonious than the developed areas of the world. They do not have a judge or a police department to constantly harass innocent or guilty people.

Life should be much more pleasant for the ones who state they are more intelligent than the ones that remain in ancient times. To me, the people who lived as ancient people showed more understanding of the things of GOD. Even though they lived in nakedness shows they did not understand that sin required man and woman to cover their nakedness.

In their poverty they remained composed. We, in our wealth and advancement, are unhappy all the days of our lives. We live lawless to death because we are lovers of money and perishable paraphernalia. We kill and hate each other. Many behave superior and treat others inferior. Some make a distinction with blacks and white or other ethnic groups.

The behavior of humanity is so difficult to understand. Why is it so hard for a person to live caring for others? Selfishness is killing millions of people all over the world. As the population increases daily we behave more profligate and cantankerous.

Since the knowledge of sexual intercourse with a woman having her monthly issues was not written about as an educational teaching, we fail to understand the danger it brings in the conception of a baby.

It normally takes seven days for a woman's issues to be completed. Why does it require another seven days, and the eighth day set for purification? Man teaches us that a woman can conceive within three days after ending of her menstruation. Yet, we find that GOD required them to be still unclean another seven days, and the eight-day was for them to purify themselves. On the eight day they could start to have sexual intercourse once more. Leviticus 15:28-30

Under a guideline such as that, a man and a woman were not capable of having a lot of sexual indulgence each month. A man and a woman would only be able to have lots of sex each month, when a woman is pregnant.

Let us analyze the body of a woman. Say there are roughly thirty days in a month. Fourteen of them require a woman to be separated from all of her activities as unclean. All things that she sleeps on or touches are counted to be unclean. All who touch anything she touches are also counted unclean. They are supposed to wash themselves and be unclean until the evening. The other thing is this; if a woman does not conceive within the first week or so, her fertility egg will start to change to waste.

Our Bible did show and teach that when a woman did not conceive, and her unfertile egg starts to change to waste, that it was unclean for sexual act. It was only when she started bleeding by issues that it became sin by death. Is it only because of the waste done to man's copulation liquid? In the Bible, it required washing, if by accident, a man's copulation juice got on the material they are using to lay on having sex.

I know that having sex is wonderful. That could be the main reason why early man, resorted to many wives as the population increased. Possible they could not stand to only have sex with their partner say seven, ten, or twelve days out of each month. The other thing that was possible, women must have been in greater abundance than men. Under such circumstances a man needed to have more than one woman as his. Otherwise, many of the ladies would return back to GOD as they came: a virgin. The other thing could be women were so beautiful and so attractive men just could not resist, they had to have more than one. Did early men know of the unclean sexual act, if they did it was not left as a legacy in teaching?

Early calendars had only twenty eight days. Every four years or so there would be thirteen months in a year. Man was the one who made twelve months in the year, so as to have the calendar we use today. We have months with thirty one, thirty, or twenty eight days. In a twenty eight day calendar, a man would only have approximately seven days or less of sex with his partner each month, if only thinking of conception, and not only for pleasure. The only time a man and a woman could have a lot of sexual intercourse was in her pregnancy.

When a woman is pregnant, a person can have sex with her all the time, day in and day out, without worrying about uncleanness. I understand that a woman wants sex more in her pregnancy and likewise in her uncleanness.

Understanding the stage of development with a woman's fertility, a person can always produce healthy babies. Allowing the woman eight more days for her egg and the blood to correlate at the precise moment will develop much more strength. When the egg is penetrated with the man' sperm, it can make a much stronger child in conception. In the early stage of a woman's ending cycle of her monthly issue, her egg and her blood do not completely develop to bring forth a healthy baby. Just as when her time is coming to start her issue, it becomes much weaker and weaker until it becomes waste matter.

Just as man teaches that a woman is fertile within days of her ending cycle, they also teach that a woman is also fertile within days of the start of her monthly period. With today's technology, mankind behaves ignorantly in many things. The fault is not with the created apparatus. It is what we do with them by making them be our controller in our life. Humanity should have been the controller of their lives.

We gave that away to live much worse than the animals that were not created like GOD. Man was created in the image and likeness of GOD, to be like GOD and rule like GOD over his own world, and constantly increase his population as a procreator. We have offspring by copulation as ordained by GOD to enjoy each other's relationship. GOD could have made us like the angels. We would not have had such sweet enjoyment with each other. We have not appreciated the wonderful things given to us by GOD. We simply abuse the wonderful things given to us by GOD.

The reason for all the various diseases that is lingering in the life of men and women today; we all have taken the laws of GOD as nothing. Because from the beginning what would have developed when copulating with a woman in her uncompleted cycle, we continue that unhealthy life style from one generation to the next creating all kind of unhealthiness. **What we have overlooked or taken for granted, is GOD created humans and He knows what is prosperous for humanity. People do not know in truth what is really healthy for people, but GOD knows.**

99.9 percent of the men and the women who keep making the statements, they are serving GOD, never receive the knowledge to teach the world all the unhealthy deadly things they are doing to themselves. The appropriate time was not yet come that we might all see and understand the evil things we have been doing to one another.

Each time a woman conceives a child in her early stage, she is subject to carry an unhealthy child. Because her transformation was not completely developed, not because she produces a fresh supply, that makes it instant for fertilization. It needs a few days to come to full strength so that the conception will bring happiness and joy at the time of birth. Immature joining will always produce unhealthy children. The lack of patience of males' and females' sexuality will bring kids into this world that will end up with one or more of the many diseases that are plaguing humanity all their lives.

Conception within the fourteen days of any woman's uncleanness will forever produce unhealthy kids with various ailments. This will bring sickness or death to the individuals at all times. Avoiding a woman when she is in menstruation can produce a healthy, beautiful child. I am not saying that all kids are not beautiful; a healthy child brings a lot more joy to the procreator. In the long run, it will be less costly to mom and dad. I do not care how much we can confess that we are genuinely in love with our kids. When they have all kinds of diseases the love is not the same. We do love our kids, especially when they are obedient children.

I know that many parents love their children although they might be ill in many ways. Still we have to all agree that parents will show much better appreciation when their children are much healthier. Having kids with good health does allow the procreator to do a lot more for themselves and their children.

Unclean Sexual Acts

Chapter (14)

In man's love for sexuality in this dispensation, he created many gadgets to keep people occupied all the days of their lives sexually. I know that we were created to enjoy one another sexually and in all things not just in sex. A very good relationship is not only about sex. Loving as we only apply sex to the word is incorrect. Sex should be part of one's relationship. It is not all. We can find many people all over the world sexually involved with one another. It has nothing to do with love. It's done either for lust, craving, or they are whores selling their bodies for money.

When a person becomes a prostitute, they do not have sex for companionship. That game is money. Men who seek those women do not seek a lasting relationship. They just need a quick fix and nothing else.

We have men and women who have an extra companion. The purpose for an extra companion is to fulfill their sexual appetite. Men have their mistresses, and women have their gigolos. Lots of women have a great sexual appetite and they are very difficult to satisfy. I know they crave sex as much as men. There are many reasons why some men are more difficult to satisfy and they need to have a lot of women daily. We can find the same in many women who are unsatisfied with a little sex here and there from a husband who is not as active as she is. Vice versa with men as it is with women.

In a world where men and women's sexual behavior is not for love, in most cases it brings children into this world that is not wanted. The children come and behave as they were treated. The trend continues generation after generation.

Humans all have to agree that sexual acts are pleasant. It is something normal people enjoy a lot. Many are unable to control their sexual appetite. Look at all the contamination there is in the world today caused by sexual encounters. Regardless of all the diseases men and women can contract, it has not deterred many. Man has made a covering for himself that he can keep right on enjoying himself with what he craves.

I am not objecting to people's fulfillment in their pleasure seeking. The thing I have to say is millions suffer yearly because of the pleasure some men and women love so much. Lots of kids born yearly have never seen a father. Some never knew their birth mother. They end up with parents who were not by birth. Sometimes they obtain much better parents than their procreator. The reason why so many kids are born that way is that we never go there for kids. Most of us go there for our own satisfaction and kids come along later.

I am not excluded in this behavior. Just because I am writing does not make me a person who has not behaved as the trend of most human comport. I am as guilty as others who chase women all over the place and make kids that were not planned for.

I had two kids with two different women, as far as I know. Only two told me or related that I am the father of their child. These two ladies got pregnant because I was getting a quickie from them. Since the place was not convenient for a pleasurable time, one was more or less hiding so that we would not get caught by the girl's parents. We were not husband and wife or boyfriend and girlfriend living together. We stole a piece here and there, thinking we could hide what we were doing without protection.

I got in trouble with two girls because of unprotected sexual acts, because I was only thinking of myself. I am a person that does not believe in wearing any protective covering. I could not stand my tool being choked to death. I did not have lasting stamina choking my tool to death. So I used it once, never again.

This came to my understanding many years later, when the LORD opened my eyes about sexual contact with women not being purified in the days given them after the issuing of their fountain. I was not taught by men or women that a woman can produce unhealthy kids not having their transformation fully developed. Until I was shown what transpired with early conception, I was ignorant of what causes so much poor health in the life of humanity.

Men and women who seek their profession in the field of research with medicine, to study and practice with mankind, have no understanding what causes most ailments in people. The responsible individuals who inform us daily with their prognosis, are still in the dark solving most of humanity's unhealthy dilemmas.

I was one of the guilty people who was not aware of the danger with men and women having sex when a woman did not wait for the days given to make herself clean. Man failed both GOD and man in this instruction, because he was not shown the complete problem that would always be in the life of people if they have sex with women being unclean.

There are many men and women who are guilty of sexual conduct with women who are not purified. To my knowledge it is still unknown to the majority of the world population. Neither did any one teach us GOD required death to all that allowed anyone to uncover a woman's nakedness when she was unclean. It was not only the man who would lose his life, it was both that would lose their lives.

GOD never handed down this teaching to the vast population of the world as incorrect and unacceptable by Him. Not knowing GOD'S requirement, we simply live very carelessly without any knowledge of what GOD required of all nations of the world. Not because unclean sexual acts were handed down to the children of Israel as death by contact, does not give the other nations the right to sin against their soul, and damn them in the lake of fire.

Israel should have been the nation that taught us the right pathway to take so that we can please GOD by walking in his commandments. The rejection of GOD by Israel, caused many other nations to continue being reckless in their behavior to both GOD and man. Because Israel was not faithful to the laws of GOD, they could not teach the other nations the way we should walk circumspect with GOD and man.

Israel's transgression, and disobedience of the laws given them by GOD, removed from all the nations of the world things that would keep many sicknesses from the world's population. Take for instance the instruction given that man and woman should have completely separated themselves from each other during the woman's unclean days.

Israel did not comply with the commandments handed to them so that they could be the head of the world in all things. They should have been the ones who showed the world that there is really a GOD that created this world and all things therein. Instead, they wanted to be like the people that GOD commanded them not to be like. All the things that GOD abhorred of other nations, Israel should have abhorred as they were instructed to. They fell in love with these things. What was commanded of them they should have done to remove ailments from them and all the other people of the world, they ignored. Leviticus 20:23. See Exodus 23:24-33

The thing we have not noticed with the children of Israel is the curse that was upon them. It caused them to scatter all over the world, and it bringing to all the other nations the same curse that would follow Israel being in rebellion to GOD. GOD made a promise with Abraham that all the nations that would bless him and his seed would likewise be blessed. All the nations that cursed him would likewise be cursed. Genesee 12:2&3.

Israel's sins caused them to be dispersed to all the nations of the world. They would be treated shamefully, with no respect and would end up bringing a curse on the nations where they dwelt. If Israel had remained in complete obedience to the commandments handed down to them, all the other nations of the world would listen to Israel. Great health and wealth they would always have within their population. Deuteronomy 28:64&65 1Kings 14:15 Jeremiah 31:10 50:6&17

To this date, many nations of the world have some kind of ill feelings towards the children of Israel. By now, the nation of Israel should not be angry with any person for the feelings of hatred they have in their heart against the Hebrews. Israel is the nation known as the chosen of GOD. GOD gave to them his laws and his statues that they should live by and teach all the other nations what said the LORD.

I see where man loves to listen to man, and the things of GOD we ignore as valueless. Possibly because man has not seen GOD, we might feel we should be left alone to do as we please without anyone having to be head over us. Man is a creature who is very difficult to understand. All the things that are suppose to be good and very healthy for man we sweep them under the rug as nothing. The things that are very bad for us, we embrace them all the time, regardless of the plagues they bring to humanity.

I am not picking on any people or nation. I am only trying to relate to humanity where we made the wrong turn at the crossroad. We should not have turned when we stood in the middle. We should have continued on the straight course we started. By stopping we failed to have impetus. Looking around brought us to a place where we questioned GOD'S authority and proceeded to be rebellious.

The rebellion found in humanity, from early development, continues to inhabit or occupy our mind, life, and everything we put our hands to do. Looking at the choices we have made all our lives, I see an evil power that harbors over mankind, with no feelings or compassion.

The evil force has become more cantankerous in this era. It looks worse than in any other generation in the past. It also seems like man behaves as if the only true loving compassionate GOD is dead and there is no more need for a person to live moral anymore. Morals seem to be a thing of the past, possibly because there is so much wealth in every developed country and Island in the world today.

I also notice that we behave like someday man might be able to create something so powerful that we might be able to place GOD in a prison where He might have to turn to man for help. This world pleasure sure has man behaving irreverent to the One that is responsible for creating us.

Israel should have separated themselves from other people, as GOD commanded them. I am in agreement with that, for this reason. If the nation of Israel did remain faithful to GOD'S commandments, they would never be abhorred by any people or nations. They would be the ones to teach the world the truth, and honesty that is pleasing to GOD. Therefore, the blessings of GOD upon them would also follow all the nations of the world. I know that many people love to have what they see other people have and what they think is outstanding.

I know that if all the children of Israel did keep all the commandments and the statutes handed down to them by GOD, and there was no sickness with them, I am positive millions would live at their doorsteps looking for the answer that they too would be able to live a sick free life. With all the ailments there are in people and nations, if one nation was able to be sick free, then the rest of the nations would want to find out why there are no illnesses with them.

I am positive if Israel was able to maintain the standard given to them by GOD, the world would be able to stay healthy by living as they live and walking as they walk. When the people who were suppose to be servants of GOD walk as the devil's servants, they give up GOD to serve the devil. GOD will never have sin occupy his kingdom. If we want the blessings of GOD to follow us all the days of our lives, we better walk as he commanded us.

In this dispensation of grace, many of the commandments in the Old Testament are ignored. We say they are not for today's people. We simply just think and say only the ten written with the finger of GOD, on two tables of stones, are important. All the others we place in the trash can or cast them into an incinerator and burn them. If the children of Israel did not count themselves unworthy, and did look at the choice made by GOD, that they would be a peculiar people above all the other nations of the world, and keep what was committed to them, they would not have suffered so much persecution from so many other nations. Exodus19:5. Deuteronomy 7:6-8, 10:15, 14:2,

What Israel and other nations possibly overlooked all these years was the type of food that was handed to them by GOD. It had to be the healthiest diet given to humanity. It was not only eating that was given to Israel. All things were given in the proper order that if they did obey all things handed down to them by GOD, they would be the example that all other nations would follow. Israel was not appreciative to GOD for the things He gave them. They wanted to be like the gentile nations that walked in sin and godlessness.

Israel should have been the head of the world to teach us the way of GOD more perfectly. They did not retain the LORD in their knowledge because they might feel that the gentile people might have had things much more abundantly. They seemed to be enjoying life to its fullness.

The nations that were not taught the statutes of GOD, they eat all the time. They never gave their systems any rest or a day off. The gentile people were not instructed to fast as was Israel. They were not instructed to abstain from a woman's menstruation for fourteen days. In those days she was counted as unclean and anything she touched while her uncleanness was upon her it was counted to be unclean. Sexual acts were forbidden by GOD within those days.

When a man or a woman would interact in the woman's uncleanness both party's lives would be eradicated.

Since the nation of Israel disobeyed GOD, all nations of the earth suffered for their transgressions. Since sin was their controller, they were not able to teach others the acceptable ways that are pleasing to GOD. Therefore all nations kept sinning against GOD. And, because the leaders saw only one sided and did not care for anyone else, they never lived up to the things commanded by GOD.

Mankind within their life on this planet seems to hate great criticism. We love when others speak highly of us. Man loves the praise of man over GOD'S exultation. Man's elevation only brings death. When GOD speaks highly of us, as say blessings, no one can change the blessings of GOD, but GOD himself.

This is what transpires in man's life today. We place such great confidence in one another. The one we should place our all with we leave at the side of the road. Man loves when another man speaks highly of them. It's as if to say we hate when another person says we are ignorant in the things we do. This could be the reason why so many of us refuse to walk in the complete commandments handed down to us by GOD.

Man does not like to feel that he is not pleasing to others. We often ignore the things of GOD, so that we can obtain self gratification with one another.

The nation of Israel's blessings should be able to bless them and all the other nations of the world. The curse of Israel also brings a curse to all the other nations likewise. GOD wanted one nation to stand holy as an example to all the others in the world. Through their faithfulness to GOD, all the other nations would be able to seek the right pathway from the people who are serving their Creator in spirit and in truth.

What the seed of Abraham did was they ignored the instruction given to them by the GOD of their fathers. They proceeded to serve wood and stone, with gold and silver, and other man made objects, things that are capable of doing nothing. The things we serve are powerless. Man in his powerless state is very great. It is mind-boggling to see one's behavior in the things we adore and esteem.

Looking at how foolishly we walk daily shows we have to have some driving force over us that makes us live in ignorance all the days of our lives. A man would go and seek one of these items: a tree, gold, silver, brass, or some kind of substance that he can use to mold an image or a statue. It could be anything placed within his mind that he desires as his idol that he can pray to or worship.

Man does not see, and does not realize, he is very ignorant in his concept. He keeps doing the same thing generation after generation. We make something with the substance we either purchase or go and cut down in the forest. We carve or mold the substance in a replica of some kind of animal or man. We place it on a pedestal or somewhere we can daily render obeisance.

Our creations can never hear, see, or speak. It will never move from the location we place it. They need to be transported by someone. They are downright powerless. Yet we bow down before these man made figures looking with expectations for an answer to what they seek. It matters not what they are seeking. It is who and what we are praying to or asking by petition. By petitioning as we do, shows that man seems to always need to speak to some other power or source beyond man. It seems to show that man is not the final authority in the universe. There has to be some other greater power somewhere in this universe

We have not learned much over the years with all the things that befall man daily or yearly since we have developed to be a multitude of people. We might not physically create images today. In the dark ages man never knew or had electricity, and serving idols was prevalent. Yet, we can find man has created a modern day kind of idol that he serves. It might not be as it was in prayer, supplication, and offering on the altar of sacrifice, looking for answers for something needed. We can find a similar behavior with modern day living. People in their walking are in rebellion to GOD and his commandments.

Israel's rebellion to GOD did more harm to people generation after generation. Even in this era, we love to express ourselves as more civilized than all other people of this earth. We can speak and show the entire world the hardship the Israelites kept going through with other nations likewise. We cannot leave out any nation of the world. No matter where we go on this earth we can find all kinds of sickness and suffering.

All the suffering comes from our rejection of the statutes and commandments that were once given to the children of Abraham. The children of Abraham should have walked in the footsteps of their father Abraham in the laws handed down to them by GOD. Abraham, being called the friend of GOD, believed the things that were told to him by the Creator of heaven and earth. Abraham walked faithfully in the commandments given to him by GOD. All the nations of the world would have been blessed through Abraham.

Since Abraham was not able to live forever on this earth, his seed should carry on where he left off. Not interested in the promises made to them and their seed to come after them, they sought the way of the ungodly. It brings death and unhappiness in the life of all nations that do not serve the GOD that created this earth and all things therein.

What should take place with Abraham's seeds? They should always be a separate people from other nations. They should not feel they are superb or inferior in human form. The only thing that should make them different is their complete obedience to the commandments they received from GOD. That was enough to make them different so that they could teach other nations to be different in their lives as they walk this sinful world. The other nations possibly did not know all that was required by GOD.

The thing that might be possible is that many fathers and mothers never teach their children the ways of GOD. If from the day they could understand right from wrong, they could talk with their procreator they would start to learn about GOD words. We have millions of people all over the world who never teach their kids anything that pertains to the words of GOD. It was the same with the population before the flood. That could be the reason so many perished in the flood.

Man always seems to keep forgetting what is good for him and the things that are deadly. We keep doing this all the time. We always need someone to constantly correct us. Why is it so hard for man to always behave himself in a pleasant, moral way?

Take the ones that should have been the head over all the nations of the world. They too just could not maintain greatness that was given to them. Adam and Eve were the same. They were the first to give up their greatness for nothing. They turned aside, just as we, and walk as our father the devil.

Abraham's seed would have been blessed if they walked as Abraham walked. I see one thing that remains faithful with Israel that was given to Abraham. The commandment of circumcision has not departed from the children of Israel to this present day. They still hold fast to that commandment with great reverence. If Israel did maintain all of GOD'S commandments with high regards as they do with circumcision, they would have remained the leaders of the world. Not taking the others with high regard will cancel the purpose of circumcision.

Circumcision alone cannot bring harmony with GOD and man. It takes complete obedience in all things given to man by GOD. It was commanded that man and woman should never be sexually involved during the days of woman's uncleanness. Man has not placed much value with that commandment, as if to say it is not as important as circumcision. Each and every one should have the same value. We should not put any above the other. With GOD all are the same, even though they were given hundreds of years apart.

All the nations of the world, in each country or Island, place harsh punishment on people for laws that are broken in their country. We do not realize that they are the same laws given to man by GOD. Today, we do not see the need to maintain the laws that GOD gave for man tomorrow. We find the majority only feel that the Ten Commandments are the only ones needed to be kept. All the others are just there as figures of speech, because GOD could not find anything better to do with His time. So He gave us words simply for us to read, as if to say, humans should always be busy reading or doing something with their time.

Many individuals love to read books. Not because they seek knowledge or because they need to update themselves. They need to have some challenge at hand for some important venture. It has to do with the way they developed themselves when they were growing up. Not many individuals, after school days, end up loving to read. They read books, at school, only because it was part of their curriculum.

It is sad to say, that's the way it seems to be with the behavior of man when it comes to the things given to us by GOD. We read the Bible like it is just another book given only for making money. Once you read the Bible, you can place it in your book shelf or some other place for safe keeping, until some more convenient day.

What of today's people that claim to be a Christian? What do they receive from GOD? Israel would have been the head, because of the blessings that would follow them all the days of their lives, if they had kept the commandments of GOD handed to them by none other than GOD himself.

Christians today were likewise chosen to be the head of all the nations of the world. They would have been the example others should follow if they were obedient to GOD'S laws. Christians behave the same as Israel and therefore blaspheme GOD to the people that are non-Christians. This shows that humans are weak and will never be able to completely obey the laws of GOD.

Christians are given greater power than Israel. They should be able to heal the sick, cast out devils, and do greater things than Jesus did when he was alive on this earth. The people that claim that they are born again behave the same as the children of Israel. Israel sins within her heart. She is not right with GOD. Christians walk the same with their lips. Their hearts are far from GOD.

Christians cannot bless anyone because they are a curse. GOD is never going to make sin overpower him, even though we claim we are born again. We need to understand that GOD does not give the people who confess being born again, the power to sin and walk in rebellion to His laws. Israel suffered greatly because of her rebellion to the laws and commandments of GOD. The people of the grace dispensation rejected the laws of GOD in the same matter as Israel. GOD will never honor sin even though we confess we have received His true spirit.

We need to always remember that GOD sees our hearts. He does not see as man sees. We can always profess with our lips to man, but not to GOD. 1Samuel 16:7 1Chronicles 29:17 Jeremiah 11:20 20: 12

In this era with Jesus as LORD of our lives, we are counted on to be a peculiar people to GOD, just as it was stated about Israel. He did give to man, after His resurrection, much greater power. We

237

gave it away just as Israel. We have been giving lip service to GOD as they were doing. Titus 2:14, 1Peter 2:9.

It is the same with Adam and Eve. They had life in the beginning. They gave away the life for death. GOD came and died, that we might obtain once more the life that we lost. Man in his love for death despises life. He continually keeps walking in rebellion to GOD, to our own hurt.

The Cause of Human Pains and Sufferings

Chapter (15)

Man has a choice in life. It's up to us what we do in our choosing as we travel this life. I do realize that all need a teacher to educate them. For someone to indoctrinate another person they have to first have some kind of knowledge in the things they are teaching others. When a person lacks the knowledge needed to instruct others, he is going to teach a lot of lies.

In this era, I observe man's behavior as they speak proudly about themselves and lookdown on early civilizations as barbaric. Do our schools and universities improve our behavior over the people we call barbaric? We need to always understand that early people were the ones who first started some of the things we do to this very day. I know that man has always placed prostitution as the oldest profession on earth. I personally cannot accept that kind of teaching.

It's not likely that prostitution can be the oldest profession in existence. Farming is the one we should place as man's first laboring job {Genesee 2: 15} Procreator, if we can classify as a profession, is the next. We can possibly use metal forging as the next. Building of homes or making of clothing could be put before procreator. If there were only two beings on the earth at first, making coverings would have to be up there as first.

Prostitution should take a back seat in profession as the last of all occupations. Prostitution became a profession only because males are very much disrespectful to women. When men dishonor ladies, they treat them shamefully. Prostitution is a stigmatized way of putting women as cheap. When a man has high regards for ladies, he would not treat a woman as a prostitute; they could be part of his family, like sisters or near of kin.

The other thing that could cause prostitution to be in the world today is, women always seem to be in the majority, and men are the minority. That could be the reason why prostitution is so popular within our society globally. I see no stopping of that kind of behavior in the world today. Women's ratio to men is on the increase seven to one. They too need comfort likewise in their life. That could be the reason why early women resorted to prostitution. They could have the sexual relations they needed and at the same time be able to support themselves in a comfortable way.

The things we also have to understand are that women are just as dishonorable to their own bodies. Why do they allow men to sexually mistreat them that way? And if a woman does not agree to sell her body for a few dollars, or something to appease as exchange for sex, the person that would like to have sex with her would have to rape the female. I do realize that a woman needs sexual intercourse just like a man. I get to understand that many parts of a woman can show when they are aroused sexually. Man only has one visible part. I know that sometimes you can have an erection and it is not necessarily, that you are sexually aroused.

We should not cast all the blame on the males for uncovering a woman's fountain to have sex with them, since it was a commandment of death. Being uneducated in many things brings heartaches and pain most of the time into human life. Who should we blame for our misconduct when men and women have sexual intercourse when a woman is unclean in her monthly cycle? That's why both parties were supposed to be executed without mercy. The thing that is very hard to understand: why would someone relate to anyone that they uncovered a woman's fountain and had sex with her?

With sexual behavior the way it is prevalent, with both parties involved when a woman still remains unclean, shows man lacks great understanding in many important things on this earth. We constantly say we are more advanced than all the previous generations, not only in technology but in education as well. Regardless of the entire claim we keep making, we still lack knowledge in the most important things there are. The wisdom, knowledge, and understanding we have obtained in this era are folly. It brings nothing more than death.

We have not advanced in the things that bring life, our educators with their tickets, feel they have advance so much in knowledge, that there is no more need to embrace GOD. We leave the Creator out of everything we do as if to say man is God, and there is no supreme being.

By not applying the laws handed down to man by GOD, we then become subjects to our enemy. Subjected to the devil, we obey his every command. We might not accept that we are being controlled by our enemy. The reason many might think that way, is they might not be riotous, because they live more honorable to all the laws of the land. They don't believe that the laws that man uses to govern all came from GOD.

People fail to understand that man's laws and GOD'S laws are completely different. The laws of man govern man with things pertaining to this earth only. The laws handed down to man by GOD have to do with life after death. On the other hand, if we would completely obey all the commandments given to us by GOD, we could live a more pleasant life on this earth in everything we do. Our health would be significantly better. Men and women would not be involved in unclean sexual acts.

The reason many of us keep having unclean sex, we have become a degenerated people all over the world. Technology has become very influential because we are in love with money and not people. Fighting for great wealth we promote evil. That makes us behave more and more immoral.

In our immoral conduct, life brings all kinds of ailments. Man has not retained GOD in his knowledge. When diseases develop in humans, we quickly seek help from man for his medication to comfort. Man fails to keep the commandments of our Creator. He goes about trying to prove his knowledge surpasses every other generation. He places GOD as nothing in his vocabulary, thereby bringing upon himself more and more diseases.

Many people that obtain their tickets from universities feel they have surpassed the laws of GOD. The things pertaining to life, they remove from theirs. If they do believe, they do not see the need of applying their life as required by Him. Many feel that at the point of death they can obtain forgiveness. Therefore, it does not matter how they live. GOD is not going to cast anyone into the lake of fire. It is the Devil and all the angels he has working with him that will be cast into the lake of fire.

Until recently I was ignorant in many things most of my life. Not knowing the error there, I did many wrong things in life just like millions all over the world who are not knowledgeable as I was. We should not be angry with anyone at this junction. I guess nothing happens before the time.

I became a little perturbed when I was awakened to many things that have been hidden from the population of the world all these years. I am not just speaking of today's generation; I am dating it back to early man on this earth.

I know the Bible teaches that "wisdom excelleth folly as far as light excelleth darkness". The reason why I became perturbed had to do with sharing the knowledge I have obtained with the world. After I was instructed to remain calm, I relaxed and maintained my composure as if I never obtained anything. At that moment I really understood the truth of the verse in the Bible that relates to us, that "wisdom does truly excelleth folly". Ecclesiastes 2:13

I apply myself to remain calm until the appropriate time comes for me to impart to the world the things that have been kept secret since the creation of humanity. Being over zealous, to learn of things never taught by anyone before or never imparted before in books or any manuscripts, can be a problem. Being impatient almost became a very bad thing in me. Most of the time more harm has been done to others being impatient.

As I maintain my composure, I realize that many will turn up their nose and plug their ears to the things I will impart in this book or the near future. Man can only teach others of the things he knows. Teaching by guessing only brings confusion and controversy. There is already too much confusion and controversy in this world. We need to try and reduce it a lot. Life is too short for us to remain being in topsy-turvy.

I have made a lot of mistakes in my life. I realize that a few people suffered for my ignorance. Looking back at the things I did wrong, they all could have been avoided if I was taught the right way to go about what I was doing. Oftentimes I hear people say that nescience never gave us any excuses for wrongdoing. We have hundreds or thousands of people yearly suffering incarceration for committing some kind of crime ignorantly. Many might be knowledgeable of the crime they committed and used nescience as an alibi to not receive any punishment for the wrong they committed.

What I am trying to do is to show some of the things that I have done that were wrong that I did in ignorance. There can be reasons why I was behaving the way I was. I was not taught or shown the correct way to go about the things I was doing. At one point I was instructed to always find whores when I needed to have sex with a woman. I was told that I should never get married. There are lots of prostitutes I could find to relieve myself when so desired.

I never thought that was not a very good thing for a person to relate to anyone, whether from a friend or an enemy. That kind of advice is even worse from one's procreator. I was never taught that a person should not have sexual intercourse with a woman when they are seeing their monthly issues. Not knowing better and loving sex as I did, going from city to city, I looked for beautiful ladies or girls to have sex with. I never knew right from wrong.

I had sex with young and old women in all kinds of locations. I spent hour after hour with them. I had married and unmarried, ones that had boyfriends and some that did not have any boyfriends. I never knew better, so I did have a few that were bloody in their uncleanness.

I never knew better and I never did what was right then. In my ignorance I hurt a few people. As I say I just recently awakened to many evil things that I did. Millions walk as I did. They are the cause, as I am, for many unhealthy kids in this world today.

Of the women I chased, two related that I am the father of their baby. Man has to take the ladies word. They know much more than the man. They are the ones who germinate. Men just ejaculate then go about their business. Once, I can recall, I had sex and I know that person got pregnant there and then. There was something that happened then, that made me aware that person got pregnant that very moment. She had a miscarriage and lost the baby. I never once had another experience like that one.

What I am trying to show the world is that both ladies that called me the father of their child, this is what took place. We did not know right from wrong; the place was inconvenient and we could not relax and enjoy ourselves. We were just hiding so that we would not get caught. So we were just getting a quickie piece. We talked to meet and hide that no one would know what we were doing. The thing was this: these women just finished their first seven days. It was about three days after they stopped their issue. They never completed the other seven days for purification. I had sex with these two ladies and they got pregnant. One is a few years older than the other. Still they had an early conception.

The first was a boy, the second is a girl. The boy was born at home by a midwife. The girl was born at a hospital. I was not there for their births. This I know and I can relate what happened because I am awakening to many people's cause of illness. We can work much harder from now on to prevent many illnesses.

What happened was this: each child at birth had a lot of problems. The boy almost died; with many ailments. At one time he would not take his mother's breast milk. She became sick. She had to pump her breasts. I can recall I would give the baby a helping hand by sucking on her breast so that she would not be in pain. It never bothered me. It was not pleasant to see her in pain and her breasts kept enlarging daily, only because the baby was sick and was unable to eat what was there for him to eat.

Poverty has its advantages and disadvantages, which is good and bad. In our poorness, the child was not able to get proper care the way the educators taught. What I found out was not everything our educators teach is correct. Sometimes ignorance pays off.

Being ignorant of many things taught by our educators has good and bad effects. The woman and I were not informed about inoculations for infants. Not knowledgeable with the procedures, we never had our son inoculated until he emigrated. The only reason we allowed him to receive that treatment was they would not allow him to attend school. If I was able back then to stop it, I would have.

When a person lives and walks in nescience, it makes someone in the end become very violent. In many cases some people lost their lives. Not everyone is able to hold their composure when they are forced to do things they do not want to.

The number two child's mother was more educated than me and the woman who had number one child. I was not living in Jamaica when the second kid was born. I emigrated before the child was born. I never spent anytime in nurturing her. I spent more time with the first child when I lived in Jamaica before I emigrated. When he joined me in America we had a great life.

The girl's mother did all the inoculations starting from when the child was an infant. I cannot speak about the girl's upbringing as much as I can of the boy. I was with the first from a baby to this date. I can relate about most of his problems. The girl I learned bits and pieces here and there.

Remember these two kids were conceived when the women did not end their period of uncleanness, which required fourteen days. They only had about ten days in their cycles. The Bible gave the women fourteen days for separation. During the fourteen days she was unclean, sex was prohibited. Death was the punishment for sexual involvement when both parties had sexual intercourse in the days of uncleanness.

The question that plagues my mind: if death was the punishment for sexual involvement when a woman was seeing her fountain, why would someone make it known, what he and his wife did in their bed, knowing that they would lose their life in the end? The question is this: how would it be known that two people were sexually involved during days of a woman's issue? We understand that fornication, and adultery was a sin of death, if Israel was being true to the laws of GOD.

If by chance I was the one that did sexual acts with my wife or girl friend, knowing what was wrong in the days it was death by contact, why would I publish the wrong I did? Is there more to GOD making things known to the population when we are in disobedience to him? Men are creatures void of so much understanding. Are we really void of understanding, or is it because we are of our father the Devil? What is it in truth with humanity why we behave the way we do?

I see we cannot get away with our wrong doing all the days of our life. I know that the Bible teaches us that the father will never bear the burden of their children; neither will the children bear any of his procreator's sin. Every tub will have to sit on its own bottom.

On the other hand, we have children suffering because of the parent's sins. The sin of disobedience in sexual conduct brings all kinds of sickness on children that have nothing to do with the kids. Children did not ask to come into this world. I know that we have to increase the population. That does not give us the right to produce unhealthy babies. We should be more considerate in our procreating responsibility and not satisfy our own sexual craving.

The thing that happens over and over, most of us copulate for self-gratification. The next thing we learn the oven is baking; a baby is on the way.

The girl's mother followed her educated background and allowed the infant to be immunized. I understand that the child had lots of problems in her infant stage. Just as our son, who is our first born; he too had lots of problems. Many times he would not eat. His mother had trouble continually with fever because the baby would not suck her breast. She would produce so much milk. I was the one that gave her a helping hand getting rid of the milk when it was too much for all the children that she had.

Her first child was the only one that had so many problems at birth. I know that it is a normal thing for babies to have colds and other normal everyday complications. When illnesses are out of the ordinary, then it is a different story.

That was the case with the first two kids given to me. One was immunized in her infant stage. The other was five when he first received any inoculation. Today he is doing great health-wise. The only problem he has relates to the injuries he obtained from school when he played football. He constantly keeps re-injuring himself all the time. He loves to play all the time, not thinking about what his future will be like if he keeps on re-injuring himself all the time. That is the only problem he has, other than getting the normal winter ailments.

The girl, on the other hand, has all kinds of problems. It is very sad to say this, but being very intelligent sometimes seems to hurt us in the long run. The reasons why I am speaking this way, the person I married was not as educated in the teachings of men. We would be counted as illiterates.

What I am saying, because we were not educated with the importance of immunizing, we never had our first child immunized until we were forced to. Otherwise, he would never be accepted in schools in America. We, being ignorant, once more went along with man's regulation, and allowed him to be immunized. I saw him have many of the ailments that he was inoculated against.

My daughter's complications started, I understand, from when she was a little child. She constantly kept having kidney trouble. The organ that pumps her blood has given her all kinds of problems all her life. Man cannot rectify any of her conditions. Physicians keep on telling her that it is hereditary.

When we do not understand, we simply refuse to speak the truth. The reason why we find it so hard to speak the truth is that the source is above our heads. Instead of letting others know that we do not know, we often use heredity to cover our lack of knowledge.

Listening to our educators most of my life, I never knew any better, so I always went along with their teaching at hand. Now that I know better, I keep trying to educate others with the truth. It has become very difficult to open the eyes of today's people. We look to the ones that obtained their tickets from higher learning, and believe they are outstanding educationally, and they are the only people we should listen to.

The other thing I see and understand is we withdrew ourselves from GOD. He is responsible for creation. We turned to the one that hates us and he keeps on making things more and more difficult for us. We just love that guy much more than we love the One that truly loves us.

These two kids that came from two different women were conceived within ten days of the woman's issues. They were still in their unclean stage; I know that for a fact. It was brought to my attention when I received the understanding from GOD of what happens to kids when they are conceived in the stage of uncleanness. I never knew anything of the kind. Neither have I heard anyone on this earth teach us that children can be born with all kinds of ailments because of undeveloped eggs. Because their organs were not developed correctly, they suffered more when they are immunized.

What I never knew was this. When an unfertilized egg is produced each month at the end of a woman's cycle, it needs to develop strength to bring a baby that will be able to grow within the mother with healthy organs. When a baby is born with unhealthy organs, their bad organs can change, if given the right environment, they can over the years remove the unhealthy organ by slowly changing the bad to good.

When we immunize babies, not knowing the total condition of the infants, we expose these children to many health problems in their life to come. Man has been playing God for a very long time. We never stop to think and ask GOD why we keep having the problems in each generation. We feel that we can keep looking for answers with the little knowledge imparted to us by GOD. We can turn our backs on GOD because we have so many gadgets invented by man, which are used daily to open our understanding. We now feel we surpassed GOD, and GOD is not needed anymore.

Man is a creature that keeps on being irreverent to the One that loves and cares for Him all the time. If He never loved us, He would not open someone's understanding and show where people have been going wrong. He could close His eyes, stop His ears, and remove His heart from us. He would not see, hear, or have any feelings towards humanity for their ignorance. He is not like that. He loves us still.

God is very merciful towards humanity. He does have a loving, compassionate heart for humanity. We are the ones that refuse to have any true feelings towards Him.

Bringing to remembrance more than thirty years of my past, He showed me what I had done wrong, so that I might open the eyes of men and women. Then they will not remain in a pattern of disobedience in the future.

In my ignorance I behaved irreverently to the laws of GOD. In turn this produced two kids that had a very hard infant life. One continues to suffer all of her life with various ailments. At the present she has not received any comfort from the physicians in either country that she lived in so far.

The oldest child was never given any immunizations in his infant days. He was five when given his first. His system was able to develop much stronger, so that his weak organs at birth were able to develop much healthier than his sister's.

In a manner of speaking this calamity, ignorance, or simply not being aware of what was being taught, became more intellectual in the end. Men that feel they are capable of eradicating illnesses by inoculating infants should make sure a baby and their organs are in perfect health before injecting them with a virus to create an antibody.

One thing we might have overlooked in the past is that with many of the various ailments that once caused many deaths and made men develop these antibody inoculations to reduce many of the viruses, did not affect every person. I never had chickenpox when I was young or anytime in my life. I was exposed to chickenpox all my life and was never contaminated. My sisters had it. My step brothers and many people I have been around had it. My last child had it when she was only three months old.

I was so hurt for her that I put her to sleep on my stomach day and night. I was told if I got contaminated at my age with chickenpox, it would kill me. I can recall I would eat after my sisters and everyone in our home when they had chickenpox. They would give them the best to eat. They never had a good appetite being sick. I would be there to help eat what they did not.

What I am trying to say is this: I recently obtained the cause of many illnesses that occupy humans today. They make the life of the people they occupy very unhappy. The men and women, who dedicated their lives to research looking for an answer to help the sick and afflicted, have been having a very difficult time finding cures for these ailments.

At one time, I believed just about all things scientists and physicians taught about the body. They are the ones who study the body. Since it is a long process to learn the body, it takes someone very intellectual to learn about the human body.

I do realize all the pain and suffering we humans go through. All can be avoided by being more considerate of others and controlling our craving for many things we crave for now. By restraining one's appetite in every area, a person can help himself and others to become very healthy.

When we allow our appetite to overpower us we bring destruction not on ourselves only but also on our neighbors, friends and our family.

Is it possible for us to create a healthy population at anytime in the course of human existence? What is it we need to do: have more understanding one towards another? Do we think if we can control our appetites it might be possible for us to have a healthy population globally?

The appetite of a person does not speak only of eating or drinking. A person's appetite is vast. The uncontrolled craving for whatever one craves can be a person's appetite. Man's behavior today needs to turn around three hundred and sixty degrees. We live our lives as if to say there is no tomorrow, that making preparation for the life to come is not necessary.

In my observations, I can be dead wrong. Still I can be right. Our appetites make us become evil. In our evil nature, we fail to love one another by the commandments handed down to man. We are so much in love with vanity and not people. The things that we love value little and last only for a while.

One thing I see that wastes millions of people's lives, and causes many to live as they are today, is that we were not brought up correctly in our childhood days. Too many procreators allow their appetites to overpower them. They leave their children to be self parented or work their children too hard. Many children learn to hate their parents. Many would kill theirs if they could get away with murder.

I know that my daughter had to feel some kind of rejection when she was much younger, knowing that her father had nothing to do with her. My daughter grew up without a dad. It had to do with my own foolish appetite and uncontrolled behavior of selfishness. My foolish way of thinking could have made this child hate me forever. In-spite of my neglect, she remains a sweet loving person towards me.

Every child born in this world should have a mom and a dad there to nurture and mold them in a perfect way that we can have a wonderful world to live in. It is not a pleasant life when children have to live without proper nurturing. I know that it is very difficult for many adults living in this world. The way things are it only seems that it is going to become much more difficult.

The Body's Potentiality

Chapter (16)

If we can address the body of humans as a machine, we can address it as one of the greatest pieces of machinery ever created. Nothing on this earth is in its class, regardless of all the doctrines or studies man does with animals stating that they are in proximity with humans.

Regardless of the teaching that animals and humans are coherent, animals are not as complex as humans. In application of living and multiplying, both animals and humans develop by the same process. Having a similar behavior, both eat to live, require oxygen, drink water, and require sleep or some kind of rest.

Animals normally do not live as long as humans, regardless of what man says about a dog's life span. None can out live man. None will stand in judgment to account for disobedience. Man is the only being that will give an account for his transgressions.

Man searches all his life for answers about health problems, more or less approximating humans and animals in their experimentation. Because of the coherent philosophy, man fails to find the answer that shows and teaches man how their body is capable of eradicating many ailments that invade the human body. It can happen without taking any medications

By separating man from animals and looking at man as an image of the Creator of this universe, man could have, a long time ago, learned what and how to make one's body work its own miracle to heal the body.

Disapprobation is not pointing at our men and women who spend their nights and days looking in every direction knowledgeable by the tickets obtained from the university where they did their studies.

I understand we can only remain in the margin of knowledge obtained from man's teaching. The last page of the book ends the journey. All we do after that will be speculation. Being skeptics, we develop doctrinal theory that brings perplexity.

Perplexity within our teaching prevents advancement from the only One that opened one's understanding that we might be knowledgeable with what we need to assist the ones that are in need of help for their health problems. All can never be wealthy. Likewise everyone was not made to be the head. Someone has to be the governor. The majority will always remain the subjects. All could not be very educated. Some have to be less fortunate. We find some that never undergo any misfortune all the days of their lives. Things happen to humans that are unanswered. Many people love to say its luck. When it is misfortune we say bad luck. Things seem to happen to us by chance. We are not able to guarantee anything.

Since stipulation is our strong point, we maintain a lifestyle like that in just about everything we do. In our stipulation we miss the key about the bodily functions that keeps us from understanding the body potentiality.

I know that people are of great value over all things on this earth that require oxygen or air to stay alive. Man would have to use something that is of less value for experimentation. What else close does man have to use than animals? They have similar body parts.

Looking at their structure, regardless of proximity, no one or nothing was fashioned like humanity. Humans, in the beginning, were the only creatures that were created to live forever. They were given the power to govern everything that occupied the earth.

We have different organizations that oppose using animals for experimentation in looking for answers that will enable man to help ailments. Sickness is not partial. It does not pick and choose its victims. Humans are the ones who walk in the pathway of sickness as long as they are alive. In death there is no need for sickness to contaminate a person's body. In death a person no longer has any faculties that remain. Sickness is a plague created by some evil source to afflict humans as long as we are alive.

Death is passing this life. There is no need to languish in the grave. When we reach the end of our journey, our enemy has no more use for us. He cannot keep us alive to maintain his torture. The control our enemy has over us removes, from man, GOD'S wisdom, knowledge, and understanding. The wisdom, knowledge, and understanding that are controlling humanity are that of our enemy.

Looking at our behavior toward our neighbors, we do the opposite as commanded by GOD. We walk maliciously daily one towards another in ignorance, not by our own will. Man's lack of foresight, maintains hindsight being controlled by evil.

Man could have irradiated many of his problems a long time ago. There is always this two letter word that plagues our mind after the fact, "IF". The constant after the fact shows that man is faithless.

I know that the majority will disagree with me by saying they are not faithless, because they by faith go about their daily life. In that concept, to man, that is their faith. That kind of faith only maintains this life. There is a life after this one. It is past time for all to awaken to the reality that we are not going to escape the one to come. That life will have a lot more languishing than this life, if we continue serving the Devil.

In this life a person's body can make all kinds of adjustments to maintain a half way pleasant life. Most people hate to die regardless of the torture they are going through. Look at all the things man is doing to keep people alive. Not every one is objecting with man keeping people alive on machines.

In this life we find out that our medical researchers spend a lot of time in research. Through persistency they are hoping that someday they might stumble on the answer needed to strengthen human bodies that sickness will no longer have that much controlling power over man. If our researchers were able to reduce man's health enigma from the majority of the inhabitants, it might create one out of these possibilities. [One] it might make life a lot more pleasurable. [Two] life can become a lot unhealthier.

Researchers feel that by the process of cloning they can produce humans that will be able to maintain a very healthy life as long as they remain alive.

Man's lack of knowledge in the body's potential, loses sight of the overall picture of the correct direction needed. Man holds the teaching that our bodies have the ability to maintain its proper health by healing itself. The problem is the medical professionals are unable to improvise a method for the body, that it can heal itself without medication.

When people are infected with the common cold it irritates in a way, which makes a person feel miserable. We resort to medications for a quick-fix when we are infected with a cold. We do not realize that most colds remain with a person for a period of fourteen days. When we visit our physicians, they normally give us a ten day supply of medication. Many times their prescriptions are written with one or more refills, all based on the strength of the medication.

Colds are not the only things that perplex man. Man does not have many ailments under his control. There are all kinds of diseases that are a great nuisance to humanity. I am sure man would love to be able to live sick free all the days of his life. It does not matter to some folks how hard life is they just love living. Most of us will do all that is within our power to remain alive.

Humans are the greatest species to inhabit this earth. They have a body like none else. However, we cannot live without being clothed. Animals have one covering. Most do not change theirs. Man has the power to make a lot of things and change many things as they journey this life.

Man's body is capable of adapting to all kinds of temperature changes. He lives pleasantly some way without great discomfort, because the body within itself is very powerful. A person's body wants to live, whether we know it or not. If a person's body was capable of speaking to itself it would speak and show what is needed to make it much healthier. Since the body does not have the ability to speak back to itself, we cannot understand the full potential of the body.

The body is unable to express itself by speech. It expresses itself through pain, discontent, or craving. When a person's body is in need, whether for water, food, or to free itself of the waste matter, or some kind of ailments, the body speaks by feelings, not by words. When we give the body what it expresses it needs, we in turn answer the unspeakable language of the body.

It is the same thing with sickness. When a person's body is infected with some kind of disease, the body language expresses itself by showing discomfort. We then proceed to do the best thing, just as when the body is in need of food or drink it speaks in more than one way. Each person's body reacts differently when it's in need of food or drink.

Daily our bodies crave good health; we should be knowledgeable to fulfill the body's hunger. Because we lack the understanding of the body's full potential, we are unable to give the body what it needs to make it work to its full capacity. We only keep giving the body things that help here and there.

Medication is a very good thing that men developed. It is not the answer. At this stage, it would be difficult to exist without the help of our physicians today. We have so many things created by humanity that it matters not how carefully we walk or behave. We are never going to stop all accidents. Many things that will happen to us in life will cause regrets. We are always going to have this two letter word in our vocabulary, "IF". No matter how cautious we walk, we are not going to prevent accidents. As long as we have so many things that can fail, we are going to have injuries.

Don't ever forget that man is not capable of seeing what is ahead, no matter how close the problem is. Man has created various instruments to detect different weather patterns. Were the instruments created to stop future catastrophe? They are still unable to stop what is about to happen.

In what way then are we going to stop problems in our daily living? Since we do not have the answer how to stop most of our problems, this should show we need each other in more than one way. Since we need one another so much, we should stop being so cruel to one another. Being more affectionate towards each other, it can make the future great. Survival depends on unity. We can move great mountains when we stand united.

In this stage of life, man should stand united with all the advancements he has made over the past several hundred years. Instead of caring one for another, we allow filthy lucre to built up a wall of division one against another. We in turn place a blindfold over our eyes and continue to live a selfish life.

In our selfishness, we have not listened to our own body language. The reason why we are not paying much attention, it is the love of money stopping many humans from being affectionate towards another person who cannot assist them in getting wealthy. The other thing is this: our schools, with our educators, do not understand the body and how it works. Not being able to understand the body, as it speaks, we continue to encounter various diseases.

Since humans are creatures that heed language by speech, we

find it difficult to perceive languages that are expressed only by feelings. Failing to understand the language our body speaks, we constantly ignore the silent speech of the body.

Looking at the body language at sleep, the teaching of our researchers and physicians is that we have to turn and toss all the time we are sleeping. Our researchers and physicians fail to understand the speech and the answer of the body at the hour of slumber.

Not hearing and understanding ones cry at slumber, we teach that we have to toss all the hours of sleeping. Man is very hard to understand. In our lack of knowledge we are unable to answer correctly the things that we do not completely understand. Many times we give an answer just to appease people. Most people place their lives in the hands of their physicians. Even when they are not being helped they continue to rely on man. They feel physicians know a lot about the human body after all the years of study.

The unanswered cry of one's body shows that physicians to this date are not knowledgeable in all of man's body languages. They think they understand all that needs to be known about the body. Still the most important cry of the body is constantly ignored.

This should open our understanding that man is a creature who we should not completely put our trust in. Man teaches that it is a normal thing for us to be restless while we are sleeping. The reason man jumps to such conclusion is the lack of understanding the bodily language.

The most important cry made by man is being ignored. We do not see the reality in the cry when a person is sleeping. The body only speaks by expression. Rest places a person's body unconscious. Being unconscious completely reduces all awareness of unspoken languages.

Snoring is a language of the body. Man has been paying attention to that speech of the body, because others suffer and complain about their partner's snoring. Man spends millions in search to reduce snoring. They have not found the answer yet. They invent the use of oxygen during the hours of sleeping to reduce snoring. That gadget can only help the wealthy because it is expensive.

What man realized is that man is not inhaling and exhaling correctly. By giving more oxygen when resting one can reduce their snoring. By not understanding one's body language at rest, we are doing harm to a person's body. At slumber people need less oxygen. All of man's internal organs should also be at rest. The body cannot fully work, as it should, because it is not resting as it is suppose to.

I found out that we should stop calling the organ in our chest, or thorax, a heart. That organ only pumps our blood. It is a pump. It does not do much more for the body, like the brains. One's brains should be called the heart or the soul. It controls all the functions of the body. Nevertheless, a body cannot function properly without its entire members. The reason I say we should change the name of the organ in our chest is too many folks misunderstand the heart that GOD speaks about.

The vertebrate center of our nervous system constitutes the organ of thoughts and neural coordination. It includes all the higher nervous centers receiving stimuli from the sense organs. It is interpreting and correlating them to formulate the motor impulses and is made up of neurons and supporting and nutritive structures enclosed within the skull. If this is what takes place in the brain, we should all agree that the head of a person where the brains are should now be called the heart.

Remember, the brain does all the thinking. The organ that we describe as one's heart does not function as outstanding as the brain. When we are able to differentiate the operation of the brain, and the organ in our thorax, we should all agree that man would then have two hearts. GOD always addresses that we should give him our hearts. We should circumcise the foreskin of our hearts. The organ in our chest does not think for us, neither does it feel the suffering pain for other organs. Deuteronomy 10:16, 30:6, Jeremiah 4:4, Romans 2:29, Colossians 2:11,

Are we in opposition with the doctrine of GOD by using the organ in our thorax as one's heart? Is that the organ GOD speaks of that we need to serve him with?

Snoring at rest is a result of unrest. Even our brains are unable to get the little rest it is entitled to. Giving oxygen in time will possibly damage the individual.

The body language at sleep: our researchers and our physicians fail to understand the speech of that cry. At the hour of slumber tossing back and froth is accepted as normal because we cannot see and understand what the body is saying. At sleep the body needs complete composure. The speech of the body is this: I am not comfortable, I need a better body elevation; I can't work as I am supposed to. The unconscious pleas of the body are being ignored. That leaves us exposed to all kinds of problems in life.

Because sleep is unconscious, we overlook one's body cry. The way we are resting, our body keeps crying out for relief. We keep on ignoring its cry. Oftentimes we seek help from our physicians for our body's nightly cry. No one that is educated by our educators realizes the deadliness there is in our neglecting of our nightly vociferation.

Because our vociferation is not an outburst, as when someone is hungry, we continue to mistreat the body plea. When we are awake, the body speaks not by words, but only by expression. We give the body what it's requesting. If we ignore the language all the time, we are going to kill ourselves. Take for instance, the normal plea of the body for food and drinks; we are able to understand that speech, and give the body what it is calling for. By long neglect, we'll not be able to live long when we do not heed the vociferation of the body. It is the same thing when the body cries to be relieved of its waste; if we should ignore the body's request, we will hurt ourselves. Someday we will reach a place of no return and death will be eminent.

Most of the time, we keep visiting physicians for our problems. It has to do with a deaf ear in the vociferation of the body languages. If for all these years we were able to understand the plea of the body at slumber, we would be able to eradicate many of the ailments that have been plaguing humanity for hundreds or possibly thousands of years.

Since we have not the knowledge of the body's potentiality, we do not know what it takes to really make the body work as it can.

The body is a great piece of ingenious creation, perplexing beyond comprehension. We are more intelligent, man says, than animals. Man has the power to work and create like GOD. Nothing else has the faculty to invent, develop, and exploit as man. All multiply in the same manner. Man, by food, controls all species. We know that many people have been eaten by some wild animals. Still man over the years used up more creatures than creatures did to humanity.

That is where we have made a wrong turn over the years. Man keeps looking at animals for an answer to solve man's problem. We are not going to find what we are looking for in that kind of research. Each species' body potential is different. Humans are all by themselves. The reason is man's life span is much longer; humans create to be like their creator. The ones that dominate being the ruler have to be supreme not only by sovereignty, but most of all in wisdom and understanding.

In the beginning man was the last thing to be created. He was given the power to be master over all things. Nothing was created in the image of man. Animals and all creatures were in their likeness. Man was in the likeness of GOD. Not one creature was in the likeness of GOD away from man.

Man's irreverence to GOD, places man as only a higher animal when in truth we are not. Man's body potential stands by itself even though we find compatibility within animals' organs. What we might fail to see and to understand, man is flesh and blood like animals. We all need oxygen, water, and whatever one eats as food to maintain their lives.

The exclusion of one of these three, water, food, or oxygen will extinguish both man and animals from this life. These three substances we need to maintain our existence on this earth.

In man and animals we can find these organs: kidneys, lungs, heart, which I call the pump, liver, and brains. We can find lots more organs within the bodies of men and animals. Then we find the bone structures, muscles, and blood vessels. We can keep on naming the body parts of men and animals. We can find similarities.

Despite the similarities in organs and blood, eating and drinking, and breathing oxygen for survival, there is none to compare with humanity. Not because our bodies are flesh and blood makes us equal so that study of animals can give the answers for ailment cures.

We know that men and animals also require sleep. Sleep is resting. We cannot live without resting our bodies. Both man and animals have to sleep. Sleep helps to retain life in man and animals.

Man is the only creature that's capable of controlling his body that he can go several days without sleep and live. We can also go without food in many cases. Animals were not made to go without sleep. Man was not created to be without sleep also. From the beginning of time for humanity, we always have night and day. Daytime we do most of the chores. Farming is not something a person can do at night. Nights were known as the time for resting. In this era of vast technologies, we have to work twenty four seven. We cannot operate only on a day shift. We design three shifts so as to make life run on an even scale.

Without three shifts it would be difficult to find jobs for the vast population. We have been selfish and greedy in this era. As we grow, we live like life is only a vapor. We waste away when death removes us from this earth.

The body's cry for long life is not heard because we cannot understand the unspeakable speech of the body. The body speaks through agony and not by words. We seek help from man each time sickness infiltrates our bodies.

Since man has not the ability to see the cause of body ailments, he cannot develop any mechanism to aid the body or to put into action the body potential that it can rejuvenate itself as it was created to do.

An animal's structure does not have the full potential as men. There is no need for rejuvenating power within their structure as man. The structure of animals was made different than men. Because all species in this hemisphere require oxygen to exist we believe man and animals are congenial.

Men keep addressing themselves as very intelligent. In our sophistication we overlook things of profound importance. Many things that man created have to use air to operate correctly. Even machines made by man in this hemisphere require the same oxygen used by man and all the rest of the species. It matters not where they live as long as they intake air to exist. They and man are not alike.

Failing to understand the body's potential creates disillusion over the power of humanity. The other thing is this: man in the beginning rejected GOD from being the only head of man. We gave up greatness for weakness. We gave up something for nothing, life for death, happiness for unhappiness, great health for poor health, long life for short life, and peace for misery. Man is truly flesh and blood. A creature that's full of misconceptions. On the other hand, man is a creature who falls away easily to evil.

It is hard to correlate why man finds it so difficult to honor GOD and to take him by His word. The person that does not have anything pleasant in life for us, we give all our life in faithfulness.

Take man out of all the other species and we find they stand alone all by themselves. Man can truly live a very long time, if we should eschewed evil and in-turn embrace good. Man once united to build a city to the heavens. It was not being built to honor the Creator. It was being made in mind to outdo GOD, just incase GOD was going to eradicate humanity from this earth by water once more. GOD, to this date, keeps showing man a much better way to take. That it might be pleasant in the Day of Judgment. Man is the one that keeps rejecting GOD'S hand of mercy.

Our rejection of GOD, all these years, holds man in vast disillusion and keeps man in ignorance. GOD is not the one we should point at. Man within himself closed his eyes, stopped his ears, and made his heart harder than a diamond.

GOD in the beginning made man coequal with Himself. Remember, GOD can never make another GOD precisely like Himself. He can only make replicas. Angels are replicas. Man is a copy. Man's ability is outstanding. We fail to understand our own potential.

Man allows the devil to place a blindfold over our face and keep us in nescience to the Day of Judgment. Man's desire should be, to have nothing to do with the one that have nothing. The Devil keeps us in bondage like slaves. Are we going to do something about this guy, or are we going to allow him to keep enslaving us for eternity?

The day man truly develops an understanding that GOD made man like Himself and anointed him with great power, it is the day he might give the devil the boot. Man failing himself gave his enemy power over him. We love misery, and is not willing to walk away from slavery mentality.

The devil is the slave master and humans the slave, for you give the wicked evil monster free contort over us. The loving compassionate caring one we despise and no reverence.

How the Body Works

Chapter (17)

In the Bible we find that we should go to the ant and consider his ways. They do not have a governing body as a sovereign head of state like a king or any other governing monarch known to man. Yet they work in harmony. Proverbs 6:6-7.

Is it only in the gathering of food that GOD is trying to make man study the ant? Is there a greater significant value GOD is trying to awaken humanity about? Why GOD wants humanity to study such small creatures, which can be so destructive? If we allow these little creatures to have their way, they might just overthrow man. Man was given the dominion over all things created by GOD. We should be able to have total control.

The ants are creatures that make their preparation for the winter in the summer. They work as a team. Observing these creatures and you will see them carrying their food to their storehouse sometimes four or five times larger than their size. In their transporting they encounter each other. Not once have I seen any opposition in their journey against another like trying to rob those that have a larger portion.

United as they are, I am sure they equally distribute all the food they gather in the summer months during the winter. The studying of the ants should have been a great lesson to man. We should try very hard to harmonize our lives as they do.

The ant does not only live in the forest, otherwise known as the woods. We can find different species of the ant family. In this era we find several types that live in man's home with man. If we are not careful these creatures will destroy our homes. We have to use all kinds of extermination methods to eradicate these insects.

Each species has their own survival mechanism built within their structure. What ever it takes for endurance: that they will do. Man has to keep making stronger repellants to keep these creatures from over populating the earth.

Man truly has a very difficult time on this earth. If we are not vigilant in everything we might become extinct. I know that ants are not the only creatures that occupy people's homes. There are rats, spiders, moths and other creatures live in man's home. Rats are another species that increases rapidly. We have men globally working constantly trying to exterminate these creatures. It seems unsuccessful in the entire effort put forth to rid people of nuisances' creatures.

We all know that the ants work very hard. We rob them of their lives either by stepping on them or exterminating them with insect repellent. We can find the same behavior throughout the world. I can remember when I lived in Jamaica. We had some ant nests built in trees so large they would kill the tree if we did not remove those ant's nests.

Many people take some of these things lightly and show no interest in the world population when it comes to ants. All we care about ants is they get in the way and become destructive. Humans love their environment to be pleasant and not to be contaminated by unpleasant species.

I am using the ant for a specific reason to open up our understanding in connection with how the body works. Ants are small creatures. They live together in multitudes. They work as they live. When you see one ant moving around, many more are not far away. Ants are the only creatures that live and behave as they do.

Study all other species that occupied this earth with humanity, they live and eat together. Every other creature on earth behaves opposite from the ant. When the ant is in trouble they instinctively come to the aid of the other ant. However, other species scramble for their lives instead of coming to the aid of the one in trouble.

Over and over, you would see different programs on TV showing the animal world and the way they survive in the wild. These programs are made for entertainment because people love to be entertained. Producing a variety increases a person's interest.

Observation of these creatures in their habitat often shows them eating together. Sometimes you see them at the water hole drinking together or sleeping in packs. The ones that eat other species regularly hunt together; they eat as a team. They do everything as a team with one exception, when in trouble they desert each other. Sometimes you can see a mother put up some kind of opposition trying to save their young ones. If they are not careful the predator will eat them. They never stand in unity to fight to save another from being eaten. Each other species run away trying to save their own necks.

The predator seeks food because they need to survive. They are somewhat fearful of their own lives because they too can fall prey to a predator or be killed by one that is more aggressive. The predator can become the prey if they hunt foolishly. In all things these animals have to be cautious. When we are watching these programs sometimes we see smaller animals work as a team to rob the aggressor of their food. They could not kill those large animals themselves as shown on the programs. They work very cunningly that they can eat and stay alive.

Each species' existence depends on what they do to remain alive. All want to live. To live was placed within each creature. Just as living is precious to humanity, it might be the same to all other creatures.

Take the domination of some males in the animal world. Is it the control they seek or is it the growth of the population they seek? Is it possible he looks forward to a strong male to continue domination as he did? Is it possible sex is what he enjoyed and he wants all the females only for himself?

Man does not have the ability to see and to understand what is in the heart of man. People can communicate with people by speaking to each other. We are unable to speak with animals. We have lots of people who try all the time to train animals for their own pleasure.

GOD is the only one that knows all things whether it pertains to man or animals. It is not only by speech GOD understands. He sees and knows what is in the heart of man. If animals have a heart like man, GOD knows what is in their hearts.

Using animals all the time to awaken man is a great thing. In the Bible, which is the words of GOD, we see GOD called men his flock, and the sheep of his pasture are men. Researchers use animals for experimentation to gain the knowledge they need to make medication for human consumption. In many cases, man's experimentation works. Man over the years, by using animals, increases his knowledge and understanding in many areas of life.

Man's research advances them so much that they by cloning can produce plants, animals, and they are hoping that they will be able to clone humans. Man's experimentation over the years brings man a long way either for good or bad. It will take time to open our eyes to know if all things in man's experimentation will be deadly or profitable. Human rebellion to GOD will hurt us in the years ahead. The impatient characteristic imbedded in the heart of mankind always brings down GOD'S wrath upon us.

The invention of voltaic current has not been with humanity for thousands of years. We can date electricity development to about two hundred years. Since the founding of electric current, man's advancement in knowledge is far beyond ones imagination. We do not think about or appreciate all the technology we have in today's society. We live from day to day like life is going to remain forever. It does look like the majority is not thinking about how unpleasant this world is, and it cannot maintain the course it is taking because of immorality.

Man with his understanding, knowledge, and wisdom that he obtained through experimentation with animals, plants, and humans makes many feel they will be able, in the near future, to make man by cloning. Men believe, through the process of cloning man, he will be able to eradicate all diseases. With a concept or belief like that, man in their ignorance places their creation far greater than GOD. GOD created man. Look at all the diseases that overpower man's body. Man now is going to take a little speck from man and make it much better. We have to be insane to believe that man is able to create a man much better than GOD. Men will always be ignorant, as long as we allow our enemy to constantly interject rebellion in our hearts.

In observation of the wild kingdom of animals and birds, you always see where fighting for food can bring death if separation does not take place. The more aggressive ones normally eat first. The ones that flee return later seeking leftovers. I see this kind of behavior in farm animals and also with animals and birds that live in the wild.

Ants are creatures we see all the time gathering their food. I have never seen them eat while they are reaping. We know that man is the only species that cultivates his food. Man's cultivation also provides for other species. Not all creatures have storehouses for their food. Most live from day to day. There are a few that store their food, but only one the Bible makes reference about that we should study. It is not only the gathering of food we need to consider about the ant.

Ants live in various locations that make it very difficult to see their behavior as they eat. We do not know if they fight while they are eating. I do not think we have ever seen the need to study the ant's behavior when they are in their homes and if there is a constructive method when the time comes for them to eat.

Do they eat within the confines of their storage area? Do they eat as if there is a dining area where one oversees the distribution of the food? Do ants have a brain like humans that they can remember where to find the food they are transporting? Is it done by telepathically messaging the body making them aware that they have found some food that needs to be transported back to home?

Ants are the only creatures that work in perfect harmony all summer long gathering their provisions for the winter. Tropical climate species should behave completely different. They do not need to alter their body or their blood for the cold weather. Most tropical parts of the world do not get that cold where plants, animals, and insects have to change to live in the months ahead. Yet, in the tropics ants do the same gathering as if to say they are expecting winter. Man knows that the four seasons cover the world. Tropical areas have four seasons in-spite that there is no snow. I can recall when I lived in Jamaica as a child; in the spring some of the vegetation was not eatable and most of the trees produced seasonally.

There is no snow in the tropics. Seasonal trees which produce food start in the spring. Just like trees in the winter climate they yield their provisions once a year then sleep until spring to bear their supply for humanity once more. We find the same in areas of the world that stay hot all year. There are some trees that produce all year. They do not yield quite as much in the off seasons. In the spring those same trees, that bear all year increase their productivity twice as much.

Ants seem to behave the same. In the winter months ants stay in their habitat or home. In their hibernation they are inactive. You do not see them moving around looking for food.

Ants in the gathering of their provisions work in harmony. When one finds an area with more than he can carry back to his habitat, he signals by telepathy to other ants that there is food that needs moving to their dwelling. The response is instant and they gather to move what is necessary.

These creatures do not only use their telepathic signal for food. When in trouble they signal once more. This time it is for saving their life. The signal brings ants in abundance to work on the predator to free the one that is in trouble. In the end the predator becomes their prey.

The ants in their united behavior in gathering their food and saving of another's life bring me to man's body. That is why I use the ants as an example to show us how our bodies work when invaded by parasites: and when an accident causes injuries to our bodies.

The human body is a fantastic creation. It is capable of great things. The only species I could use to awaken man to understand how our body works is the ant. Ants are the only living entity that can send for help when in trouble and a complete response is obtained within seconds.

The message sent out is received with directions that bring the others together to the direct location within seconds. When there is danger, time is essential. One cannot panic. Split second timing is very important at that moment. A delay in response will bring injury or death.

The quick responses to the telepathic signal of trouble work to free the troubled member of the family. The body of ants does not reply that you are only one, and the loss of one is not important. They do not, at that moment, think of their life by saying they might not be able to kill the predator. All the body of ants will become prey instead of one. The value of one is as great as the whole body.

Understanding the unity of the ant's family regardless of danger brings me to understand that man is a very evil, selfish being. Little insignificant creatures as the ants harmonize themselves with greater intelligence for survival than man who is created with far more wisdom, knowledge, and understanding. Yet, we find these little creatures, that we have been trying to annihilate for years, behave more compassionately one towards another than humans behave one towards another.

Man from the beginning of the fall to his present day is unable to help one another to be free from the strong hold the enemy has over them. When we understand the behavior of the ant, as the Bible recommends the study of the ant, we should be able to see that we have not walked in the footprint of the ants. In truth Christ Jesus is the only One that disregarded His life for the saving of human lives, because we are always in trouble from the day we fell in sin. The colony of ants does not fight their same species. Ants are creatures that colonize when anyone member is being invaded as prey and they call for backup.

People never colonize to fight their predator. Man has always fallen continually as prey to the devil. We have not once seen the need of colonizing to make our predator become the prey. Man's plunders colonized against a lower creature in the beginning and humans have remained the Devil's prey continually. Not all have fallen prey to the enemy. Less than a handful has been freed from the predator through Christ Jesus.

What has transpired in the life of humanity is that we have not seen the need to behave like the ants. Can we save another person's life, like the way the ants save another ant? The signal an ant sends out when they are in trouble saves the troubled ant. Has man been sending out signals for a very long time? Yes we have. We have fallen prey to the predator and the predator is unmerciful. He is able to stop our comprehension so that we are unable to receive the signal sent out by the one that has fallen prey.

Because we are fearful of losing our lives we refuse to help others that are fallen in the snare of the predator. The ant's instinct knows nothing else than to rescue one of their comrades when in trouble. Man seems to always work with the predaceous that we never will be able to reverse the predator to be the prey like the ants do all the time.

The predator's strong hold is so great that we are unable to free ourselves in all the things the destroyer holds us in. Man's body is very powerful. It was created to eradicate all ailments. Not able to see and understand the beckoning of one another, we cannot free ourselves in anything. It is very difficult to understand why man loves to remain a victim.

Is it possible someday we might fight to reverse the predator to a prey? So that he will be no more predaceous over humanity. We know that the ants have obstacles, yet not all the time. The few they encounter they are able to become the aggressor and feast in the winter on the once predators.

Before we proceed in opening man's eyes to the way the body reacts when in trouble, just like the ants' does when they are in trouble, I would like you to take a look at some of the members that make up the body. You might not be able to see each member completely as I would like you to. It is vitally important for us to learn a little about the body parts and the way they work. It might make you fight harder to nip the predacious enemy in the place that hurts the most.

FROM PAGE 270-283 YOU WILL FIND THE ANATOMY OF THE BODY. THE COMPUTER TAKES A FEW SECONDS TO BRING UP THE PORTRAIT OF THE BODY. THEREFORE YOU HAVE TO WAIT A FEW SECONDS FOR EACH PICTURE OF THE BODY TO POP-UP.

Your torso consists of two parts — the chest and the abdomen. The chest contains your heart and lungs; your abdomen contains the digestive and urinary systems. Your chest and abdomen are separated by a dome-shaped sheet of muscle called the diaphragm.

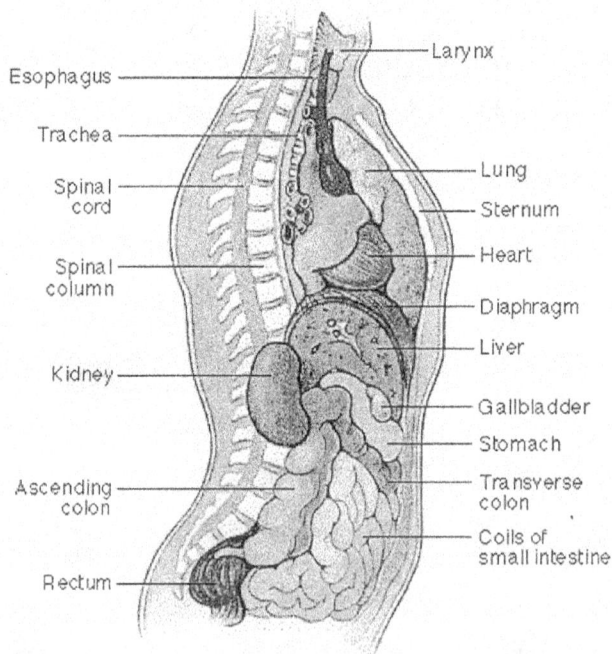

270

Your urinary tract is the body system involved in the formation and excretion of urine. The kidneys filter out waste products from the blood. These waste products in combination with water are urine. The urine passes out of the kidneys through two narrow, muscular tubes called ureters. The ureters empty the urine into the bladder, and the urine is then excreted from the body through a tubelike structure called the urethra.

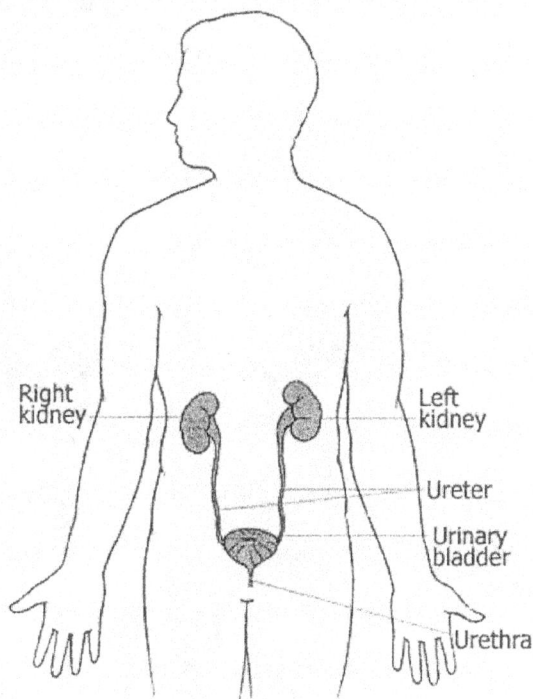

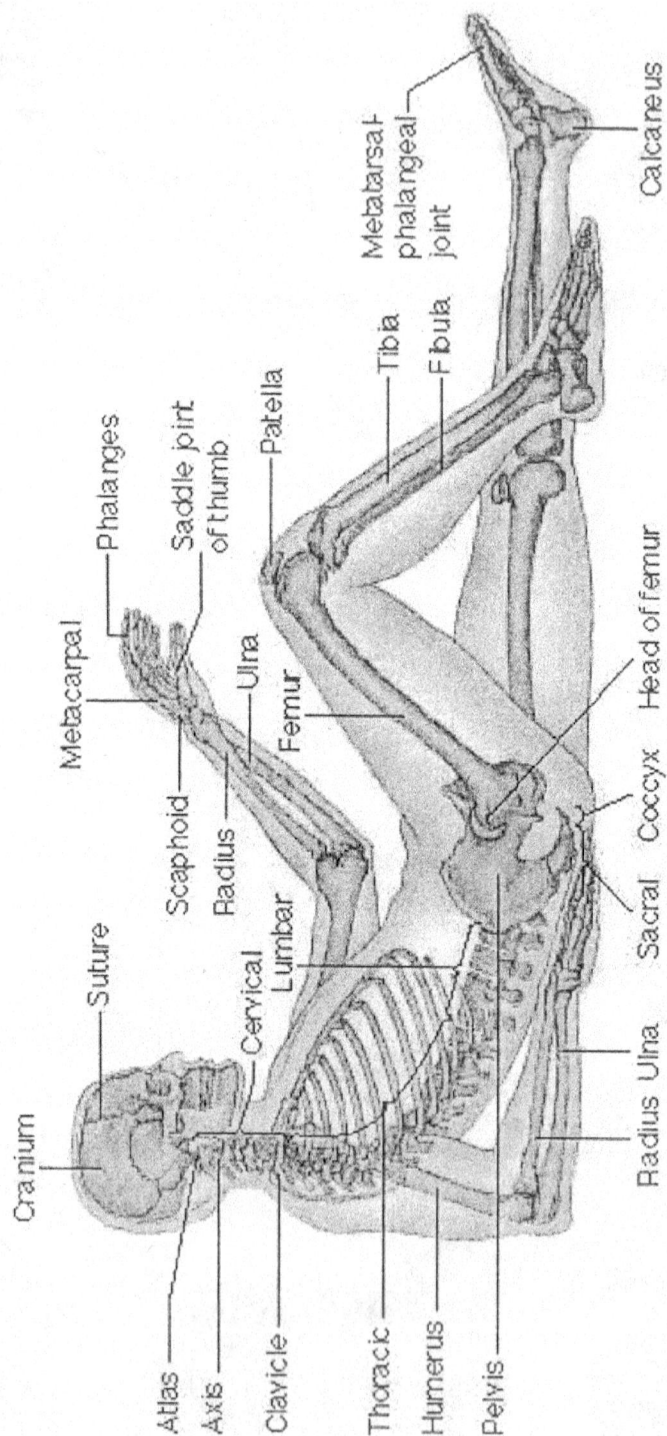

Cranium

Suture

Atlas

Axis

Clavicle

Cervical

Thoracic

Humerus

Lumbar

Pelvis

Radius Ulna

Sacral

Coccyx

Head of femur

Metacarpal

Phalanges

Saddle joint
of thumb

Scaphoid

Radius

Ulna

Patella

Femur

Tibia

Fibula

Metatarsal-
phalangeal
joint

Calcaneus

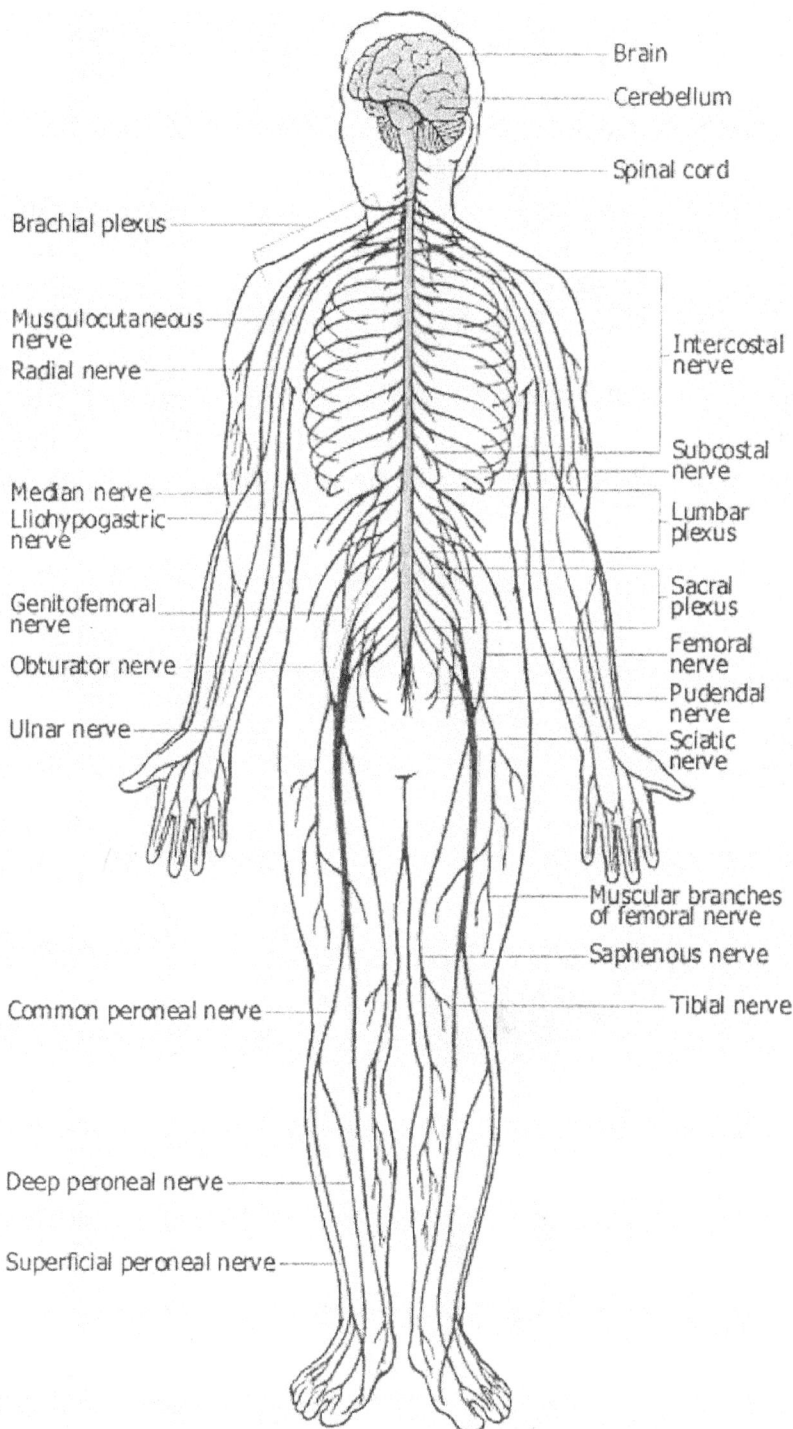

Brain

Cerebellum

Spinal cord

Brachial plexus

Musculocutaneous nerve

Radial nerve

Intercostal nerve

Subcostal nerve

Median nerve

Lliohypogastric nerve

Lumbar plexus

Sacral plexus

Genitofemoral nerve

Femoral nerve

Obturator nerve

Pudendal nerve

Ulnar nerve

Sciatic nerve

Muscular branches of femoral nerve

Saphenous nerve

Common peroneal nerve

Tibial nerve

Deep peroneal nerve

Superficial peroneal nerve

portion of the body. Not that the outer layer is not important. Every part of the body is vital. Nothing should be ignored.

Each body portrait was given just to make you have a little more knowledge of how the body is made up. Then you can understand what the colonizing of the body will consist of.

Because I did not show pictures of the skin, fingers, ears, eyes, or, other parts of the outer layer of the body, we should not feel that they are not necessary. The reason I placed more emphasis with the human's internal organs, was they do much more for the body revitalization. We still have to give the outer layer great honor. The inner organs will lose a lot if the outer portion of the body has all kinds of problems. We need to have good health all the days of our lives. When the body stands in unity, the whole body will remain strong and healthy.

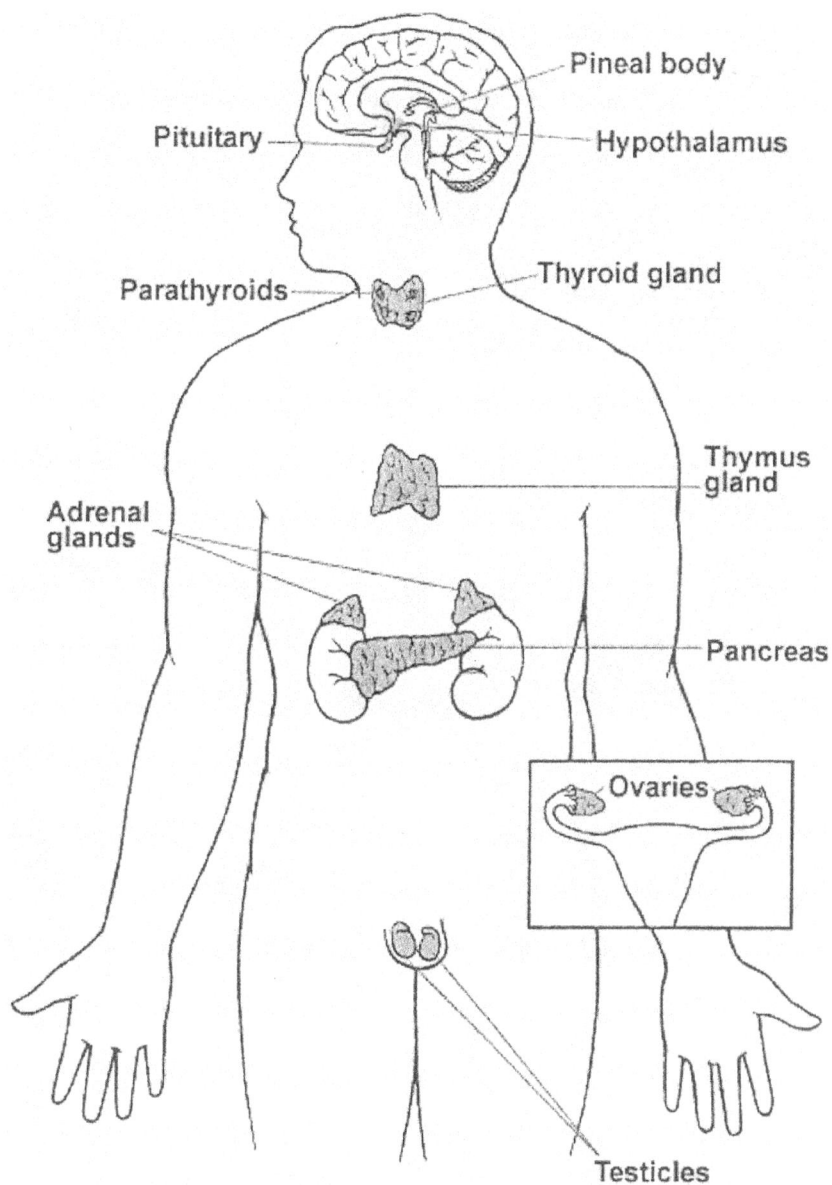

Pineal body

Pituitary

Hypothalamus

Parathyroids

Thyroid gland

Thymus gland

Adrenal glands

Pancreas

Ovaries

Testicles

Your respiratory system provides the energy needed by cells of the body. Air is breathed in through the nasal cavity and/or mouth and down through the throat (the pharynx). The throat has three parts - the nasopharynx, the oropharynx, and the laryngopharynx. The air passes down the trachea (the windpipe), through the left and right bronchi, and into the lungs. Oxygen in the blood is delivered to body cells, where the oxygen and glucose in the cells undergo a series of reactions to provide energy to cells, and the waste product of this process is carried out of the lungs.

The larynx is your voice box; the epiglottis, a flap of cartilage that prevents food from entering the trachea; and the esophagus, the tube through which food passes to the stomach.

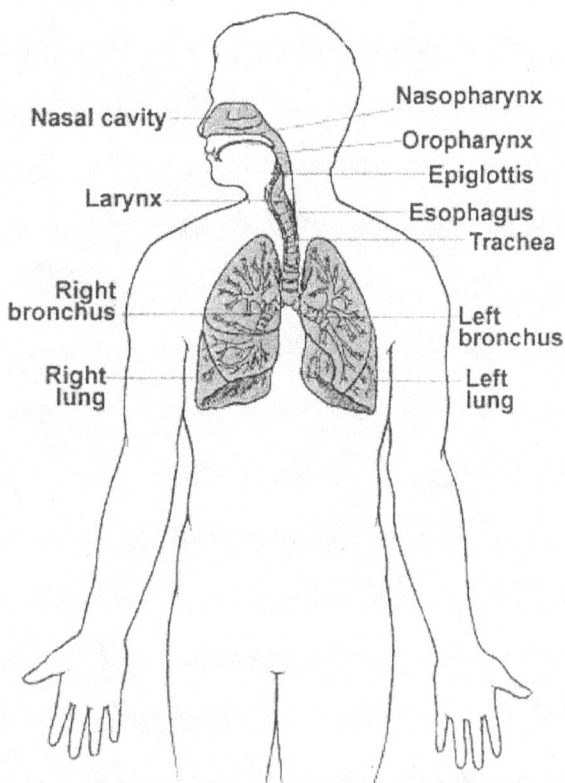

Each of your muscles is made up of thousands of thin, long, cylindrical cells called muscle fibers. The muscle fibers' highly specialized structure enables the muscles to relax and contract to produce movement. Muscles vary greatly in their shape and size, depending on their function.

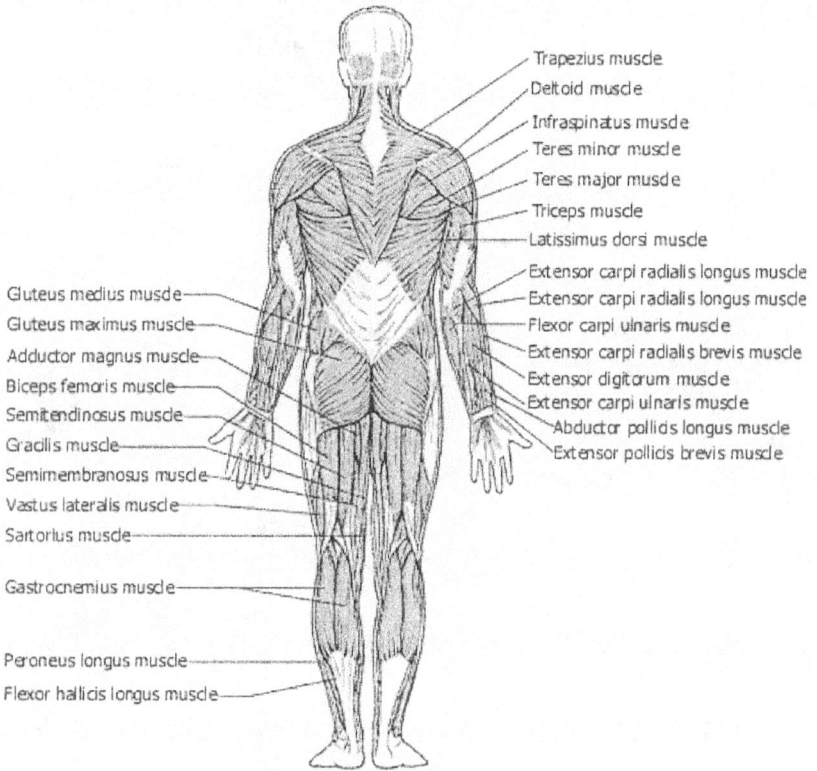

Trapezius muscle
Deltoid muscle
Infraspinatus muscle
Teres minor muscle
Teres major muscle
Triceps muscle
Latissimus dorsi muscle
Extensor carpi radialis longus muscle
Extensor carpi radialis longus muscle
Flexor carpi ulnaris muscle
Extensor carpi radialis brevis muscle
Extensor digitorum muscle
Extensor carpi ulnaris muscle
Abductor pollicis longus muscle
Extensor pollicis brevis muscle

Gluteus medius muscle
Gluteus maximus muscle
Adductor magnus muscle
Biceps femoris muscle
Semitendinosus muscle
Gracilis muscle
Semimembranosus muscle
Vastus lateralis muscle
Sartorius muscle
Gastrocnemius muscle
Peroneus longus muscle
Flexor hallicis longus muscle

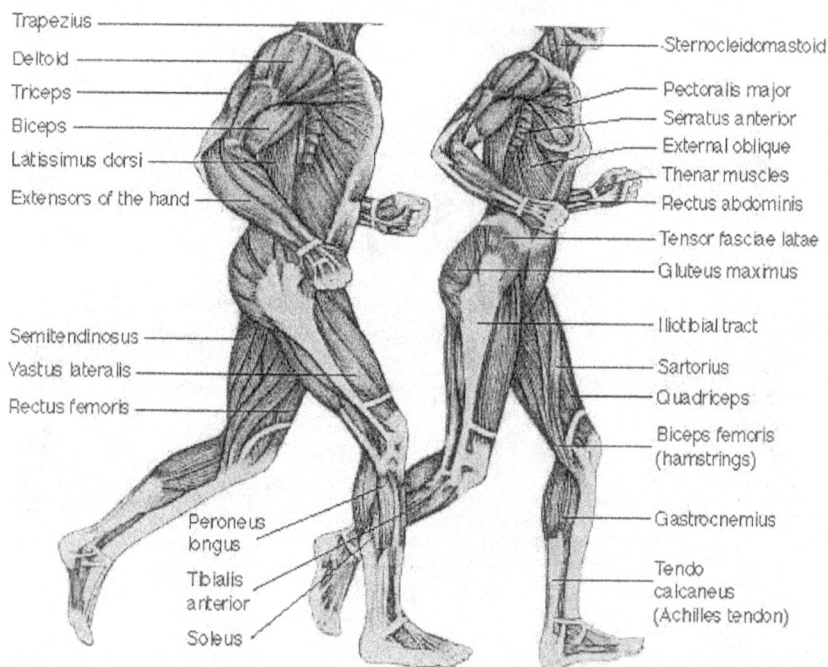

Trapezius

Deltoid

Triceps

Biceps

Latissimus dorsi

Extensors of the hand

Semitendinosus

Vastus lateralis

Rectus femoris

Peroneus longus

Tibialis anterior

Soleus

Sternocleidomastoid

Pectoralis major

Serratus anterior

External oblique

Thenar muscles

Rectus abdominis

Tensor fasciae latae

Gluteus maximus

Iliotibial tract

Sartorius

Quadriceps

Biceps femoris (hamstrings)

Gastrocnemius

Tendo calcaneus (Achilles tendon)

Each of your muscles is made up of thousands of thin, long, cylindrical cells called muscle fibers. The muscle fibers' highly specialized structure enables the muscles to relax and contract to produce movement. Muscles vary greatly in their shape and size, depending on their function.

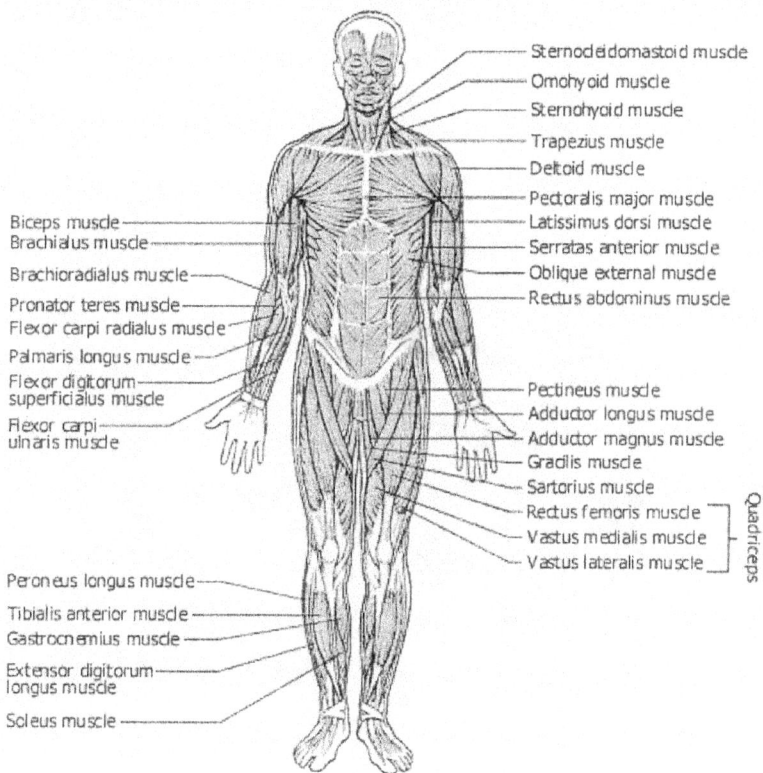

Sternocleidomastoid muscle
Omohyoid muscle
Sternohyoid muscle
Trapezius muscle
Deltoid muscle
Pectoralis major muscle
Latissimus dorsi muscle
Serratas anterior muscle
Oblique external muscle
Rectus abdominus muscle

Biceps muscle
Brachialus muscle
Brachioradialus muscle
Pronator teres muscle
Flexor carpi radialus muscle
Palmaris longus muscle
Flexor digitorum superficialus muscle
Flexor carpi ulnaris muscle

Pectineus muscle
Adductor longus muscle
Adductor magnus muscle
Gradlis muscle
Sartorius muscle
Rectus femoris muscle
Vastus medialis muscle
Vastus lateralis muscle

Quadriceps

Peroneus longus muscle
Tibialis anterior muscle
Gastrocnemius muscle
Extensor digitorum longus muscle
Soleus muscle

Your brain has three main components - the cerebrum (which consists of the left and right cerebral hemispheres), the cerebellum, and the brain stem. The cerebral hemispheres of the brain make up the largest part of your brain. The cerebellum is the structure located behind the brain stem, and the brain stem is the lowest section of the brain and is connected to the spinal cord.

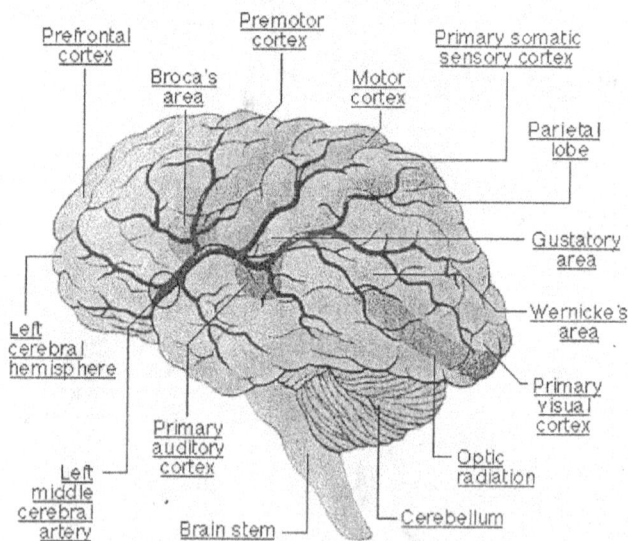

The other reason I decided to show some of the anatomy of the body is when you know the cause of most illnesses' development, then you might learn to value or appreciate your body more than we have. Many might think more about the sweetness of life when they are able to maintain good health. For the first time in life we can have the power to do something about our health.

All that we knew about our body for years was not enough to make us not spend so much time and money at the medical facilities. The knowledge that our medical professionals have been giving us about the body, will remain as unanswered answers because our national health organizations themselves do not truly understand the colonization of the body, and how the body stops diseases.

Man keeps saying that he does not know in truth how cancer and many other diseases formulate in the body. As you read what is written in this book you may not completely understand it. In the next one you will learn how all diseases develop in the body and how you can easily eradicate these plagues.

Many things that we were indoctrinated about regarding the causes of many diseases are incorrect. It is not a good thing to always accept everything taught by our medical educators. Life is too precious to remain in ignorance a lifetime.

Give me a little time. You will know the causes of many sicknesses. You will have the wisdom and the understanding within your hands, and what it takes to make your body work as a colony that when an invader infiltrates the body and tries to become a parasite, otherwise known as the predator, the body will then be able to annihilate the predator and eject the invader.

I do not have time to waste. Each person's life is more valuable than all the wealth of this world. We should value each other much more than we have in the past.

One more thing I would like you to know. I understand the unspoken, unconscious language at slumber. You will also know the answer to why all are restless while they are sleeping.

The other thing is this: I will also elaborate more about exercise, and I will show you how to make your body exercise for you. You do not have to do anything. When your body is doing the exercise for you, it is not likely you will have any injuries at all. I know and understand the body so much. That is why I can teach you how to make your body exercise for you instead of you exercising your body. A person does injury to their body when they exercise their body, especially the way we exercise these days.

Look for the answers and the directions in the next book.

If you would like more information about the body please do not be impatient with yourself and others. Look at it this way: if you never purchased this book your understanding would not have been opened. You would keep walking as a blind man all your life being ignorant of the truth. Another several months will not kill you. You are not going to be cured instantly being knowledgeable about diseases.

What you need to understand, even when you are knowledgeable enough with how to make you body annihilate any intruders, it is not going to do it overnight. It is going to take some time. A person's body has to make a complete round about turn of three hundred and sixty degrees.

Please be patient with yourself, especially if you have taken all kinds of medication all these years because you have been suffering with various diseases. There are doctrines that teach a person should take an aspirin a day or a, none prescription drug to keep you from having heart failure or other ailments that can develop within your system by not taking precaution before they develop.

You need to know that your body has to readjust itself so that it can work as a colony for the first time in your life. What you have to do is very simple. So sit back and allow your body to do the driving for you when you receive from us, the ultimate understanding.

Each picture shows a different profile of the body. The body is made up of many members. Each member serves its proper function without interference. Confusion is not part of the bodily operation. Daily, all the members work in harmony.

Not one member of the body ever worked in opposition or refused to perform its operation. The body parts work in harmony. Not once did any organ complain they were inferior, or behave as superior. Each organ works hand in hand to make the body retain life.

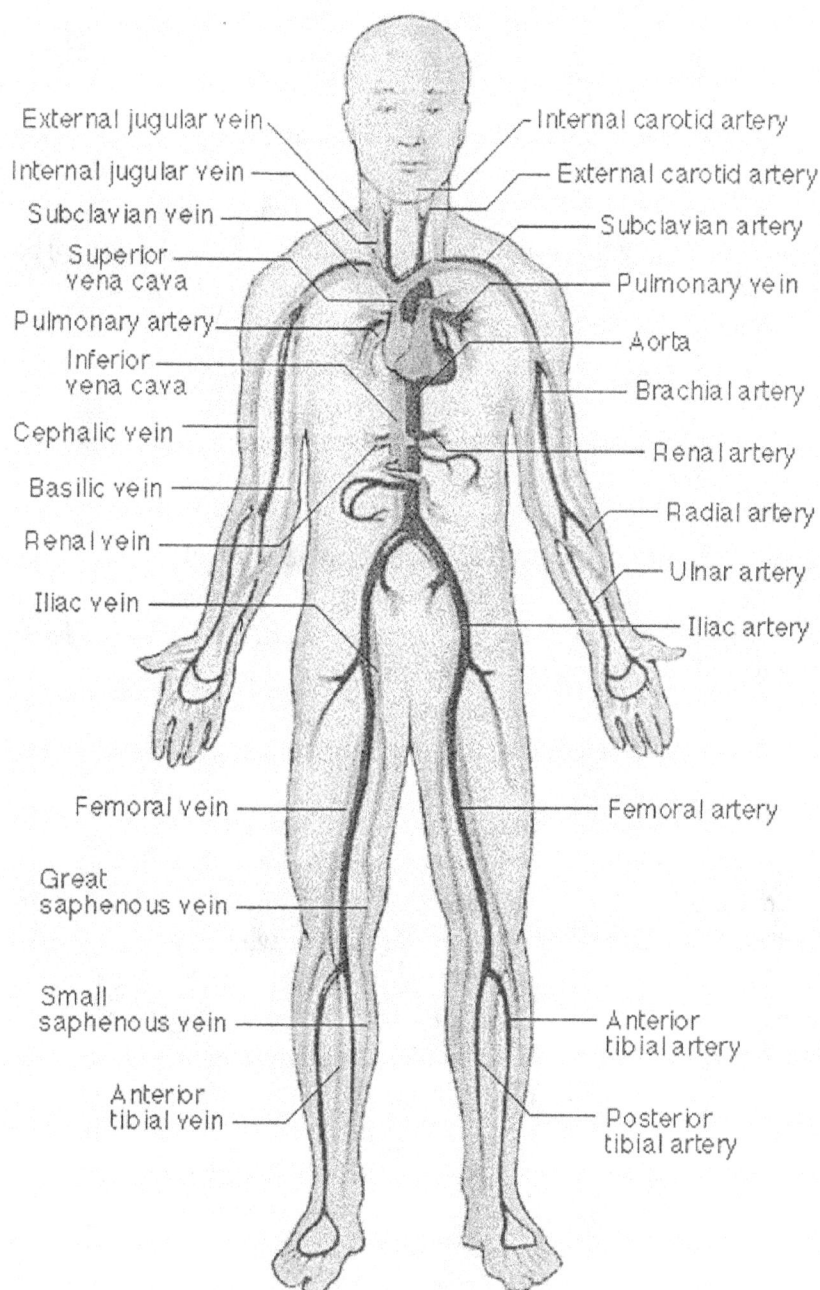

External jugular vein
Internal jugular vein
Subclavian vein
Superior vena cava
Pulmonary artery
Inferior vena cava
Cephalic vein
Basilic vein
Renal vein
Iliac vein
Femoral vein
Great saphenous vein
Small saphenous vein
Anterior tibial vein

Internal carotid artery
External carotid artery
Subclavian artery
Pulmonary vein
Aorta
Brachial artery
Renal artery
Radial artery
Ulnar artery
Iliac artery
Femoral artery
Anterior tibial artery
Posterior tibial artery

body language is not yet understood by each individual. Obtaining the understanding, it will enable us to work daily with what it takes to make the whole man work in unity. At the present we lack the understanding with the language our members are speaking. The problem is we are unable to see or hear the cry of our body daily, because it was always hidden from our understanding.

Man's studies of animals and plants awaken us to understand many things. Regardless of all the wisdom, knowledge, and understanding we have obtained through many years of intensive research, it has not given us the understanding about the body. They still have a very far way to go. I have the answer in my hands that our researchers are looking for.

Take the ant family and their behavior. They never behave inferior or superior. They always work hand in hand. The gathering of their food to the storehouse is vitally important for their survival in the winter. With controversy, preparation will be hampered. They will run into a shortage of supplies in the winter.

That is why when any ant is in trouble and calls for help, the colony marches with one determination to conquer their predator that it will become the prey. They never stand reserved like losing one would not affect the colony. Their behavior shows that each and every one is vital for their winter survival. Shortage of food for the winter can bring death possibly to the complete body.

I am not sure if they would eat their own for survival. I know that a few species will eat their own to maintain their own existence. That could be the reason these creatures work so hard in harvesting their supply. They are not going to make anything stand in their pathway. So there will be no shortage in the winter.

Man's lack of knowledge with the body's beckoning prevents giving the body what it is crying for. Take the ants that are not in trouble. If they were not able to understand the signal of the one that cries for help, death would be instantaneous. When the cry is heard, help will be obtained. If the cry, was not knowledgeable neither will there be any answer. The one that sends out a signal for help would lose their life. Understanding and caring is vitally important for survival of all species. The ant signal is used for two purposes. One, when an ant comes across a large supply, they signal the body for help. Two, when ants are in trouble they also signal for help.

Look at all the nerves, muscles, veins, tissues, organs, and bone structure that makes up a person's body. We can categorize the body as a colony. The colonizing of the ant gives them power over their predators. If there was no unity in the hive, we all would have to agree, there would be no establishment. Building for the winter requires each and everyone to be in one accord with one goal.

Variation brings shortage. Shortage in the end will bring death. In the Bible when man set out to build the tower of Babel, man was working united with one common interest. They were going to build a city that would reach the heavens. Because man is a powerless being to his Creator, man's Creator did just one simple little thing. Changing man's language divided man so that they were unable to accomplish their ambition. The mightier will be the master at all times. Genesee 11:1-9.

Man will never be able to rise over GOD no matter the strength we have if all stand as one. Just like man with ants, it would take a very large multitude of ants to be the aggressor over humanity. Man can always out smart those insects. I have experienced standing in their habitat. Those creatures sure bite viciously.

Man's body when colonized works the same as ants. Ants do not only work in harmony to gather their future supply. They work like a strong military that conquers their enemies.

Man's body, with all its internal organs, muscles, nerves, tissues, cells, and bones works to fulfill its purpose. The pump, not only pumps blood, the kidney not only separates the waste, the digestive system, not only digests the food placed within the body. The brain is the most complicated of all. There is so much the brain does for the body and it gets the least rest.

What happens to a person when their brains malfunction? Look what man has created. They developed a machine to sustain man's breathing in their nostrils even though they are unconscious. Man's brain controls all the bodily functions. Man teaches that the organ that pumps our blood works independently, that you can remove the pump and it will continue its pumping action for a time. Still the pump is no good without the brain. A person's body cannot function correctly with missing parts. Man has been removing organs from a person's body, when they are unable to make corrections. Doctors are just doing a cover up job because the medical professionals do not know any better, or they lack the knowledge and the source to correct infections of human's organs. Unable to make correction to infected human organs, our doctors only other choice is to remove the disease controlled organ.

The brain receives all the signals about whatever ails the body. I was taught that when you accidentally hit your fingers, toes, or any part of your body, before the location that got hit feels the pain, the brain first feels the blow. It then averts it to the area that got injury. The brain is the vital point of all humans. Regardless of the necessity of the brain, there cannot be a human with only a head. The brain needs each and every organ placed in the body to maintain a healthy life. Remove one organ from the body and many more sicknesses will follow the individual because their body is not wholesome anymore.

Take the blood that runs in our veins. If we should lose too much within seconds, without quick restoration, we would die instantaneously. All our members and organs were placed proportionally equal within our bodies from the first day we were created. It will remain that way until the end of time.

For humanity to live and walk this earth healthy, we need to stop the cover-up job doctors are doing. The health professionals just love to remove organs from our bodies when they are infected. Our bodies need all its organs for healthy living. We need to stop the infections, and the removal of infected organs is not the answer.

I hear many men say that their life would not be worth living if their sexual gratification would fail them before their death. Our researchers see the importance of sexual pleasure. They develop drugs so as to give longer endurance when sexually active.

Why is it, man can make things to increase sexual relations, but is not able to restore other health problems? Oftentimes I hear people say correction will never stand satisfactory to people that are suffering because man's true feelings lie elsewhere. The understanding I obtained in the last few years shows me that we need to reweigh the facts of life in a perfect balance. Let perfection have its free course in our life. I know that when our understanding opens up, there will be people loving the pathway of great health. Some will not have any interest for their own good.

The unity of the body performs much greater than the knowledge and the understanding we have acquired by man's teaching. Not knowing the way the body operates, most ailments remain a nuisance to humanity for generation after generation. If GOD does not give us the greater understanding about the body, we are going to maintain the unhealthy teaching and practice given to us, and the unhealthy teaching and practice will never be able to truly help our fellowman.

Most humans are knowledgeable with the bodily organs. The complete potential of the body still remains a mystery, not only to the unlearned, but also to the ones that study the body. Man recently began to update many things they were taught during the age when there was no electricity. The knowledge and understanding that has been increasing daily is phenomenal. The power in man's hand by voltaic current makes man behave overbearing in our walk of life. I am not saying that we should not make plans for the future. I feel we should always place GOD first in everything we do. In a way that will be much brighter for the ones that will continue seeking knowledge, not only on behalf of human's health problems but living on this earth.

The advancements we have in this era, through voltaic current, make life far more pleasant for this generation than all the previous civilizations. What we have overlooked might have been careless on our part, simply because of pushing a button or flicking a switch. I am glad that I am alive in this epoch. I personally do not think I could make life very pleasant without electricity.

I know that tropical climate adjustment is much easier than winter climate. Hot weather does not require artificial heat within houses, offices, or any other kind of business that encounters complete enclosure. Dating back within three hundred years or less, when there was no electrical power, life in just about every situation was difficult. Man's working days were far more extended than our working days. I know that we have more jobs and greater opportunities for excelling than the people that lived in the era without electric.

I also know that most of today's population will agree with me that life is outstanding having all these conveniences. Man has become very lax, because we no longer live in darkness. I also know that man has not completely eradicated darkness. Night will remain as long as man lives on this earth. The occupation of earth requires day and night. Night was for resting. Days were for men and women to work hard providing what was needed for existence.

Advancement in technology has its advantages and disadvantages. We have not differentiated either. We maintain a life that is perplexing. Being perplexed brings dysfunctional behavior in many things we do in life that could lengthen pain and agony.

All the educators in the world, with all the modern technology today, have not given man the understanding needed to change his practice in removing infected organs from a person's body. People love their life. They visit physicians because they are suffering. The reason for visiting doctors is they claim they understand the human body organs and are the ones that know how to treat ailments.

A person would not seek a carpenter to repair their TV or other mechanical devices. Neither would we call a physician to correct our drain. Each profession requires that all be trained in that skill. That is why, when a person is sick, they seek a physician. This era, with all the sophisticated gadgets there are, still leaves man in the dust of ignorance. Millions all over the world claim to be intellectual and knowledgeable with the body. They can skillfully remove infected organs from a person's body and use many electrical gadgets to help regulate affected organs and tissues.

What we have taken for granted might be much more serious than we think. Men and women do not like when their sexual craving begins to lose its zest or drive. We have both men and women working night and day looking for ways and means to increase people's sexual stamina. Not all care for long lasting sexual acts. Many would be much happier if they could have a much healthier body.

The Body's Daily Opposition

Chapter (18)

Daily our bodies encountered various oppositions. When it's not work related, it's other problems. Man does not seem to truly love real happiness. We talk a good talk all the time in relation to changes. Looking at yearly resolutions made in the beginning of the year most seem to forget within hours of their speech. The other thing that is possible is the majority of humans are undisciplined in their behavior. Therefore they are unable to maintain their resolution.

The reason for resolutions, people realize that their lives are going in the wrong direction. Therefore millions feel they need to alter their lives in a way that they think is much healthier. The reason why most people try to change their lifestyle, it usually has something to do with today's philosophy of this life. People are unhappy with themselves because of the pressures being forced on society for healthy living. Looking and listening to the trouble in society about the future is going to be unpleasant, if people do not start to change their unhealthy habits for a healthier lifestyle.

Man's doctrine keeps him searching for physical health, which profits little or nothing. The emphasis we place on healthy bodies and minds is because we think it can bring a bright future with happiness. When we examine man's philosophy for a healthy body and mind, it does not address everyone. The poor are in a class all by themselves. They constantly encounter opposition daily. We have more poor people than rich or middle class. The majority of ailments will be more noticeable in the largest of the population. The other thing we have in our society, are people who are wealthy, they can afford seclusion; they are able to keep their ailments less noticeable in the eyes of the public.

The poor have to visit where their pockets can take them, or what the government provides. It's the same with vacations or just traveling for pleasure. People that do not have much can't enjoy much even in their daily ration. Much of their clothing is secondhand either from used clothing stores or hand-me-downs. Regardless of the poverty that many people have been forced to live in, it has not removed pleasure and happiness from them. In most cases, a poor person can be more composed knowing that they will never have to worry about losing a fortune. The poor man's poverty is his wealth. Can we find a lower class than poverty? Therefore, it is much easier for a person that lives in poverty, to be exposed to more contamination over the years.

Contamination is often generated by filthy surroundings. Look at the poor people's conditions of work. Many times the government has to put their foot down for large corporations to clean up their acts in the reduction of their pollutions. Exposure too long to filthy surroundings will bring later in life, pain and suffering.

It should not matter with man. Whether rich or poor, black or white, we are all flesh and blood. The lives of the ant show more concern and understanding one for another, than what humanity shows for one another. When in trouble they work harmoniously to save one ant. Man's behavior lacks correct discipline when it comes to caring for each other. We should value one another's life the way the ant does. The way they fight to save one life, man does the opposite. Man will take the life of another for one dollar or even less. Some will do it for nothing. Within man's heart there is bitterness and hate.

Man's comportment also brings great opposition upon him because he lives by hindsight. Looking at the picture before our face with love, understanding, and caring, we might behave like the ant who values the life of another ant when in trouble.

We know that mankind is the only creature that buys and sells the products of the earth. All others live and eat freely. Man purchases food and other products for their domesticated animals, whether at home, zoos, or other entertainment purposes.

Man could live on this earth without buying and selling. Opposition brings atrocities. Division remains continually in the human race. Regardless of all the people we see that die daily, and end-up in the cemetery, it has not done much for the living to awaken us to be more affectionate. What I have observed in man's behavior globally, is we place vanity over flesh and blood. I know that many might feel I am including animals in vanity craving. Since they have no use for vanity I am not addressing any other species but man.

As I write, I am not including animals in the craving of vanity. We have hundreds of people globally who care more for their pets than they do humans. We should have more love and affection for people than animals.

All the atrocities to gain gold, silver, and precious items that man has acquired have not given one person good health or an extension of life. We die whether rich or poor, good or bad, loving or hating, caring or despising. It's a constant battle we have daily. Why is it so hard for man to change and be affectionate one to another?

As we travel this life, we have to encounter opposition only because we have one that continually stands in our way and keeps us in rebellion against ourselves. This makes man live antagonistically not only with each other, worse of all with our own selves.

Many people will claim that they are not at enmity with themselves. The reason we acknowledge we are not at enmity with ourselves, is we do not know that our bodies can work as a colony. We look at our bodies as one with many members, with each organ fulfilling its general purpose. Not knowledgeable with the bodily function, we lose insight that the body colonizes when a predator intrudes seeking a habitat to live.

The predator of the ant is not seeking a habitat to occupy as with man's predators. One seeks food and the other looks for a place to live knowing that death will be eminent if they do not find a place to dwell. After taking residence-if no opposition or ejection, they will remain alive. A predator is an entity that lives by finding a prey or becomes a parasite.

A prey is food for the plunderer. A parasite needs a place to live which in-turn becomes his prey as his life sustainer. This will end both lives in the future if something is not done to eradicate the intruder. The ant's intruders will waste the ant instantly if the message calling for backup does not reach in time. If the predator is able to devour or crush the ant instantaneously, they won't be able to send any message out trying to alert his colony that he is in trouble and needs help. If the message is received in time help will be on its way. If that ant gets killed the colony will over power the predator that he will end up as the prey.

What is man's bodily intruder that's making havoc of people?

Is it the culprit we call or know as a microscopic organism? Where does this organism come from? There are all kinds of theories on microscopic culprits and their origination. Do we have any choice with the doctrine imparted to us about development of microscopic organisms?

The doctrine of our educators makes us knowledgeable that these culprits exist through grass or flowers. Upon their opening time they scatter pollen in the air. Man teaches that when the day is fine and clear, as the temperature rises, air carries the pollen up through the atmosphere, sometimes to the height of cumulus clouds. When convection currents cease as the earth's surface cools in the early evening, pollen grains fall in concentrated clouds. It should not matter the time the pollen mixes with the clouds that makes them become an organism. Placing microscopic organisms under a microscope, to enlarge it hundreds of times, makes it look like an entity from the sea or a dried up orange.

Should we accept that pollen reaches the clouds by air and then descends to earth to join with a little piece of cloud undetected by man's naked eyes? Is this culprit only bringing allergies and nothing else? Do we have more than one kind of microscopic organism? Does a parasite develop by pollen, ascending to the clouds, returning alive to the earth, penetrating man and contaminating him?

Is it only affecting humanity? Why do allergies more or less ascribe to infect ones sinus? Is it because the mucus would be the first thing the microscopic organism would encounter when entering the body when being sucked into our bodies through the nostril? As the microorganism finds its way into the body it creates an infection because each person has this mucus in their septum. It, by some unknown procedure, is able to escape ones nasal cavity and enters into our mucus to contaminate and infect it. Then it turns into a cold or other problem that develops into allergic symptoms.

Take the common cold how miserable it makes a person feel when the mucus in ones head is contaminated. We often hear that colds are the cause of microscopic organisms. Allergies also link with these entities.

I am bewildered with the teaching that these entities only seem to stay in one location when they enter or penetrate the body. Let us speculate for a little bit. The parasite, known as a microscopic organism, man always teaches us, infiltrates the human body. What if there are hundreds being inhaled as they descend from the heavens? Possibly there are billions of microscopic organisms descending to earth's atmosphere continually. As we inhale these particles, which are alive, our bodies now become its prey unbeknown to us. When it settles in the mucus in our head, not strong enough to contaminate our mucus, is that called a common cold?

Allergies are a cold that is not infected severely. Since it is not completely tainted and cannot exhaust freely from the body, it makes a person itch. In that case they have to scratch, to relieve the irritation or discomfort, or medicate. Physicians know no other way to treat man when they are sick.

The air we inhale, as we have been taught, enters our bodies through our nostril, mouth, and possibly our pores as stated by our educators. Here we find three locations of the body where oxygen is able to enter the body. Two take the oxygen to the lungs, the other, if it truly enters the body, would go directly to the bloodstream. Speculation, is only used when we are perplexed because we do not have the answer.

With all the grass and flowers there are that release pollen in the air, we have to always have a contaminated atmosphere. Having contaminated air, it is more than likely, we have to always have millions or billions of organisms descending daily that we keep breathing in all the time when we are outside. I do not think this makes sense according to the way we have been educated. What about all the other ailments that have been plaguing humanity even worse since we have electricity, cars, and factories?

We have more flowers and grass in this era than in any other generation before us. We also have more people globally than any other generation. I do not think ever before in the history of man that the population has ever grown to what it is today. We have the largest population in history because man is somewhat unrestrained in today's society and all the violence by killing is not as prevalent as it was.

As we inhale oxygen tainted with entities, they do not stop in the mucus in our head. Are we to say that the mucus in our head is our bodily air filter, and it is suppose to trap all intruders? When it is more than the mucus can handle does it cause infection? What if some escapes to the lungs and takes up lodging and starts to grow or stops at the pharynx and become a residence as a parasite?

By this time I believe each person above the age of six knows what a parasite is. If this organism is capable of moving from one area to another and taking up residence, they can bring great bodily harm.

For sometime now I know that millions all over the globe remain perplexed with many things our educators keep teaching. They have no way, nor anyone, to bring some kind of tranquility to their lives. Prevarication keeps people living a topsy-turvy life. You can find many have no interest in advancement even if they are being paid. To me it is very sad to see so many people who are content to remain living a sinful life.

As we inhale these little unseen monsters that we are not aware of, they cause lots of problems to humanity. Because we are unable to see them, or touch them, we are unable to prevent infiltration being so small. Man cannot see them with his natural eye. They can only be seen under a microscope. What is seen does look like some living entity. The thing is this: they do not enter the body and exhaust when people exhale. Because the body's inner temperature is more adaptable than the air, these organisms become inquilinous by changing their body properties.

In the atmosphere they have no rest. They simple drift all over until someone inhales them. Entering a person's body brings them to rest. They now can seek a place to live. The microscopic organism then becomes a parasite to the body it occupies. A parasite is an organism that feeds off others without self-sufficiency.

The potentiality of the body is outstanding. If the body is unable to eject the intruder, which has become an inquiline's, it will remain a menace to the person they are attached to. Because the body is unable to overpower the now indwelling habitat, it will be harmful to the body as it ages and others join as they infiltrate.

What happens in the body when an intruder enters is it capable of sounding an alarm that an uninvited guest is present. We, as humans, know when someone or something enters where they are not invited: they are going to try their best to remain, especially if they think things can be outstanding where they are.

The first thing many will do is: they will pretend they are invited by looking for an invitation or looking to see if they know someone that's there. Then it might look like he was truly a guest at that affair. Many times all one has to do, is get the guest list and go over it, name by name, to see if that person's name is on the visitor list. If he is not, they can have him arrested as an intruder.

The body of a person behaves the same way. The organism does not want to leave. He likes where he is, and is going to do all that is in his power to remain where he thinks he's found a home. Who wants to keep being blown around all the time? Finding a habitat that has all you need, why change it for nothing? The microscopic organism is going to put up a fight to stay. It will travel the whole body seeking a weak organ to become an inquilinous. Finding no abiding city they have to leave. It exits the body completely or seeks help from other organisms as they enter the body.

What is wrong with anything wanting to remain in a comfortable environment without any cares in the world? Knowing that if all people of the world could be at a place where they do not have to do anything and all things will be there when you are in need; why would someone walk away to go and labor and never have anything?

The microscopic organism will keep searching the body until it finds a place where it will remain inquilines. If the body rejects that species it will not be able to survive. It cannot move from body to body. It will die when ejected from the body it has been trying to inhabit.

Microscopic organisms are small light entities that remain in the air until they're inhaled, as long as there is oxygen in the atmosphere. These particles will keep floating. If landed by chance where they are not able to taint the object, they will be air bound another time much stronger than before. Infiltration of a person, they will have it much more difficult, especially if they are contaminated with insect repellent other wise know as insecticide.

A person's body has to put up a horrendous fight daily. There is so much opposition we encounter as we travel this life. Our bodies are made with great will power for existing for a long time. It matters not how powerful we are. We cannot remain very long with all the obstacles in our pathway.

I think we have said enough in speculation. Since speculation leaves man perplexed we should dive right into the truth without delay.

Illnesses are one of man's greatest enemies. We have many foes. We should know that sickness is not the greatest. Man's greatest enemy is the devil and his confederates. We are our number two enemy. I know that it is very hard for us to acknowledge ourselves as our foe. One of these days many will realize that they themselves are their own nightmare.

In the world today we have hundreds of sicknesses making havoc with humanity; common people are not the only one's that have these ailments. The men and women that dedicate their lives in search of answers trying to eradicate as much of these sicknesses as they can, they too get infected with diseases. These people choose research as their profession. It is a very hard, mind-boggling job. In this case we have people troubled over ailments; when it's not the physicians it is the patient or the researchers. Today, we have our sovereign heads of state trying to ease the agony that millions are going through daily. By allocation of funds many can be thankful with what the government is trying to do because they care somewhat.

I should stop saying that sickness is impartial. Somehow do all have to be sick with one thing or another as long as there is humanity, which is flesh and blood? Is sickness compulsory? Death is the only thing in life that is appointed to man. Since death is the only thing, we should be able to escape all others.

Before we proceed any further, I would like for all to ask themselves this question. Where is the pollen from grass and flowers in the winter? Is pollen, from grass and flowers in the summer, the culprit that causes allergies, flues, and colds in man? In the winter in areas of the world that get icy cold, there is no grass or pollen to ascend or descend. They are sleeping for the winter. What then makes pollen or microscopic organisms remain in the parts of the world that are icy cold?

In wintertime I see more people get sick with colds, flues, and more ailments than in the summer. I see a few people here and there are infected with colds, flues, even pneumonia, when the temperature is warmer.

One of the many reasons a person is prone to contract ailments in the winter, a person's blood property changes, and becomes thicker. This exposes us to more contamination in many areas. And don't forget that one's temperature is not as stable as it is in the summer when the temperature is not as variable.

That is one of the main reasons why so many people are affected with back trouble that live in the locations where it is cold. Many of us are disrespectful of the four seasons and we dress foolishly either by pride or because we are poor. There is not much other choice or our educators lack the understanding of good and bad in our apparel for good health. The other thing that might be possible is man keeps thinking he is running out of supplies and has to make preparation for longevity. Making plans forever makes man go to inferior substances that expose a person's body to the cold weather.

The other thing it can be is the population is much larger today than it was a hundred years back. There are more jobs and much more money in circulation. This can also be the possibility that competition and fashion bring out many things that are beautiful and very cheap because people are disrespectful to their own bodies.

The other thing I see in the behavior of humanity is immorality; immorality is the controller in this era. Within the last fifty years men and women, boys and girls dress disrespectfully to their own bodies. As if to say they do not care what the future will be like. When we pass the age where our procreator does the dressing, we follow the population. The parents who once nurtured the child from their birth now become old fashioned. What makes humans feel their bodies no longer need proper attire? Did this start from the first day they started going to school? I see this behavior all the time in kids, especially in the people that live where the temperature is cold.

What a person does when they are young oftentimes follows them to the grave. Not many change their lifestyle when they are young. The reason many never make any changes is they like when other people speak highly of them. Humans often feel unwanted when other people do not praise them. Even when we are doing evil things, we love to hear people find a way to exult us.

To maintain a healthy life from birth to death is like an impossible task. First of all, we never know how to copulate that each pregnancy would bring healthy children. We are involved sexually so much, we never think of the consequences. I know that most of us never plan our children's future. When we start getting involved sexually, we love to only think of ourselves and never think of children. Many think only of children when they are sexually active in a financial way. They do not want the girl they are having sex with to have a child for them because they do not want the commitment. There are many reasons why people wear protection when copulating.

I am not speaking about fear of commitment when sexually implicated; I am speaking of self-control when sexually committed with the child's future that is possible. Not many know the Bible's requirement for monthly implications. It is not as much, as we have been doing. Since we never knew the consequence, we continue to live immoral all of our lives not knowing the pain and the agony it will give the nation.

Not knowing what takes place when a man and a woman interact during the unclean days of a woman's cycle, we continue to be sexually involved unhealthily. Because we would like for our children to have a better life than we did, we should know the proper time for sexual intercourse.

In all my life, that I live on this earth, not once did I learn or was I taught by anyone, that sexual involvement with a woman in her days set aside for her uncleanliness would bring unhealthy children. I recently obtained this knowledge from GOD with all the things I am showing the world how the body behaves.

What happens each monthly cycle with women: we are not aware of the consequences. A woman can get pregnant within days after the end of the first seven days of her menstrous cycle. Yet, the Bible gives fourteen days of uncleanliness. If a man and a woman are sexually implicated, they should be cut off from the land; that is to say they should die. This was an important factor that GOD was teaching Israel; they should not allow people that were involved in unclean sexual acts to remain in the congregation alive. Leviticus 18: 19. 20:18 go to Ezekiel 18:6

In this era with all the technology we have, we ignore the teachings of GOD as if they are outdated. The majority only accepts the Ten Commandments as guidelines. The rest of the commandments we put little or no value on. On the other hand if we look at some of the laws of the land that are used to govern our society, these are some of the same laws that GOD gave the children of Israel in the wilderness.

Take for instance the abuse of fathers and mothers against their children. Our government imposes imprisonment for the crimes that are committed against parents and children. These laws are used to govern our society. We accept a few of the laws given to us by GOD. Many things commanded by GOD we ignore. These commandments could remove painful heartaches later in life.

Man, in his rebellion against GOD and His commandments, injures none other than man. Take all the ailments we have globally; man is the one that is in agony continually. The enemy that keeps us in rebellion has not suffered any pain and agony all the years that he has been going to and fro in the earth, and going up and down in the earth. Job 1:7 2:2 Humans are the ones that keep suffering all the time, and not only with all kinds of illnesses. We have poverty, wealth, and killing one another as things that plague man all the time. All the things we go through in life, there is no need for things to be that way. By rejecting the one that keeps us in rebellion and turning to the One that loves and cares for us we can eliminate many of our enigmas.

Man just loves to suffer. All the things we hunger and thirst after all the days of our life seem to keep us in bondage. Our bodies would appreciate an environment to colonize, so that our bodies can work to protect itself from inquilines. Not knowing the power of the body and its potential, we live daily with many inquilines occupying our bodies not knowing that they are killing us.

When our bodies no longer can tolerate these menaces it cries out for help. Sometimes it is too late, because the parasite takes over the internal organs. The cry or message that the body keeps sending out all these years was not able to work for the body because there is too much opposition we encounter daily.

If given the right environment the body can discharge or eject all the invaders that are trying to be inquilines. A person's body at sleep, being unconscious, is capable of doing a much better job for the body than when it is conscious. The unconscious stage, when at rest, can eradicate all the parasites that invade the body to destroy ones internal organs.

When a person is awake their faculties are not as sensitive to detect the invasion of an organism as when at rest. When we are awake our telepathic signal device cannot operate because of constant agitation. Normally the body needs the brain to concentrate on making the body function normally.

If the brain behaves the same way when a person is sleeping as when they are awake, we would not be able to have a regular activity during the day. At rest the body behaves opposite than when it is awake.

When a person is awake their brain is much more active than when they are resting. The body does not need to think, feel, or do anything because it is unconscious. When the body is vigilant it needs all its senses for normal daily routines. Sleeping does not require anyone of our senses to be in motion.

Man needs a good environment at all times. We need one when we are awake and we need one when we are asleep. When we are slumbering, if we give the body the right surroundings it is capable of not only detecting the invaders, it has the power for expelling all uninvited guests that are trying to use the body as their life sustainer.

Understanding the characteristic of the ants, we see that they are the only species we find that we can use as a perfect example to teach man how the body operates when it is in trouble. The body does not only behave that way when an uninvited predator seeks dwelling. When a person, by accident, injures their members, the injured member sends out a cry the same way it does when an unwanted organism infiltrates the body.

The ant when in trouble finds they are not strong enough being alone. When they colonize they are very powerful and oftentimes they are able to overpower their predator. The predator ends up being the prey.

The body colonizes not only because of the invasion of organisms but injuries also bring the body together to alleviate the enigma it encounters. For the body to perform as it is capable of doing, we need to create environments so that the colonization can work in harmony.

At this crossroad we reach in life, with all the technology at hand, our educators and intellectuals fail in answering the unspeakable languages of the body as it cries for help.

We can eliminate many of man's problems when we change our surroundings. Take cancer of the lungs. We make cigarettes as the culprit. Junk foods man keeps saying causes obesity. Chemicals we also accredit as the cause for many of man's ailments?

I am trying to make people aware that a person's body has the power to work a miracle for the body in dispersing anything it picks up that would be harmful to the body without the use of medication. Billions are being spent yearly looking for answers in areas where in truth there are no answers. I feel the only reason why man keeps heading in that direction can be because we are a proud people in the educational achievement world today.

The devil's controlling influence makes us place GOD as nothing and makes us behave foolishly. From a child I heard someone keep saying this: "send the fool a little farther." That is what seems to be taking place in our lives in this era. The Devil is making fools of us and sending us much farther from reality.

The ants, when in trouble, telepathically notify the body that they need help. When the message is received, action is taken immediately to rescue the party that is in trouble. It is the same thing with the human body, whether by invasion or injury. A person's body does cry for help from the other members. If nothing jams the signal, they will colonize to free the area of the body that either just suffered an injury or the invasion of an entity. Or!

I promise each and everyone the truth in the next book, that they will have the answer about how the human body truly develops all disease. A microorganism is not the cause of man's many sicknesses. You will know how to stop all infections.

All way remember and know that GOD alone knows human body, He made man and He knows what is best for man and how to teach us the proper method to be health all our life while living on this earth.

Errors in Today's Dogma About how the Body fights off Diseases

Chapter (19)

This chapter is placed in the book to help educate and to open peoples' eyes and understanding regarding the erroneous concepts of our medical professionals. I realize that most individuals are not aware of many findings published by the medical association of the world. Because of the increases in health problems, people should be made aware more through our major mass media of what the medical association's research reports are that are being furnished to the world.

Our major medical institutions need to address to the general public more correct information on how the body works. A person's body works completely opposite from the way we have been taught by our medical educators. The immune system is the one that medical researchers teach as the fighting mechanism for diseases. They place most of their research on the immune system.

There are many articles that have been written about man's immune system. It is not necessary to elaborate on each of those publications. There are too many. The ones we will present should suffice.

The report that you will read about the immune system, most of it came from the internet. I needed the information as a vehicle to show you the error in our medical research teams. I did not see any names, or any copyrights; that is why I used the information. They are not my words.

"The immune systems job is to recognize potentially harmful invaders {pathogens} and then destroy or neutralize them. "Transfer factors" are tiny protein molecules which are produced by immune cells called T-cells.

Transfer factors are the key to the immune system memory of previous pathogen exposure; and thus, are an integral component for maintaining immune system integrity and effectiveness.

302

Transfer factors allow the immune system to remember conditions for which immunity has already been established. When, a person has been infected with the chicken pox in childhood. For example; the body develops a memory of that illness which prevents the person from becoming re-infected later in life.

In the future the specific immune transfer factor molecule for chickenpox will endow the immune system with the exact "blueprint" of what the chickenpox looks like; and the body will be able to quickly recognize and respond to any possible re-infection before it cause disease. So then, why do people get the chicken pox, bad cases of it, after they have been inoculated, some will get a mild case?"

"Over fifty, 50 years of research, producing more than three thousand, 3,000 articles in scientific journals; confirms transfer factors ability to support the bodies, immune system response mechanism.

When a mother breast feeds her baby, transfer factor in colostrums has the sole purpose of transferring immunity from the mothers to the baby immature immune system. This imparts the mother's immunity to the baby while the baby immune system matures.

There are world-renowned medical experts who formed a professional organization dedicated to the study of transfer factor. {Don't forget they also dictate to people.}

They now have transfer factors on the market. There are several products. Immune transfer c6 and immune factor 2 product designed for enhanced activity for herpes virus 6; Epstein - Barr virus, Chlamydia. Both products utilize chicken derived transfer factors with added bovine colostrums.

The goal is to destroy the specific pathogens through supplementations, with the appropriate transfer factor molecules. This may be the missing link allowing the immune system to target and destroy the offending pathogen, and mitigate the symptoms of the disease.

{<u>Researchers words</u>} The factors that regulates the level of t-cells in the body.

T-cell is disease fighting white blood cells that play a central role in the capacity of the immune system to fight off harmful invaders. {Infection decreases the t-cell production.}

{Crucial Chemical} Using the HIV Patients researchers found that a chemical called *interleukin-7 [IL-7]* appears to a crucial role regulating number of t-cells. IL-7 Stimulates the production and expansion of the T-Cells. Researchers found that IL-7 levels rise in HIV patients after the virus has begin to kill off T-Cells. They believe this is the body's way to restore T-Cells to their proper level.

It appears cells within the lymph nodes of the immune system are able to detect a drop in the T-Cell levels, and to respond by stimulating IL-7 production. Researchers hope it will be possible to increase T-Cell numbers in patients with weakened immune systems by boosting their IL-7 levels artificially.

The use of IL-7 may prove to be a weapon against the effects of Diseases. Researchers believe it has the potential to restore types of T-Cells that have been completely diseased. The researchers warn that IL-7 may pose problems if administered to the HIV patients as it can increase the replication of the H I V virus. The immune system is an amazing *Protection Mechanism* it is designed to defend you against millions of *Bacteria Microbes Viruses Toxins and Parasites,* that would love to invade your body.

The immune system what is it, how does it works? {Example} Cancer research institute. How the immune system works to avert cancer and other diseases. Components of the immune system *{A}* Lymph system, *{B}* Thymus, *{C}Complement system, {D}* White Blood cells, *{E} Leukocytes".*

"Example, of your immune system at work when you get a cut. Bacteria enters your body, your immune system responds and eliminates the invaders. When you get a mosquito mite; you get a red; itchy; bump, this is a visible sign of your immune system working. Each day you inhale thousands of germs; bacteria that are floating in the air. If your immune system did nothing; you could never fight off these germs. Example: colds and flues. Each day you eat hundreds of germs, most germs die in the acids in your stomach. Vomiting and diarrhea are {2} common symptoms that your immune system is working.

There are all kinds of ailments caused by your immune system not working properly. *Allergies:* immune system over-reacting to certain stimuli. *Diabetes:* caused by the immune system inappropriately attacking cells in the pancreas and destroying them. _Arthritis:_ immune system not functioning right in the joints. Diseases is an immune system error.

Basics of the immune system. What does it mean when someone says I feel sick today. Your body is a multi-cellular organism made up of trillion cells. Each cell has a nucleus. Bacteria is a single cell organism, they have no nucleus. When the bacteria is able to reproduce and start causing problems, your immune system is in-charge of eliminating it. Viral and bacterial infections are the most common causes of illness. The job of the immune system is to protect your body from these infections. The immune system protects you in {3} ways. {1} it creates a barrier that prevents bacteria and viruses from entering the body. {2} the immune system detects and eliminates bacteria and viruses before it can make itself a home and reproduce. {3} if the virus or bacteria does reproduce and starts causing problems, the immune system is in charge of eliminating it.

Immune system detects cancer and will eliminate it; if it is in the early stage. Virus is not really alive. A virus particle is a fragment of D N A. When virus comes in contact with a cell, attaches itself to the cell wall and inject its DNA into the cell. The DNA uses the machinery inside the living cell to reproduce new virus particles. Eventually the cell dies. The cell is like a factory for the virus. The viral particles may bud off the cell so it remains alive.

Components of the immune system. Your immune has been working for you; your entire life and you know nothing about it. Skin is an important part of the immune system. It acts as the primary boundary between germs and your body. The skin secretes antibacterial substances. Your nose, mouth, and eyes are entry ports for germs to enter. Tears and mucus contain an enzyme called logotype that breaks down the cell wall of many bacteria.

Saliva is also antibacterial. Since the nasal passage and the lungs are coated in mucus; many germs not killed immediately are trapped in the mucus and soon swallowed. Mast cells line the nasal passages, throat, lungs and skin. And bacteria or virus that wants to gain entry to your body must first make it past these defenses. Once inside the body a germ deals with the immune system. The major components are Thymus, Spleen, Lymph system, Bone marrow, White blood cells, Antibodies, Hormones and the Complement system".

"Lymph system is a clearish liquid that bathes the cells with water and nutrients. Lymph is blood plasma, the liquid that makes up the blood, minus the red and white cells. Each cell has to get food, water, and oxygen to survive. Blood transfers these materials to the lymph through the capillary walls, and lymph carries it to the cells. The cells also produce proteins, and waste products, and carry them away. Any random bacteria that enter the body also find there way into this inner-cell fluid. One job of the lymph system is to detect and remove bacteria; to drain and filter the fluids.

Small lymph vessels collect the liquid and move it toward lager vessels so that the fluid arrives at the lymph nodes for processing. Lymph nodes contain filtering tissue and a large number of lymph cells. When fighting bacterial infections, the lymph nodes swell with bacteria. Swollen lymph nodes are an indication that you have an infection. Once lymph has been filtered through the lymph nodes it re-enters the blood stream.

The thymus lives in your chest, between your breast bone and your heart. It is responsible for producing T-Cells. Without a thymus a baby immune system would collapse and the baby would die. The thymus becomes not as important as an adult. You can remove it and you will live. Other parts of the immune system will handle the load. The thymus is important to the white blood cells, and T-Cells maturation.

The spleen filter the blood looking for foreign cells, the spleen is looking for old red blood cells in need of replacement. You can live without a spleen.

The bone marrow produces new red and white blood cells. The red blood cells are full formed in the bone marrow, and then enter into the blood stream. White blood cells are produced somewhere else. All blood cells are produced in the marrow from stem cells. Stem cells branch off and become many different types of cells. Stem cells change into actual specific types of white blood cells.

Anti bodies are produced by white blood cells. They are Y-shaped proteins that each respond to a specific antigen. {Bacteria virus or toxin} Antibodies come in 5 classes, immunoglobulin. A, D, E, G, M. Each antibody has a special section at the tip of the two sections of the Y. That is sensitive to a specific antigen and binds it in someway.

When an antibody binds itself to a toxin, it is called an anti-toxin; the binding disables the chemical action of the toxin. When an antibody binds at the outer coat of a virus particle or the cell wall of a bacterium it can stop their movement through cell walls. A large number of antibodies can bind to an invader and signal to the complement system that the invader needs to be removed.

The complement system is a series of proteins. There are millions of different antibodies in your blood stream. Each sensitive to a different specific antigen. There are only a handful of proteins in the complement system; and they are floating freely in your blood. Complements are manufactured in the liver. The complement proteins are activated by and work with complement. The antibodies hence the same, they cause bursting of cells and signal to phagocytes that a cell needs to be remove".

"The hormones, there are several hormones generated by components of the immune system. These hormones are called lymphokines. Certain hormones suppress the immune system. Steroids and corticosteroids components of adrenaline suppress the immune system. Tymosin a hormone that encourages lymphocyte production a form of white blood cell. Interleukins hormones generated by white blood cells, example interleukin-1 is produced by macrophages after they eat a foreign cell. Interleukin-1 has a side effect when it reaches the hypothalamus it produces fever and fatigue. The raised temperature of a fever is known to kill some bacteria.

The interferon this interferes with viruses and is produced by most cells in the body. Interferon like antibodies and complement are proteins and there job is to let cells signal to one another. When a cell detects interferon from other cells it produces proteins that help prevent viral replication in the cell.

The white blood cells are the most important part of your immune system. And it turns out that white blood cells as actually a whole collection of different cells that work together to destroy bacteria and viruses. Here the different types; names, classifications of the white blood cells. Leukocyte, lymphocyte, Monocytes, granulocytes, B-cells, Plasma cells, T-cells Helper- T –cells, Killer- T-cells, Suppressor T-cells, Natural killer cells, Neutrophils, Basophils, Eosinophols, Phagocytes. Macrophages.

{The leukocytes} all white blood cells are known as leukocytes. White blood cells are not like normal blood cells in your body. They actually act like independent living single- cells organisms able to move and capture things on their own. White blood cells behave very much like amoeba in their movements and are able to engulf other cells and bacteria. Many white blood cells cannot divide and reproduce on their own, but instead have a factory somewhere in the body that produces them. That factory is the bone marrow.

White blood cells are used as a measure of immune system health. In a blood sample a normal white blood cell count is in the range of 4ooo- 11000 cells per micro-liter of blood. How does a white blood cell know what to attack and what to leave alone? There is a system built into all of the cells in your body that makes the cells in your body. Any thing that the immune system finds that does not have these markings, is therefore eliminated. The system that is built into the cells is called human leukocyte antigen. {HLA}

There are two types of MHC, protein molecules, class 1 and class 2 that span the membrane of almost every cell in the organism. MHC is the same meaning as human leukocyte antigen; called M A JOR Histo compatibility complex. MHC molecules are important component of the immune response. They allow cells that have been invaded by an infectious organism to be detected by cells of the immune system called T-Cells".

"The MHC molecules do this by presenting fragments of proteins or peptides belonging to the invader on the surface of the cell. The T –Cell recognize the foreign peptide attached to the MHC molecule and bind it; an action that stimulate the T-Cell to either destroy or cure the infected cell. An uninfected healthy cells the MHC molecules presents peptides from its own cell to which T- Cells do not normally react if the immune mechanism malfunctions and T-Cells react against self peptides; and autoimmune disease arises.

Once a particular disease is recognized by the specific B-Cell; the B-Cell turns into plasma cells. Clone them-selves and start pumping out antibodies. The second set of B- Cells remains in your body for years; so if the disease re-appears your body is able to eliminate it before it can cause harm to you. Many diseases are not cured by vaccines.

{How antibiotics works.} Sometimes bacteria is producing a toxin so quickly, your immune system cannot activate fast enough. In this case it would be nice to help it along. Antibiotics work on bacterial infections. Antibiotics are chemicals that bill the bacteria cells but do not affect the cells that make up your body.

Many antibiotics interrupt the machinery inside bacterial cells that builds the cell wall. Human cells do not contain this machinery; so they are unaffected. Different antibiotics work on different parts of bacterial machinery; so each one is more or less effective on specific types of bacteria. You can see this because a virus is not alive; antibiotics have no effect on a virus.

A problem with antibiotics is it loses its effectiveness. The bacterial off spring will contain a mutation that is able to survive the specific antibiotic. This bacterium will then reproduce and the whole disease mutates. Eventually the new strain is infecting everyone, and the old antibiotic has no effect on it.

The immune system makes a mistake when your immune system attacks your own body. The way it would normally attack germs, called autoimmunity. Two common diseases are juvenile onset, and diabetes. When the immune system is attacking and eliminating the cells in the pancreas that produce insulin. Rheumatoid arthritis is caused by the immune system attacking tissues inside the joints.

Allergies; the immune system reacts to the allergen that should be ignored. Allergen is food and animal fur.

Transplanted tissue is made nearly impossible. Immune system attacks the tissue. You are given immuno- suppressing drugs to try to prevent an immune system reaction. By suppressing the immune system these drugs open the patient to infections.

The anatomy of the liver is very important because of many teaching with the immune system".

"The liver is located in the upper right hand portion of the abdominal cavity. The organ weighs 3 pounds. There are two distinct sources that supply blood to the liver. {1} oxygenated blood flows in from the hepatic artery. {2} nutrient rich blood flows in from the hepatic portal vein.

The liver holds about one pint of the body's blood supply at any given moment. The liver consists of two main lobes; both of which are made up of thousands of lobules. These lobules are connected to the small ducts that connect with larger ducts to ultimately form the hepatic duct. The hepatic duct transports the bile produced by the liver cells to the gall bladder and the first part of the small intestine called the duodenum.

The function of the liver is to regulate most chemical levels in the blood, and excretes a product called bile, which helps carry away waste products from the liver. All the blood leaving the Stomach and intestines passes through the liver. The liver processes this blood and breaks down the nutrients and drugs into forms that are easier to use for the rest of the body.

More than 500 vital functions have been identified with the liver. Some of the functions include production of the bile; which helps carry away waste and break down fats in the small intestine during digestion. Production for certain proteins for blood plasma. Production of cholesterol and special proteins to help carry fats through the blood. Conversion of excess glucose into glycogen for storage. This glycogen can later be converted back to glucose for energy.

Regulation of blood levels of amino acids which form the building block of proteins processing of hemoglobin for use of its iron content. The liver stores iron. Conversion of poisonous ammonia to urea. Urea is one of the end products of protein metabolism that is excreted in the urine.

Cleaning the blood of drugs and other poisonous substances regulating blood clotting. Resisting infection by producing immune factors and removing bacteria from the blood stream. When the liver has broken down harmful substances it's by products are excreted into the bile or blood.

Bile by-products enter the intestine and ultimately leave the body in the feces. Blood by products are filtered out by the kidneys and leave the body in the form of urine. The live can lose three quarter of its cells before it stop functioning. The liver is the only organ in the body that can regenerate itself.

{The liver disorders} {1} Wilson's disease: copper intake. {2} Hemo chromatosis: absorption of two much iron in the blood. {3} Liver failure: from food Liver cancer, liver disease. {4} Autoimmune *liver disorder, an autoimmune disorder is any reaction or attack of a person's immune system against its own organs and tissues in the liver. The immune system can destroy liver cells and damage bile ducts. {5} Alcohol induced liver disease. {6} chronic liver disease: cirrhosis. {7} Virus induced live disease- hepatitis, hepatitis A an B. {8} Liver tumors. {9} liver birth defects".*

Leading the charge: White blood cells

"The identification and elimination of germs and other foreign invaders in perform by white blood cells, or leukocytes. Friend is distinguished from foe by monitoring the shapes of protein molecules on the surfaces of cells and foreign substances. The body's own cells have proteins that mark them as friendly, while the proteins on foreign substances mark as foes, or antigens. White blood cells can be divided into two main groups: those that defend against a large variety of invaders and those that are tailored to look for specific antigens.

{General Defenses}

Several types of white blood cells defend against a large variety of germs. Attracted to the site of an infection by chemicals released by dead and damaged cells, these white blood cells help in different ways. Some stimulate inflammation, allowing fluid and defensive agents to reach the injury. Others destroy invaders by enveloping and then digesting them. Others produce proteins toxic to certain parasites.

{Targeted defenses}

Specialized white blood cells, known as lymphocytes, deal with only one particular antigen. These cells have receptors on their surface that match up with a particular antigen. Although each cell interacts with only a particular antigen, the body is capable of producing lymphocytes that match to millions of different antigens. There are two types of lymphocytes: B-cells and T-cells.

{The foot soldiers: B-cells and antibodies}

Each B cell is a small factory that turns out a specific antibody. A "Y"-shaped molecule meant to defend against a specific antigen. When a B cell is stimulated by its matching antigen, it divides and creates a plasma cell and a memory cell. The plasma cell continues to divide, producing additional plasma cells; all produce and release antibodies.

The memory cell divides but does not produce antibodies. It stays inactive until a new infection appears, preparing the body for future attacks. An antibody has two receptors that bind with the antigen, these molecules either bind several antigens together, making them easier to eliminate, or cover an antigen, inhibiting its proper function.

{Command and control: T cells}

T cells regulate much of the immune system's response to the specific antigen. There are four types: {1} Helper: many B cells cannot make antibodies until the meet both the antigen and a helper T cell. {2} Suppressor: these regulate antibody production by turning off other immune cells. {3} Delayed hypersensitivity: these attract other white blood cells, which consume antigens. {4} Cytotoxic: they kill foreign cells by poking holes in and deflating them.

{Eating the enemy} Several white blood cells that provide general defenses can be phagocytic, meaning they consume intruders. {1} the cell first encircles the intruder, forming a bubble inside the defender. {2} the bubble then merges with small packets called lysosomes. These contain enzymes that digest the intruder. {3} after digestion, the remaining particles are expelled from the cell".

"{The parts of the immune system} White blood cells reside in the lymphatic system, a network of vessels and nodes that returns fluid [lymph] to the blood and helps remove foreign material such as bacteria from the body. White blood cells are also found in the blood and will move to infected areas of the body. T cells mature in the thymus, which stops functioning at puberty. The spleen helps filter both blood and lymph system. Many white blood cells congregate in the lymph nodes. These nodes filter microscopic invaders from the lymph. Located all over the body, lymph nodes often become swollen during an infection. All blood cells- white, and red and platelets- originate in the bone marrow".

This section of the immune system came from the U.S. News & World Report. The body on fire, published Oct. 20, 2003 By Katherine Hobson, it seems her information came from Lisa Coussens of the University of California- San Francisco's cancer research Institute.

"When the body is injured or infected by a germ, t6he immune system's first line of defense is a process called inflammation. It's

sometimes painful, often itchy- and certainly familiar to anyone who has a sprained ankle or been bitten by a spider. While its effects may be uncomfortable, inflammation in these instances is a good thing. It is helping the body get rid of the trespassers and heal from trauma. But this same natural healing process, if it spins out of control, can become an adversary and cause serious health problems. Indeed, researchers are now tying inflammation to a host of common but serious diseases, including cancer, diabetes, heart disease, and even obesity. This new avenue of research is not only illuminating the nature of these diseases; it's also offering new hope for ways to prevent and treat them.

While the external symptoms of inflammation are easily recognized- the pain, redness, swelling, heat- the biological process going on beneath the skin is very complex and still not totally understood. We do know that blood vessels dilate and become "leakier" to allow infection- fighting white blood cells to reach the damaged tissue. This initial inflammatory response unleashes a cascade of chemical messengers that can in excess have damaging effects on the body.

Doctors have long suspected a connection between inflammation and disease, based on their clinical observations. For example, when the bacterium helicobacter pylori invades the gut, it cause inflammatory ulcers in some people; those same people are also move likely to develop stomach cancer. Similarly, ling cancer is now thought to develop at least in part from the body's inflammatory response to the tiny foreign particles contain in cigarette smoke.

But researchers are just beginning to tease out exactly how inflammation encourages tumor growth. There are at least three likely pathways {diagram}. "We know that inflammatory cells are full of growth factors that used by various cell types to help them proliferate." Such regeneration would obviously be helpful in healing damaged tissue. But by increasing the rate of cell division, it might also speed up the development of cancer. Second, molecules called oxidants, also produced by inflammation, can damage DNA and produce malignant cells. And finally, tumor cells can hijack certain inflammatory cells and in effect force them to labor on behalf of the tumor- building a blood supply, for example".

"Inflammation is also suspected as the culprit behind another big killer: heart disease. The fatty plagues that gum up arteries were once thought to be the result of too much low density lipoprotein-LDL, the "bad cholesterol"- hanging around and clogging the vessels, much like a hairball in a drain. Now there's a more complex theory, involving inflammation. When those LDL particles sit around for long enough, they oxidize and cause the blood vessel walls to become "sticky." The sticky walls in turn attract specialized white blood cells- monocytes and T cells- and suck them into the inner wall of the artery. A complicated cascade of chemical events follows, but the bottom line is that it's the immune system's inflammatory response- not just the bad cholesterol itself-that gums up the works, causing strokes and heart attacks.

This new view of heart disease is already changing the way doctors look for warning signs in their patients. According to a study released last year, a person's level of CRP, a protein released by the liver during inflammation, is a better predictor of heart disease than the level of LDL itself. Intriguingly, doctors have also found higher levels if CRP in people with type 11diabetes, a disease that often travels in the tandem with obesity and heart disease. In fact, Type 11 diabetics have two to three times the risk of atherosclerosis that nondiabetics have.

Such correlations have researchers rethinking the like between heart disease and diabetes. Hospital in London, theorizes that both heart disease and diabetes are connected to the activation of the immune system associated with inflammation. So rather than diabetes causing clogged arteries or vice versa, he says, "they occur in parallel."

Obesity most likely plays a big role as well in the inflammation underlying these diseases. Researcher conjectures that the fat that accumulates around your middle- the proverbial spare tire- produces the same damaging chemicals seen in an inflammatory response to infection. An excess of these chemicals could exacerbate diabetes, heart disease, or both. This would also explain why obesity can be a vicious circle.

A University in N.Y. "To counteract that local inflammation, the same fat cells also begin to produce the anti-inflammatory steroid cortisol," which makes you hungry, he says. So the more belly fat you have, the more food you crave. The list of theory goes on, and on". You need to be the judge.

Medical research reports on the immune system are misleading. Within the medical research reports you can find many controversial and contradictory findings. It tends to point only to the immune system and you have several types of immune systems within the body all through the blood. Looking at how they present the body mechanism to eradicate diseases from the body, I see a very poor understanding in their reports. The foundation placed on the immune system by the medical research teams of the world is a foundation that has never properly been laid.

The operation of the body works differently from the medical professionals' teachings. In a section of this book, you read that the body is capable of colonizing itself. That kind of operation is completely different from the immune system as the fighting mechanism taught by the medical researchers of the world. Therefore they are working without a solid foundation, which constitutes continual errors in their search for answers as how to stop invasion of diseases in the human body. All that the human research teams have been able to give to the people, in my estimation, are unanswered answers about how the body protects itself against invading diseases.

Leaving the driving all these years to the medical association, they continually are feeding us deceptive theories. We have only one source without any recourse, leaving us vulnerable. Being venerable removes other options. We are like prisoners snared in the traps of our educators.

The understanding man seems to have about the body tends to lead them onto the wrong pathway in their research for many years. The possibility why man centers his course of studying the blood so much, and accredited the blood as the link to find all the answers for fighting diseases that invades human's body, might stem from what is said in the Bile about the blood.

In the book of Deuteronomy 12: *23 it says. "Only be sure that thou eat not the blood: for the blood is the life; and thou mayest not eat the life with the flesh".* The Bible required man not to eat the blood of animals because it is stated that the blood is the life.

Another reason why man studies the blood so much is they are unable to develop other sources to correlate infiltration of invaders.

The other possible reason can be ancient medical legacy remains intact. Unable to develop other avenues leaves us in the same misconceptions of the body as ancient medical professionals. Although we have advanced with machineries that shorten our daily activities, these machines have not given us any more understanding about the body.

Concentration on curing diseases seems to rest profoundly on cell research. The process that is used today in regards to finding cures for sickness does make the structure of the body appear weaker to fight off diseases, thus showing man's body is not all that complex. Researchers of the human body express their knowledge, detailing the body accomplished from man's teaching.

The knowledge given by GOD will out weigh men. Men have been making up names for the body as GOD allows. We are at their mercies, simply because they made us to believe they know the body. Being ignorant we go along with their teaching. I am not saying that these men and women, who spend so many years in educating themselves about the body, are completely ignorant of the body. The medical professionals do know quite a lot about the body.

The other possibilities might be the health professionals might know more than they are making us aware of. Or in truth, the game is not all for money; it might be power and control. I realize that more people are becoming evolutionist. I do not know the quantity of evolutionists who are responsible in searching for answers for good health and longevity in life. Looking at the power of ailments over human life for centuries, are we really in love with each other, or is selfishness the greatest controller today?

Our society is so demanding these days that we are selling our souls to the devil for death. We spend long hours with in-depth research, because of today's life demands for survival. It might not have anything to do with love and caring. We have to make provisions for this life. It requires a job. Many will take the life of their procreator so that they will have a job.

I am not here to reduce the work force; I would love to see the economy improve where everyone has a good paying job. It hurts very deeply to see so many folks sick, and unable to enjoy the fruit of their labor, especially when they reach retirement age. Life is not a pleasant thing when you see suffering everywhere you turn.

It is time to stop, look, and listen for men do fail men. We need to see what GOD is trying to do for us. He knows the future: that it is going to be worse. He knows that it is not going to be pleasant for mankind; He uses man to help man. GOD opened my understanding about the body, and I have to give you what He has given me. If you reject the knowledge of the body that GOD has given me it will be to your loss. You are the ones that will suffer in the time of hardship.

The knowledge that GOD gave me about how the body works, is completely opposite in dispersing invaders which will become a menace in your body as taught by the health professionals. I promise to give all the answers in the next book. A person learns in stages. I keep hearing that people do not like to read too much. It is always best to do things in stages. Man does not have the ability to retain all things at once. Please be patient with yourselves and us. It could be worse, knowing that our researchers keep promising years ahead for answers for curing diseases.

The way medical professionals treat their patients has side effects. When we give the answers, and show you how to stop many problems, there will be no side effects. The power of your life will be in your hands. What you do with your life from that day onward will be up to you. Life no longer has to be perplexing. Life can be a lot more pleasant, because there won't be anymore need to keep visiting doctors, for every little thing that ails us. I know that not everyone is going to be thankful to GOD for the knowledge that He imparted to someone.

I do not want to influence you to be thinking negatively that I am being belligerent against doctors, scientists, researchers, who have been trying for years to educate us with the insights concerning our bodies. I am not that kind of a person; I am simply trying to give you what I was given. The devil takes over this world in a way that should never happen. Man in his weakness is unable to pull himself out of the pit he falls into. GOD, being merciful to us, once more sends help. Let's be thankful and try to do better by showing our appreciation for GOD'S hands of mercy.

People in the developed world incarcerate folks for ignorant mistakes made. The courts and our government do not give much lenience when someone does a crime through ignorance. What is it that our doctors are doing? Yet, we pay them enormously for their theory practicing on humans.

The emphasis on healthy body it profits very little. The emphasis should be on having a spiritual body. Death is not the end of a person, so why do we fight so hard to have a healthy body alone why not do it more sincerely for a spiritual body. Having a healthy spiritual body will make your natural body also healthy.

Better Health through Better Understanding

Chapter (20)

We have developed two books to educate each and every person in the world if possible. I know that it might be difficult to open everyone's understanding in the world. The first book will be great. The second will be much greater. The reason why the second book will be of greater value is that it will be able to give the understanding of how diseases formulate in the body. It will also help to correct many things that we have been doing wrong all our lives that have been erroneous.

What we have been doing wrong for a very long time is we have been paying attention to teaching which says that we can control our health problems if we eat right and exercise. How can we correct our health problems by watching what we eat and drink? There are teachings that we are able to stop disease from infiltrating our bodies by what we eat and drink, and how we exercise; this is incorrect. Stopping diseases from developing in the body is completely opposite from the teachings that are publicized.

It is imperative for each and everyone to read book number one first and book number two later. Book one relates to many things that we have been doing wrong for many years. It also helps to pave the road, like the first step a baby would make when just starting to walk. A baby is unable to move along normally at first. Over time, they eventually will.

The point to emphasize is to read each book more than once. Regardless of the comprehension ability that one might have, even above normal, it is beneficial to read each book more than once.

The books should also help people to understand that it is time to stop listening to our medical scientists for a significant reason. They have been leading the majority of the people astray.

I know that just about everyone would like to live very healthy without any kind of diseases. I would like for you to know that it is possible for that to happen. I am not here to rob you of your money. I am here to be truthful to you. That is why I was instructed to develop two different books, as educational tools, so that you might learn the truth.

Please allow me to elaborate a little so that you might see and understand that I am not here to play games. Each person's life is priceless and should not be robbed of its treasures for monetary reasons.

We have hundreds or thousands of formulas given daily for making people healthy as they claim. When it is not through diets, it is exercise.

The words of how to be healthy are everywhere. People are becoming confused and do not know which way they should take.

Each month someone says this or that food is healthy to stop the clogging of your arteries. They say drink this fruit juice and you can also clean your arteries.

We also hear that a person can defeat many ailments, such as type 2 diabetes, arthritis, or heart disease, by eating many of the delicious products on the market today.

ARE WE BEING USED BECAUSE WE ARE FEARFULL OF SICKNESS AND DEATH?

I know that sickness makes people suffer in a way that is unspeakable, especially in light of what cancer does to a person's body before they die.

The fact of the matter is this. Where do we find the fruits, vegetables, nuts meats, herbs, and water potent enough to be able to handle Alzheimer's, heart problems, or cancers. Just about all the sicknesses that man keeps telling us that various fruits, meats, and vegetables can rid us of our plagues that have been making havoc of people's lives for thousands of years.

Think about this for a few days and you will find this creates many questions. I have been hearing for sometime about certain foods, that if we should feed on those products they would be able to make us healthy. I have been eating most of the foods they claim will make a person healthy. So far it has not done what they claim the food is supposed to do. People still have all kinds of problems with their health.

The truth and nothing but the truth: it is not likely that what we are eating is able to solve our sickness problem.

What kinds of fruits, in any part of the world, can we find in the winter that is fresh and healthy for human consumption? What fruits are able to supply all the nutrients for a person's body to be healthy and strong so it can overpower diseases?

For a person's body to be healthy, as we have been taught, we have to supply it with all kinds of vitamins daily that are supposed to be found in our daily ration. Our medical professionals teach that we are unable to get the correct amount of vitamins in our normal daily food supply. Vitamins are manufactured according to what they think a person should consume daily.

The thing I see that needs to be pointed out, that has not been taught by anyone, is the following. Take the fruits we purchase in the stores. We are instructed that we need to have so much fruit daily to get the necessary vitamin supplements needed to make our bodies strong and healthy.

This is what we have not been shown. When we eat any fruits that are immature, they have not reached their proper maturity. An immature fruit lacks the correct nutrition, flavor, and quality. How can the undeveloped fruit have the powerful ingredients within its contents when it never reaches its full growth?

How much nourishment can the undeveloped fruits supply to a person's body? Are we just eating fruits because we are instructed to eat them because they are nutritious? Do we eat fruits because our souls keep lusting after them, and we just love to satisfy our craving? If the immature fruits are not capable of supplying the daily supplement it is stated as being needed to help us fight off diseases, why are we finding all kinds of doctrines around us that fresh fruits are very healthy for human consumption?

VALIDATE THE FRUITS FOR YOURSELVES. I AM NOT SURE IF ALL PEOPLE UNDERSTAND THE SPOILAGE OF FOOD?

The shelf life of fully developed fruits and vegetables is very short.

The handling of food from one point to the next requires days or weeks. The time span has to do with the area the food is being shipped from.

It is not every fruit that's picked green that is capable of ripening and having a long shelf life, especially if it is coming from a distant country.

We need to know that only a handful of fruits that are picked off a tree green are capable of ripening.

I would like you to know that I am not speaking of fruits when they pick it off the tree and it is still young. I am speaking of mature fruits.

In most cases, the products that are shipped from one state to the next, the majority are being harvested immature so as to have a longer shelf life. The demands are so great, that it would be too costly for fully mature fruits to get to the markets. To have the abundance of supply to feed the vast population that exists today, a greater percentage of the foods have to be harvested immature.

If the produces are being distributed unhealthy, why are we teaching people that they are able to eat unhealthy fruits and vegetables that are still able to make us healthy?

What is taking place is this. The demand is so great because many areas of the world are unable to produce food in the winter seasons. The people who live in the areas that are cold are unable to cultivate foods in the winter.

There are many kinds of food products that are being kept in cold storage. Also, wax is placed as a covering to retain freshness and to stop spoilage.

What I have noticed is lots of people who never knew what healthy sweet mature fruits taste like; they only know to enjoy unhealthy immature fruits and other half-grown products that get to the market weekly. I have seen lots of folks just love to eat fruits that are not ripe. They say that they do not like when the fruit is too soft.

We do not only get fruits and veggies unhealthy, the majority of the meats are

in the same category with fruits, veggies, and nuts. Juice is another thing that we need to analyze. How should we address milk, cheese, eggs, and what about the water that we drink daily? Do we use them daily because it's a natural thing for us to without any examination? Look at a deadly poison that is in the drinking water. Arsenic! Scientists today are developing a majority of the food products in their laboratories through genetic engineering.

Today you can find several food stores that are carrying food that is labeled as organically grown.

Where can a person find land that has not lost its strength so that it can produce foods without being fertilized? The cost and the demand are factors for fast quantity, plus the time the weather allows for growth. Take all the vitamins that are being pushed as healthy for a person to take. Do we think they have the potency within the content as stated?

The soil lost its strength many years ago. Whatever the earth produces today, the quality is destroyed because of the pressure placed on it by society wanting to be healthy. When the demand overpowers the time of growth, man is going to fertilize for fast growth to meet the demands.

You be the judge. How healthy do we think our drinks are? We have water, sodas, coffee, juices, and various teas, hot or cold.

Juices that are sold in the stores are made from concentrated juice being diluted with water and other added ingredients. Many things are added for various reasons. For people who make their own home juices, when compared to those that factories manufacture, what is the difference? Homemade substances do not add any preservatives. Therefore, they are unable to have a long shelf life. They have to be used up faster.

Now that you have learned a little about what you are eating, and that which is not helping you to be healthy, why not start to learn more about your body that has kept you alive this long. If it were the food alone you needed to truly sustain your life in good health, you would have been a dead person long before now.

The more you know about the power of your body, the better off you will be. Then, you will know that you do not have to rely on the teachings that our educators have been passing along to their students for years. Your body, within itself, is able to work wonders for you. But, you have to know how to make your body work that way for you. It has never been taught before by anyone because the knowledge has been hidden all these years. It will soon reach the pages of a book or on the screen of your computer.

Have we examined medications that so many people consume these days? Do all know that the manufacturing of medicines is not being done with product from another planet? All the substances come from man's habitat. They are not being made in any other place away from earth. So evaluate the quality and potency that you are getting in the medication you are taking for your health problems you are having. The substance use to make all medicines come form earth's depleted soil.

The ball is in your court. If you have to see lightning strike as evidence before you believe, and start to learn from this book, then you do not care for your health or that of any other person. How many people have contributed to the many organizations that keep promising answers for ailments? They keep telling us the answers are years ahead. Your good health now is up to you. When you purchase both books, you will be receiving a million times more for your money than all you have gotten by giving to researchers over the years. The books' answers, and the power that will be in your hands, should be worth millions to you.

Stop being a procrastinator just because we have a society that is only motivated by statistics. I know that the Bible teaches that

324

we should trust no man. However, I am asking everyone to have some faith in me because of what I have received from GOD. GOD instructed me to come to you for your help to make all things work much more pleasant for all. When it takes effect, you will see for sure that it was not from man.

In previous chapters you read of many problems I encountered in Jamaica and in America. All people of the world need to stop paying attention to erroneous teaching to be healthy by eating organic foods. I have this to say; when I live in Jamaica all I ate was organic foods. We grow our food supply. There was no pesticide no fertilizer and even the water I grow up with had no chemical within the content.

The latest teaching is organic is the way to go to be healthy. Organic foods in the store these days are more expensive than fertilized and pesticide foods. It is sad to see people are being brainwash only because we are simple minded. I grow up on the foods that are now portraying to be best for humanity consumption. If that is true why was I so sickly? It too is then just propaganda.

What we all fail to see and to understand, the people who take the responsibility to teach and to educate people first need to be knowledgeable before they should take it upon themselves to teach anyone. Having poor knowledge error will always remain in humanity life.

The Only True Lover of Humanity

Chapter (21)

I do not need to say much in this chapter. On the other hand this chapter should be the longest of all. It addresses the Creator of all things. Yet, in two words we can find the greatest joy and happiness all can address.

Can we ever find the words to address GOD? Man will never be able to understand their Creator fully. We constantly keep misunderstanding Him. The more He tries the harder it seems for humanity to get closer to Him. And the problem is not GOD nor with GOD.

In this world affair we can find three governing bodies, one that is GOD the Creator, the ruler of all and the only true power of the universe. The second is man that was given dominion of this earth, which did make man god of this planet. The third is the Devil, the one that outsmarted humanity, stole man's kingdom from him, and treats us shamefully being over us as a god.

Two out of three is not bad. There is only one bad guy -and he is inhumane. His only ambition is to waste the human race. He does not have any good thing in-store for flesh and blood creatures known as humans. They were made lower than him and given their own world or kingdom. He was only a second fiddle to man.

GOD created man in His image and His likeness. He always loves and cares very much for His perfect likeness. I was not taught that angels were created in the likeness of GOD, knowing that GOD is a spirit. Angels are spirits just like GOD. Since we were not taught, whose effigy angels came by, we only get a glimpse of them through the scriptures.

Man is a species that GOD gave their dominion and power over all things created by GOD on the earth. We learn from the Bible that angels are ministering spirits for GOD and man. Hebrew 2:14.

The Devil is an intellectual being. Yet, he is very foolish in his behavior and his thinking. The ways he thinks and behaves, he is able to control man, his children, from the day when man fell. Now the disobedient man thinks and behaves like Satan.

Look at how the Devil keeps us. Mankind is always unhappy and continually complaining. Nothing ever seems to go right for us. We are impatient in everything in life. The behavior of man shows that he has never taken GOD serious at His word and His promises. Our master, the Devil, is cantankerous. We live as he lives. GOD wants to remove our cantankerous living from us. We refuse to give Him the opportunity

Man gives the Devil just about all the years we live on this earth. What does he have to offer all the people that listen and obey his every command?

Let us analyze for a short space the foolish pride that causes envy and jealousy within Satan and at the same time look at GOD and humanity.

Did Satan give up heaven because he was only a servant? He was not created to be lord over anything that GOD created. He could never be GOD in heaven. He had to be a servant forever to GOD and man. The Devil, within his feelings and thinking, was displeased with what GOD did. He rebelled and stepped down from heaven to earth.

GOD the mightiest power of the universe often leaves his throne or His mansion in heaven to come down to humanity to serve us. Are men so mighty that GOD would honor man with such great honor, that He is the one that keeps serving humanity?

The Devil rejected a fantastic place, only because he felt that man was beneath him. Man was the creature he thought should fall down to him and serve him. He was not going to make an insignificant being like man stand tall over him.

GOD at no time behaves like the Devil. GOD made man. Man is a creature that lives by breathing from their nostrils. Angels: what is it they live by?

The understanding we should obtain, as we read or learn, is that GOD is the One that keeps serving humanity. It has never been the other way around, where man is the one that keeps serving GOD. We need to be more thankful to GOD knowing that He is our true LORD and master if we honor and obey Him. As we honor and obey Him, He takes time out with us to make sure all things are comfortable for all the people that are willing from the heart to walk in His statutes and commandments.

Take what the Devil did. In his envy he wanted man to be under him. GOD never wanted man to be under Him. It is not likely that GOD is going to make a GOD like Himself. He made man and angels like Him-self. There can only be one GOD.

The sweetness and greatness of GOD: He never once behaves like man or the Devil. When man gets the job to exercise GOD'S authority he can become partial and evil like the Devil. Satan, as the reigning entity, is not capable of caring with love and compassion. He can only reign with the desire of his heart and what he is. Since Devil evil and wickedness, he can only behave according to his character and no other way.

The god of this world plagues humanity with sickness, because he cannot do anything else. He has to always keep plaguing humanity as long as he remains going up and down in the earth, trying to show that he is God. By the time the world population awakens to this guy's deceptions, it will be too late. If we should ever become knowledgeable with this guy's antics, we should work much harder to stay away from being like the devil. At anytime, if any kind of evil dwells within our hearts, that's not very good. It shows that our enemy still has some control over us. We need to stop allowing the enemy to have complete control over us. I know it is not easy for that to happen, because we are sinners by birth. We have to put forth great effort to win in this fight, if we want to become GOD'S sons and daughters. The power of self control we can be victorious over the wicket evil one the Devil.

Looking at the constant pain and agony we encounter daily, it seems to be increasing more and more with no chance of stoppage. If something does not happen soon, to decrease the immoral behavior of this world, it is going to be a very despicable place to live.

I have an idea what the future will be like. When I look at the way things are going my heart does pain immensely.

What can man do for GOD? Even when the offerings to GOD were on the altar of sacrifice, the things offered burned on the altar. The truth of the matter is smoke is what GOD would receive.

When we analyze humans that inhale smoke, as their comforter, tranquilizer, or addiction, what is the titillation that one can obtain from inhaled smoke?

Smoking the way man does, it is not likely we can compare a sacrifice offered to GOD for a sweet savor. Whatever offering was offered to GOD in ancient times, burned up, only smoke ascended. National health officials teach that smoking is unhealthy. Smoke kills many through fire. There is no nourishment in smoking to man. However, is smoke is of greater value to GOD, when offered from an altar of sacrifice as a memorial in obedience to him?

GOD is not in need of any earthly possession of man. He let us know that if He was hungry He would not need to inform us. If there was anything He needed, there is no need to inform us. When we call Him, and we are pleasing to Him, He answers, and gives us the desire of our hearts. Psalm 50:8-15. In this generation, what can we offer GOD, since there is no more physical altar of sacrifice?

GOD keeps stretching His hands of mercy to man. Man is the one that keeps ignoring his master- servant. Take Jesus Christ. When He walked this earth He made us aware that He came to serve, not to be served. He did serve while He was here.

Look at what He did. At the last supper with His disciples He served them. "When supper was ended He took a towel and He washed His disciple's feet. He used the towel and wiped their feet. He proceeded by saying, ye call me master and LORD: and ye say well; for so I am. If I then your LORD and master, have washed your feet; ye also ought to wash one to another's feet. For I have given you an example, that ye should do as I have done to you. Verily, verily, I say unto you, the servant is not greater than his lord; neither he that is sent greater than he that sent him". St. John 13:9-19

What a GOD. He sure does not behave like the Devil. The Devil, not once, has he ever tried to be pleasant to man. I can be dead wrong with my opinion about the Devil. To me Satan is not intelligent being a god. He reigns over the population by cruelty, instead of conning deceptively by not being cruel, that all would confess that they are the servants of GOD, when they would be under the control of Satan. The Devil remains harsh to his loyalists; he is unable to have any compassion. GOD is compassionate and very sweet; He will never leave us or forsake us, as long as we remain faithful to Him, in-spite of all the opposition of the Devil.

The question we should all ask ourselves, did it make sense for the Devil to give up heaven to become god of this world? The few years that he reigns over humanity as god, is it worth a life living in torment forever? It might not matter to the Devil that he is going to be cast into the lake of fire for eternity, because he was able to fulfill his desire for a short time. Man is the creature that will regret living in the lake of fire. All we can do about the Devil is speculating. Either he will regret or he will have no regrets. At this juncture, is it too late for humans and the Devil to change that the future can be pleasant?

I personally have a very hard time understanding why it is so hard for us to always see, and walk with someone who is so loving and compassionate towards humanity. We find it so hard to heed to a great relationship that is not evil. I need to always try my best to remain faithful to GOD, and help others that they might stop from serving the Devil and all his companions or confederates that he has going around the world working on mankind in many areas of life. When it is not sicknesses it is many other plagues, such as death, nakedness, losing one's job or a member of your family or ones car, home, or business. There are so many things today that the Devil has at his disposal. We just keep looking at the many things we have like they are outstanding, because we cannot see the distraction there in. These are the things I am trying to make us aware of. The Devil keeps the weak and the unbelievers in bondage with vanity. We need to get away from this evil being.

GOD is the only true lover of humanity; it matters not to Him that He has to serve us. GOD finds great pleasure in serving people that honor Him. On the other side of the coin, look at all the wicked people that GOD allows to be rich and famous with this world's substance. We had the psalmist, who GOD stated was a man after his own heart; David wrote that when he saw the wicked accelerated over the righteous, it almost corrupted him to change from walking with GOD. David looked beyond with foresight, and with the power of self control was able to keep him from falling. He realized that all that is in this world is nothing: why give away something for nothing. Psalm 73:1-28.

If it pleases GOD to serve humanity, why are we not showing greater gratitude for the mighty GOD as our servant? Oftentimes when man has a faithful servant who obeys his every command he speaks highly of that servant. A good servant makes a happy master. GOD is both master and servant. He would appreciate us if we did appreciate Him the same way He does us.

Look at GOD'S love for us and His compassion. He opened my eyes and understanding about many things that are necessary for us to know about our bodies that we can live a healthy life on this earth, in-spite of the Devil's opposition. He could have allowed us to continue in our ignorance until the transition passes.

GOD, knows the horrendous plagues that are about to come upon the entire world. He, in-turn has given man the knowledge to try and see if people will listen and change before the needs arrive. We are going to need some kind of consolation sooner than we think. Not many people are knowledgeable or care, about the up coming plagues that will hit the world before the transition.

The other thing that GOD has done, He did not give the intellectuals the answers that they have been searching for, so that they would be able to eradicate ailments. They still keep looking to the future to obtain the answer they have been searching for all their lives. Our men and women who keep looking for answers, in connection with sicknesses, they are not looking with the expectation of GOD to come. They believe all things will continue forever. GOD begins to show us a better way. He put the answer in the hands of a person that never obtained a diploma from man.

It does not matter what many believe, or even when they speak evil about GOD; it will not stop GOD from being loving and compassionate to all. He will never change and become evil. We might as well just make up our minds and try to become like GOD.

It pays to serve the LORD. He is the rewarder of all: from the devil to the last human that will lives and walks this earth. Not one individual will be able to escape Him. It matters not the depth or how high we proceed in life we will have to stand before GOD someday to account for what we did in this life. If it is bad, we will be the recipient of death. When walking in righteousness in complete obedience to GOD, death will have no power over us. Life will be our portion. We will live forever with GOD in his kingdom.

Why not serve who serves us and love the One that loves and cares for us? The only One that's able to give us all things to enjoy.

Looking at GOD in His faithfulness to humanity, we should appreciate Him much more than we have and try much harder to be like Him. GOD is not biased in His treatment to man. Take the words of David about the prosperity of the wicked. He realized that GOD'S rain also blesses the sinners as the righteous and the wicked seem to excel financially over the righteous.

Man needs to conduct himself the same way one toward another like GOD. GOD who is the highest, yet He humbled Himself to the lesser and always served man. Too many feel others are below them and they should continue being their servants, and continue to keep those they hold as servants in contempt.

If we are going to be perfect like GOD, we need to serve like Him, love like Him, honor like Him, and in all things we need to be like Him. In that way, we will be perfect just like Him.

May GOD help us? Human beings have become very evil creatures. If GOD, by His power, does not intervene on behalf of man, man is going to regret every moment he lived and walked this earth. What I have seen in the behavior of men and women today: the true lover of humanity has been ignored, as if He does not exist.

As I observe man's actions today, I see that not even our doctors and psychiatrists are listening to their patients. What seems to be happening is they are treating people according to how they are being taught in the universities. It looks like they treat people the opposite from the way the patient addresses their doctors or psychiatrist.

Our intellectuals must have developed a new method of how to treat people or they are experimenting with something new. Maybe they have some kind of a drug they are trying out. They seem to ignore what their patients are saying to them. They are more apt to take the word of someone else and try to treat the patient according to what the other person is saying.

If that's the case, may GOD help us? We are in big trouble with our medical professionals. If they begin to treat us on how they feel things should be and not according to the patient's complaint, what are the chances; will we survive or live a healthy life? They will forever have our life in their hands to do with us as they please.

At the present, they are the ones that seem to be the controller. They keep telling us what to eat and what we can drink. They are trying to make a healthy society, they claim. Whether its paint, or cigarettes, as long as they put their stamp of approval on it as unhealthy, they force the issue that it needs to be removed from the population of the world. We need to stop listening to the carnal man, because that man is very much a failure. He sold out to the devil many years ago and we gave him full control of our lives.

We need GOD to stand by us, to open our eyes and our ears, and to give us a heart to perceive. We lose sight of reality, because we fail to see the things that GOD keeps showing us daily. It is the same thing over and over with humanity. We claim we are making progress in research with various diseases that exist today, but the way treatment is being done is not by hearing the patient's complaint. The doctors are more inclined to listen to the companion and not to the patient.

It is the same response we find with our diets. They are teaching us that we need to always keep eating and we should always drink a lot of water. Water is not a cleansing agent to use to flush your system. Whatever goes through your digestive system is transformed into the necessary substances required by the body for maintaining your life.

GOD that loves and cares so much for us, created us. As with all things man creates, man also manufactures an instruction manual to go with their products, so that the equipment you purchase will be able to give you satisfactory service. GOD keeps doing so much for humanity in-spite of us ignoring His instructions. We keep looking to man for the answer as to how to be healthy.

Taking GOD'S directions, we can live healthy in this life and in the life to come. When we ignore the instructions of GOD, we are hurting none other than our own selves.

May GOD help us, because we are not in love with ourselves, henceforth can we love our neighbors in an appropriate way? This lack of love brings on acts of deception one towards another, and brings us to a place where we belittle each other. We cannot remain belittling each other if we are going to have a pleasant life in this world and the life to come.

The reason for my analogy, I see the conduct of today's society that I never knew existed before. I was flabbergasted when I saw, and learned what we are doing today to make a dollar to exist or to survive. This takes me back to the One that really loves and cares for humanity. As I travel each day and see how people are acting, it shows that the Bible does stand alone.

Man lacks discipline in his life. We never think of others when we are on a quest for pleasure. People will trample on other folks as long as they are receiving their arousal. It is not only sports or sexuality that people pleasure in. People take great pleasure in their jobs or in the area where they are making their livelihood. They will kill you if they think you are in opposition with them and their jobs.

The pressure of life to eat and to clothe oneself is outrageously despicable. We sell ourselves to the devil for nothing, because we do not care what happens to our fellowmen. I know that we are unable to survive without eating and sleeping. We need to be clothed. The problem with the way life is going, is we place lots of pressure on none essential items and the essential things are not important anymore.

As I keep saying, may GOD help us? The reason for me to keep saying GOD help us is we need His help. The reason why we need His help is we are failing one another, and ourselves. The more we fail, the more difficult life will become.

I keep seeing and hearing so many folks say they are unable to pay their monthly bills, although they have a job. Today, most families have two people providing for the family. One no longer suffices. In-spite of two people working in a family, their bills are still very high. It's not necessary that they are placing their basket higher than they can reach. It's the rapid increase of commodities that make lots of folk's baskets rise higher than they are able to reach.

What is happening these days is the cost of living keeps rising higher and higher. Man is unable to change the course and the way things are going. That is why we need GOD'S help. If GOD does not remain loving and affectionate to humanity, all are going to have things much more difficult than it is right now. Even the people that keep praying and seeking GOD'S help are going to find themselves in a situation that they might believe that GOD no longer exists.

Can we analyze the things that man has been doing for man all his life? Where has it brought us thus far? Does man truly love man? Does man truly care for himself? Do we walk daily with foresight over hindsight? What are we looking for out of life? The other thing we should ask ourselves: does life end in death? Oftentimes we hear people say life ends at the grave. What about the millions of people that never parted this life the way of the grave? Over the years, many folks end up being eaten, or something happens to them that cause them to end up somewhere else away from the graveyard. Today lots of people are being cremated.

That is why I would like to know how we feel about life if it ends in death? If we feel that death does not completely end man's existence for eternity, where are we going to spend eternity? The other thing is this: do we believe what GOD stated about all the people that do not love and care for themselves?

There is a section in the Bible, it is found in St. John 3:16, For GOD so loved the world, that He gave His only begotten son, that whosoever believeth in Him should not perish, but have everlasting life. To me, this is where a great deal of controversy begins in this era. Most people I see and hear address that they believe the Bible to be the words of GOD. Yet, in their beliefs they are not willing to walk as it is stated for us to walk.

I have to accept the section of the Bible that is found in St. Matthew 7:13-14. The Bible is telling us that we are to: "Enter ye in at the strait gate: for wide is the gate, and broad is the way, that leadeth to destruction, and many there be which go in thereat: Because strait is the gate, and narrow is the way, which leadeth unto life, and few there be that find it".

Understanding these verses of scripture, I think that they are showing us that it is going to take much more than belief. It is saying that we have to enter in the strait gate and only a few people will be able to enter the strait gate. Not that GOD is partial saving humanity. The verse in St. John says that GOD so loved the world that he gave His only begotten son to die, that whosoever believeth in Him should not perish, but should have everlasting life. It never says GOD'S son died for the minority of the population or only for the majority. The world means everyone. It is not addressing the physical dirt, the earth, the trees, or vegetation. It is only speaking about humanity.

The only problem is: humanity does not appreciate the goodness and love of GOD. People lightly esteem what GOD has done and what He is going to do. Humans are very difficult to please, because we are not willing to close our eyes against the things we can see. The way man visualizes things it has become detrimental. For the present time, it's glorious. In the future, it is going to be weeping and gnashing of teeth.

In the Bible we read that GOD made us aware that our bodies should be His temple where He can dwell. He let us understand, whosoever defile the temple of GOD, him will GOD destroy. It is found in 1Corinthians 3:17. GOD keeps showing humanity a much better pathway to take in life. We are the ones that keep rejecting better for worse.

We behave, as if to say, it is much more pleasant for the Devil to occupy our body as his temple. We give him all the space and time he desires continually. We are not being positive in our walk of life. Why are we allowing an enemy to take full control of our bodies for nothing?

The one that has nothing to offer us, we give him all our entire needs, such as the best years of our lives. The One that still supplies our entire needs daily, we constantly reject Him. He has not stopped providing for us. If GOD should stop the rain for several years, man and the Devil, with all the technologies at hand, would not be able to make it rain.

Life would be much more pleasant if we were able to keep our temple undefiled that GOD would be able to inhabit it continually. We behave like it is impossible to live a sin free life and to keep our tabernacle spotless that GOD, the Creator, will be able to find a place to rest His head peacefully.

Our temple is contaminated beyond acceptance with GOD, because we have not taken the time to keep it clean. Humanity has become a sluggard. Even in our sinful walk, we are unable to feed ourselves correctly. We keep hurting ourselves, because we are too lazy to clean our temple correctly.

The more we ignore the laws and statutes of GOD, the more we are going to encounter pain and agony. We are going to feel it worse in the years ahead. We need to try much harder than we are doing for the good of humanity in the near future. The longer we remain being faithful to the one that hates us and despises us, the longer we are going to suffer in pain and agony. Not only in this life, also in the life to come. It will be more horrendous than all the things we can imagine with the human faculties.

Man is limited in his thinking when it comes to the things of GOD and the ways of GOD. We behave daily without foresight for the real future. The future living on this earth is nothing, because man does not live very long on this earth. The life span of all humans, born and created on this earth is not eternal. The life to come will be. To whom we serve, him will we inhabit.

GOD loves all of His creation. Humans love the things they created. GOD will never fall prey to anything that He has created. GOD will never allow what He has created to have any kind of advantage over Him. Men have created lots of wonderful things that give great pleasure to the vast population.

Man's invention is able to bring pleasure to the one who is the creator, when it generates lots of cash. Do we think GOD'S invention is pleasing to Him? Is GOD pleased at times with His creation? Was GOD displeased at anytime with His creation, and why was He displeased? What causes people to become displeased with their creations?

All of man's creation does not have the ability to think or reason. When GOD created man, He put a lot of Himself in man. Men can create, and love like GOD. Men are compassionate and forgiving like GOD. GOD can change from spirit to be like man. He can change back to spirit. Man does not have the ability to make those transformations as GOD can.

Men's inventions deteriorate. No matter what man creates, it is unable to remain without deterioration. Humans are unable to develop a protecting source that can stop their creation from destruction. The trend of today's population is to keep buying new Products all the time; patience is something that is needed to be written in the vocabulary of humans. The other thing I notice, most of the manufactured items, are not made to last.

Older cars, homes, and furniture have better restoration quality. Not every person has the time, money, and patience to restore a car, home, and furniture. It takes lots of time, with hard labor, and lots of cash to restore an older car. Restoration is only required when it is deteriorated. To stop deterioration, the car owner has to work hard in many ways to keep what they are in love with, immaculate. A properly built home can last many more years with proper maintenance, and holds its beauty at the same time. Furniture made of good quality wood can give excellent service if proper care has been taken.

Transportation vehicles give the most problems in deterioration. When a vehicle is badly rusted away, a better job requires welding new pieces of material in the areas that's rusted out. Short cuts only bring dissatisfaction sooner. People love to restore the things they are in love with.

Restoration takes place when men and women see the need of their possession to be restored. Contemplating renewing ones treasure, the individuals will factor in the advantages, and the disadvantages. Restoration is needed when deterioration causes disfigurement. Disfigurement of ones treasure requires drastic measures.

Take the three monarchs, GOD, Man, and the devil. Two are disfigured. Lucifer was the first one that became contaminated, then mankind. GOD the Creator is all powerful; He can make restitution better than the beginning when He created both the Devil and man. The question we need to ask ourselves: can GOD by His power regenerate the devil and man without their approval? Would mankind and the Devil live faithful and true to GOD without sinning? Both were flawless in the beginning; they were unable to maintain the beauty which is obedience. We need to be appreciative to GOD for all the time and effort He spent in helping man to transform from a life of sin and death.

GOD created man in His image and His likeness. Man and angels have the effigy of GOD. Nothing man ever created has their effigy. GOD has the rights to love His creation. GOD can do as He pleases with His invention whether we like it or not. GOD will not do that because He gives us knowledge of choice. Man is the one that will have to make the choice to turn from sin and walk with GOD in spirit and in truth. Does GOD know that the Devil and man will revert? Yes! Would GOD leave restoration in the hands of the both disfigured creatures only? No!

I am not GOD. I do not have the power to help man regain perfection. Speculation generates rebellion. GOD in the beginning gave man and the Devil and the angels the power to choose. Two of the monarchs take death over life. We are the ones that need to fall in love with GOD. Falling in love with GOD, means that I love myself. We have to bring ourselves to a place where we weight the advantages, and the disadvantages. Are we willing to pay the cost of deterioration? We are disfigured by sin and death. We need to understand that GOD will be there for our every need when we are determined to make GOD our choice: restitution! If we are not willing to work hard to restore our selves to where we were before we sin, death will be ours someday.

GOD'S source of supply will never run short, even when over two hundred billion folks are using GOD'S source all at once. GOD will be there to encourage us when we desire restitution. It gives great titillation to GOD and the entire heavenly host when someone is given restitution.

It brings greater pleasure to GOD when someone works hard on their preservation. GOD is the one that has all the supply and the necessary ingredients for restoration, and preservation. We need to count the cost of regenerating before we start the process and fail.

Sin is the destroying source in humanity's life. It is like salt to metal. Salt slowly eats away metals. Mankind will go through a lot of trouble trying to prevent disfigurement to the things that they love so much. Stopping erosion especially to motor vehicles is a very difficult task. Stopping sin from erosion in our lives is even much more difficult than automobiles. It is not cheap to keep our pride and joy from contaminations. It is a constant battle daily. The Devil is the salt, man is the automobile. GOD is material supplier for restitution. Man has the ability to work on himself to remove disfigurement. Most of man's creation ends up in the junkyard. If people do not stop to count the cost of being cast in the junkyard, which is the lake of fire, it will be their own fault. Wake up people, fall in love with me, myself, and I. Time is getting shorter every tick of the clock that it makes.

So much I could say, yet it simply ends up like this: GOD is love.

In the next book you will learn how and what to do to be free from many ailments. It is not far away as long as you work with me and exercise patience.

If you do not obtain the next book, you never purchased the original. Someone made a replica and you purchased it from an outsider. That will not enable you to receive the one that will show you how to make your body work as a colony.

I will not hold it against you if you obtained the book another way. As long as you are able to get some help that is what is important. If you would like to obtain the next book please feel free to contact me if you can. All the people that obtained this CD or book by me will always know how to contact me directly.

Bibliography

Scripture quotations in this book are from the Old King James Authorized version of the Bible taken from a Scofield Reference Bible.

Pictures of the anatomy of the human body in this book, on various pages 270-283 are from different medical books.

Information about the immune system, italicized section from page 302 to page 315, came from two different internet sources.

Italicized section from page 311 to page 315 came from U. S, News and World report Oct. 20, 2003 issues.